Treatment Plans and Interventions for Mental Health Disorders

Treatment Plans and Interventions for Mental Health Disorders

Editor: John Dalvi

AMERICAN
MEDICAL PUBLISHERS
www.americanmedicalpublishers.com

AMERICAN
MEDICAL PUBLISHERS
www.americanmedicalpublishers.com

Cataloging-in-Publication Data

Treatment plans and interventions for mental health disorders / edited by John Dalvi.
p. cm.
Includes bibliographical references and index.
ISBN 979-8-88740-536-0
1. Mental illness. 2. Mental illness--Treatment. 3. Psychology, Pathological. 4. Mental health.
5. Psychiatry. 6. Psychotherapy. I. Dalvi, John.
RC480 .T74 2023
616.891 4--dc23

American Medical Publishers,
41 Flatbush Avenue,
1st Floor, New York,
NY 11217, USA

ISBN 979-8-88740-536-0 (Hardback)

Contents

Preface

The purpose of the book is to provide a glimpse into the dynamics and to present opinions and studies of some of the scientists engaged in the development of new ideas in the field from very different standpoints. This book will prove useful to students and researchers owing to its high content quality.

Mental illnesses are health conditions involving changes in emotional, thinking, or behavioral patterns. The most common forms of mental disorders are neurodevelopmental disorders, obsessive-compulsive disorder, bipolar disorder, and schizophrenia. Factors such as a traumatic brain injury, use of alcohol and recreational drugs and chemical imbalances in brain can lead to the development of mental disorders. There are several signs and symptoms of mental disorders such an inability to cope with daily problems or stress, suicidal thinking, major changes in eating habits, fatigue, low energy, and sleeping problems. Patients with mental health disorders can be best managed with the help of a mental health treatment plan or mental health care plan, which involves three basic steps, namely, assessment, planning, and referral. The assessment step involves assessing a patient's mental health condition and making a diagnosis. Planning includes preparing a mental health treatment plan. The last step, referral, involves referring a patient to psychologist, psychiatrist, or other occupational therapists. This book addresses the treatment and interventions for mental health disorders. It will help new researchers by foregrounding their knowledge in this branch.

At the end, I would like to appreciate all the efforts made by the authors in completing their chapters professionally. I express my deepest gratitude to all of them for contributing to this book by sharing their valuable works. A special thanks to my family and friends for their constant support in this journey.

Editor

1

Exposure to a Standardized Catastrophic Scenario in Virtual Reality or a Personalized Scenario in Imagination for Generalized Anxiety Disorder

Tanya Guitard [1], Stéphane Bouchard [2,3,*], Claude Bélanger [1] and Maxine Berthiaume [3]

1 Département de Psychologie, Université du Québec à Montréal, Montréal, QC H3C 3P8, Canada; tanya.guitard@videotron.ca (T.G.); belanger.claude@uqam.ca (C.B.)

2 Département de Psychoéducation et de Psychologie, Université du Québec en Outaouais, Gatineau, QC J8X 3X7, Canada

3 School of Psychology, University of Ottawa, Ottawa, ON K1N 6N5, Canada; mbert094@uottawa.ca

* Correspondence: stephane.bouchard@uqo.ca

Abstract: The cognitive behavioral treatment of generalized anxiety disorder (GAD) often involves exposing patients to a catastrophic scenario depicting their most feared worry. The aim of this study was to examine whether a standardized scenario recreated in virtual reality (VR) would elicit anxiety and negative affect and how it compared to the traditional method of imagining a personalized catastrophic scenario. A sample of 28 participants were first exposed to a neutral non-catastrophic scenario and then to a personalized scenario in imagination or a standardized virtual scenario presented in a counterbalanced order. The participants completed questionnaires before and after each immersion. The results suggest that the standardized virtual scenario induced significant anxiety. No difference was found when comparing exposure to the standardized scenario in VR and exposure to the personalized scenario in imagination. These findings were specific to anxiety and not to the broader measure of negative affect. Individual differences in susceptibility to feel present in VR was a significant predictor of increase in anxiety and negative affect. Future research could use these scenarios to conduct a randomized control trial to test the efficacy and cost/benefits of using VR in the treatment of GAD.

Keywords: Generalized Anxiety Disorder (GAD); virtual reality; exposure in virtual reality; cognitive exposure; standardized scenario; personalized scenario

---

1. Introduction

In the treatment of anxiety disorders, exposure is defined as "any procedure that confronts the person with a stimulus which typically elicits an undesirable behavior or an unwanted emotional response" [1] (p. 121). This stimulus can take an animate form (animal, insect), inanimate (heights, storms), a situation (public speaking), or even a thought (memories of a traumatic event, anticipation of a catastrophe). Regardless of the stimulus, the purpose of exposure is to learn new mental associations between the stimuli and lack of threat [2,3]. Considering that exposure requires confronting feared stimuli, the confrontation is associated with an increase in anxiety [4]. Studies have demonstrated that, compared to people who do not suffer from an anxiety disorder, immersions in virtual reality (VR) can elicit anxiety in people suffering from specific phobia [5], and from obsessive-compulsive disorder characterized by fear of contamination [6] or by checking behaviors [7]. Several studies, summarized in literature reviews (e.g., [8]) and meta-analyses (e.g., [9–11]), have documented the relevance and efficacy of using VR to conduct exposure (also called *in virtuo* exposure, [12]) in the treatment of anxiety disorders.

VR is defined as the product of using computer and behavioral interfaces to simulate the behavior of 3D entities that interact in real time with each other and with a user immersed via sensorimotor channels [13]. VR systems are designed so images viewed in a head mounted display (HMD) change according to the user's head movements. When immersed in VR, individuals can explore different environments, allowing them to feel as if they are physically in this synthetic environment [14]. This feeling of being "in" the virtual environment is called ''presence" [15] and is considered an important feature of VR.

Conducting exposure *in virtuo* in the context of cognitive behavior therapy (CBT) has several benefits when compared to in vivo exposure. First, *in virtuo* exposure allows a greater control over the environment, which can be practical for both therapists and patients [16]. Unanticipated events (e.g., poor conditions during an airplane flight or unexpected animal/insect reactions) are less likely, allowing a more controlled exposure session. *In virtuo* exposure also provides greater standardization of the exposure cues, which can be useful for researchers as well as clinicians. Finally, using VR is considered more attractive than in vivo exposure for some patients [17].

However, creating virtual environments for *in virtuo* exposure for the treatment of generalized anxiety disorder (GAD) could be more complex than with other anxiety disorders. GAD is defined by excessive anxiety or worries almost every day for at least six months and concerning a variety of themes. It is characterized by fear of negative and uncertain future events [18–20]. As opposed to other anxiety disorders, people suffering from GAD are not essentially afraid of specific and concrete stimuli. They are afraid of uncertainty accompanied with a broad range of situations. In the cognitive-behavioral treatment of GAD, exposure is often conducted in the imagination, where patients have to repeat mentally or write down a scenario depicting one of their worst catastrophic worries [21,22].

Using VR for exposure with GAD has its share of advantages [23]. For example, not all patients are good at imagining or visualizing feared situations, yet exposure in imagination is often used with GAD patients. It may be difficult to know what patients are thinking about, if they are engaged in avoidance or neutralization behaviors while doing exposure, or if the right stimuli are included in the scenario. With respect to neutralization, subtle avoidance and safety seeking behaviors, using standardized scenarios reduces the risks of avoidance because the content of the scenario is known and visible to the therapist during the immersion in VR.

Previous work has been conducted to identify common ingredients in the exposure scenarios of actual GAD patients [24] and to proposed standardized scenarios that can be used for exposure [25]. Empirical data collected with GAD patients exposed in imagination to their personal worry scenarios or to the standardized ones showed that standardized scenarios can elicit anxiety (as measured with self-report and heart rate) and negative affect [25]. In their research, Guitard and her colleagues [25] demonstrated that the effect size of exposure in imagination to the individualized scenarios was slightly higher than the standardized ones on the measure of heart rate but, nevertheless, the results were positive enough to warrant transposing the scenarios used in imagination into VR scenarios and testing them with people suffering from GAD.

Accordingly, the goal of the current study is to document the potential of virtual environments adapted from catastrophic scenarios to induce the anxiety necessary to eventually use VR as an exposure strategy in the treatment of GAD. Three exposure scenarios are compared: (a) exposure to a neutral virtual environment; (b) exposure in imagination to a personalized scenario (IM-Exp); and (3) exposure in VR to a standardized scenario (VR-Exp). Each participant was exposed to all three conditions, first to the neutral environment and then to exposure in imagination or in VR, in random order. The hypothesis was that exposure in VR will induce more anxiety than the neutral scenario. Power estimations were performed before the study, with medium to large effect sizes expected for this hyposhesis based on results from other studies [5,6,25]. To prevent having to prove the null hypothesis (i.e., *in virtuo* being as effective as in vivo) without justification, no formal hypothesis was expressed for the comparison between exposure in VR and in imagination, and no power estimation was conducted a priori.

2. Materials and Methods

2.1. Participants

Inclusion criteria for this study were as follows: (a) primary diagnosis of GAD, (b) aged between 18 and 65, and (c) never having experienced VR before. The Randot Stereo™ test from Western Ophtalmics was used to assess if participants have stereoscopic vision. Exclusion criteria consisted of: (a) suffering from an anxiety disorder other than GAD as primary diagnosis; (b) suffering from claustrophobia, because the experimentation was held in an immersive CAVE-Like system, a rather confined area; (c) use of benzodiazepines, because of the impact this type of medication might have on the variables measured; and (d) suffering from any of the following health issues (due to potential interactions with VR): diseases related to the inner ear or vestibular system, cardiovascular diseases or circulatory disorders, migraines, blood pressure disorders or diabetes. The final sample included a total of 28 participants who all met the criteria.

2.2. Procedure

Participants were recruited through the Université du Québec en Outaouais (UQO) via email and posters. The project, conducted in concordance with the Declaration of Helsinki and the Canadian Tri-Council policy statement for ethical conduct for research involving humans, was approved by the Ethics Committee of UQO and participants signed a free and informed consent form. All individuals who wanted to participate in the study were first briefly screened by phone in order to assess whether or not excessive worry seemed present. In cases where anxiety was caused by another disorder, they were referred to another service. When GAD seemed probable and exclusion criteria were screened, a first meeting was scheduled to proceed to the complete evaluation using the ADIS-IV. The participants included in the study were randomly assigned to one of the two conditions: (a) exposure to a standardized scenario in VR followed by exposure to an individualized scenario in imagination (VR-Exp/IM-Exp; $n = 13$) or (b) exposure to an individualized scenario in imagination followed by exposure to standardized scenario in VR (IM-Exp/VR-Exp.; $n = 15$). At the end of the assessment session, all participants were given a battery of questionnaires to complete alone at home (without consulting other people) and return at the following meeting. In session 2, participants were asked to identify a worry theme and write a catastrophic scenario based on their worst fear. The writing of the scenario began during the session to allow time for the therapist to review the content and give feedback to the participant. Following this, participants were asked to further improve their scenario, if needed. They were told not to read their scenario at home to avoid habituation. A third and final session was scheduled in which the exposures took place. Each participant was first immersed in a neutral non-catastrophic virtual environment for 5 min that consisted of a quiet and empty room with a glass door and the sun shining in from large windows. Participants were asked to physically walk around the room to familiarize themselves with VR. Following the first experimental exposure scenario (either in VR or in imagination), a distraction task was performed where participants were asked to dash the A letter each time it occurred in a random and incomprehensible text. Following the distraction task, the other experimental exposure session took place. At the end of the third session, debriefing was completed to ensure the well-being of the participants following the brief exposure to the anxiety provoking scenarios and offer relevant clinical referrals, if necessary.

2.3. Virtual Environments (VE)

The three standardized exposure scenarios used in imagination by Guitard et al. [25] were recreated in VR and the experimenter selected one based on the main worry theme as reported by the participant: (a) VE 1: an emergency room (used with 11 participants), (b) VE 2: an apartment (used with 15 participants), or (c) VE 3: a student room (used with 2 participants).

2.3.1. VE 1: Emergency Room

This environment was created with the intention of eliciting worry in participants suffering mostly from worries related to health. The participant was immersed in a hospital emergency waiting room. Other patients are nearby and display symptoms of sickness (coughing) or fatigue. One is wearing a disposable face mask. Sounds are heard, such as a mother crying after receiving bad news concerning her child, and a wife is told that nothing can be done to save her husband, etc. Other patients are called to see the doctor, but not the participant. At some point, doctors come into the waiting room and discuss a case while looking at the participant, who cannot, however, understand what they are saying.

2.3.2. VE 2: Apartment

The setting for this scenario is an apartment that participants are invited to visit. Participants first overhear a conversation taking place behind closed doors suggesting that an accident has occurred. Afterwards, a special announcement is made on the radio regarding recent burglaries in the neighborhood. At the same time, a rock is thrown at the window, and when the participant looks out the window, a group of men is seen roughing up another individual. Finally, a brief message is left on the answering machine. Seven message options are available to choose from: (a) the police calling because a loved one was involved in an accident, (b) the doctor calling regarding test results that were previously overlooked, (c) the participant's spouse, either male or female, is saying that they have met a new lover and are leaving, (d) the bank needs to be called back regarding several late payments and is threatening to take action, (e) a receptionist from work calling regarding recent budget cuts and a problem involving the participant, (f) the university calling regarding unpaid tuition fees and the impossibility of registering for the semester, or (g) the school is calling regarding the participant's child's recent behavior and academic problems.

2.3.3. VE 3: Student Room

The third environment, created for students, alludes to both academic difficulties and social isolation. The participant is in his or her room having to study for upcoming exams. Scattered unpaid bills are visible and suggest financial difficulties. Voices are heard coming from the hall, talking about a student who is failing out of the program. Roommates heard from another room are planning a party to which the participant is not invited and that might, furthermore, disrupt his or her study time.

2.4. *Measures*

2.4.1. Diagnostic and Clinical Measures of Severity

An initial diagnosis of GAD was made using the ADIS-IV at the first session. Questionnaires were then given to each participant to be filled out at home and brought back at the next session. Those questionnaires were used to further assess each participant and assess the clinical severity of the sample as well as describe VR factors that may influence the results.

Diagnostic Measure: Anxiety Disorders Interview Schedule for DSM-IV (ADIS-IV)

This semi-structured interview allows for a thorough evaluation of anxiety disorders as well as mood disorders, substance-abuse disorders, and somatoform disorders as they hold the higher comorbidity rates with anxiety disorders. The ADIS-IV [26] was used for diagnostic purposes and the severity score on the diagnosis of GAD is reported to describe the sample.

Clinical Measure: Penn State Worry Questionnaire (PSWQ)

The French translation of this questionnaire [27] comes from Ladouceur et al. [28]. This 16-item questionnaire measures the level of worry typical to GAD on a scale of 1 to 5. The psychometric properties of the English version are very good, with good internal consistency (Cronbach's alpha ranging from 0.86 to 0.95) and test retest reliability (ranging from 0.74 to 0.93) [29,30]. The same was found for the French version (see [30]) indicate equally good validity and internal consistency. The PSWQ was used to describe the sample.

Clinical Measure: Cognitive Avoidance Questionnaire (CAQ; Original French Version)

Cognitive avoidance plays an important role in maintaining excessive worry in GAD. This measure [31] was therefore used to evaluate the degree of cognitive avoidance in the sample. Studies have indicated good psychometric features for this scale with a Cronbach's alpha of 0.95 for the totality of the items on an adult sample and of 0.92 on a sample of adolescents, both non-clinical samples.

2.4.2. Measures of Users' Experience in Virtual Reality

These questionnaires measure important concepts in clinical applications of VR. They allow comparing reactions of participants from one study to another.

Users' Experience: Presence Questionnaire (PQ)

The PQ is a French-Canadian translation (validated by the Cyberpsychology Laboratory of UQO [32]) of the Witmer and Singer Presence Questionnaire [33]. This questionnaire contains 24 items in the form of closed-ended questions, on a scale of 1 ("not at all") to 7 ("completely"), and as a measure of presence it is useful to describe how participants perceive the properties of the virtual environments and the technology used. Cronbach's alpha reaches 0.84. The duration of administration was approximately 7 min.

Users' Experience: Gatineau Presence Questionnaire (GPQ)

This questionnaire was created by the Cyberpsychology Laboratory as a brief supplement to the PQ to address the experience felt by the users while immersed [6]. It includes four questions, on a scale of 0–100. The GPQ has a Cronbach's alpha of 0.69.

Users' Experience: Simulator Sickness Questionnaire (SSQ)

This questionnaire is a French-Canadian translation (validated by the Cyberpsychology Laboratory of UQO [34]) of the Simulator Sickness Questionnaire [35] designed to measure the level of unwanted negative effects induced by the immersions in VR. It consists of 16 items, rated on a four-point scale. This questionnaire was administered to participants for the first time at the beginning of the meeting involving virtual reality, in order to know their physical state well before the first immersion (results not shown) and after the immersion in VR. Cronbach's alpha reaches 0.87. The SSQ was scored according to guidelines from Bouchard et al. [34] and the raw total score is reported.

2.4.3. Dependent Variables

The following questionnaires were used as dependent variables to assess the level of anxiety and negative affect throughout the experimentation process of the third session. Participants had to fill out these questionnaires after each exposure session.

Dependent Variable: State Scale of the State Trait Anxiety Inventory—Form Y1 (STAI-Y1)

The French version of this questionnaire [36,37] was used. Only the Y-1 version (state form) was retained for the present study because the goal of the project was to assess anxiety levels at different times during the experimentation rather than evaluate anxiety traits in the participants. The French version of this measure has excellent psychometric values, with a Cronbach's alpha of 0.94 and 0.86 for men and women, respectively [36].

Dependent Variable: Negative Affect Scale of the Positive and Negative Affect Schedule (PANAS)

The French-Canadian version [38] of the questionnaire developed by Watson, Clark and Tellegen [39] was used. It consists of two scales; one measuring positive affect and the other negative affect. Only the negative affect subscale is reported here, given the study's focus on anxiety. Items represent different feelings and emotions that are rated on a 5-point scale ranging from 1 ("very slightly or not at all") to 5 ("extremely"). Internal consistency of the negative affect subscale is adequate, with a Cronbach's alpha ranging from 0.80 to 0.84.

2.4.4. Predictors of Levels of Anxiety and Negative Affect During the Immersion in VR

Predictor: Intolerance of Uncertainty Scale (IUS; Original French Version)

This questionnaire [20] rates the degree of intolerance to uncertainty using 27 items that describe uncertainty as negative and something to be avoided. Participants have to rate each item on a 5-point Likert scale ranging from 1 ("not at all characteristic of me") to 5 ("entirely characteristic of me"). This measure possesses very good internal consistency (Cronbach's alpha of 0.91) and good convergent validity with the PSWQ. Also, the main advantage of this measure is its good sensibility and specificity to excessive worry that allows it to be administered more than once during treatment to assess progress [21]. The IUS, and the following two questionnaires, were used to describe the sample and explore potential predictors of patient's reactions in VR.

Predictor: Why Worry-II (WW-II)

This questionnaire is a revised version of the original Why Worry [31]. It assesses positive beliefs about worry with five different subscales: (1) worry as a problem solving tool; (2) worry helps motivate; (3) worrying protects and prepares in the face of a negative outcome; (4) worrying can, in itself, prevent a negative outcome and (5) worry is a positive personality trait. This self-reported measure contains 25 items ranging from 1 ("not at all true") to 5 ("absolutely true"). This questionnaire possesses good test-retest reliability ($r = 0.81$) and internal consistency (Cronbach's alpha of 0.93) [40].

Predictor: Immersive Tendencies Questionnaire (ITQ)

This questionnaire is a French-Canadian translation (validated by the Cyberpsychology Laboratory of UQO [32]) of the Immersion Tendencies Questionnaire [33] and contains 18 items calculated on a scale of 1 ("never") to 7 ("often"). This questionnaire aims to measure the predisposition of the individual to experience presence. It was administered only once. Cronbach's alpha reaches 0.78.

2.5. Experimenters and Hardware

Four experimenters, all doctorate students with training in CBT for anxiety disorders, conducted the study. Supervision was made available to them and provided by a licensed psychologist. The immersions in VR were conducted in a 6-side CAVE-Like system using retro projected stereoscopic displays and wireless motion tracking (see Laforest et al. [6] for a technical description and a picture).

3. Results

3.1. Sample Description

The sample ($N = 28$) consisted of 24 women and 4 men with a primary diagnosis of GAD. They were all francophone with a mean age of 38.33 (SD = 12.78). According to the PSWQ, participants scored within the range of adults suffering from GAD. Comorbid disorders were diagnosed in 64.3% of the sample—social anxiety being the most frequent ($n = 8$) while others were specific phobias ($n = 4$), panic disorder ($n = 3$), obsessive-compulsive disorder ($n = 1$), and other diagnosis ($n = 2$). Further description of the sample is provided in Table 1. No differences were found between the two conditions on the GAD severity (as assessed with the ADIS-IV and the PSWQ), on how they perceived the quality of the VR system (PQ), and in unwanted negative side effects induced by the immersion in VR (SSQ).

Table 1. General description of the sample.

Variable	*N*	%	Mean (SD)
Nationality			
Canadian	25	89.3	
Senegalese	1	3.6	
Level of education			
University (some or completed)	18	64.3	
College or professional diploma	5	17.9	
High school diploma	3	10.7	
Some high school	2	7.1	
Socioeconomic status			
High	9	32.1	
Middle	15	53.6	
Low	4	14.3	
Marital status			
Married	10	35.7	
Single	8	28.6	
Common-law partner	8	28.6	
Divorced	2	7.1	
Descriptive clinical measures of generalized anxiety disorder			
Anxiety Disorders Interview Schedule-IV severity of GAD			5.7 (0.93)
Penn State Worry Questionnaire			59.88 (8.89)
Cognitive Avoidance Questionnaire			68.32 (20.35)
Descriptive measures of users' experience in virtual reality			
Presence Questionnaire after the VR-Exp scenario			61.17 (19.05)
Gatineau Presence Questionnaire after the VR-Exp scenario			89.90 (14.32)
Simulator Sickness Questionnaire after the VR-Exp scenario			9.57 (6.65)
Predictive measures selected for exploratory analyses			
Intolerance of Uncertainty Scale			68.61 (21.62)
Why Worry-II Questionnaire			47.29 (17.93)
Immersive Tendencies Questionnaire			70.88 (16.81)

3.2. *Statistical Analyses*

Prior to analyses, all variables to be used in further analyses were examined for accuracy of data entry, missing values, normality of distribution, and univariate outliers. After ensuring that there were no errors in data entry or missing values, we screened for extreme kurtosis and skewness values (below 1.5 or above −1.5), which would indicate non-normal distributions. The negative affect scale of the PANAS (neutral scenario and second exposure) had extreme kurtosis values. We also screened for univariate outliers on the state anxiety scale of the STAI and the negative affect scale of the PANAS. When univariate outliers were found, they were winsorized to the next most extreme but acceptable value in that condition (with a z-score less than 1.96 or above −1.96). To do so, z-scores were first obtained for all variables to be used in further analyses. When a z-score was greater than 1.96 or less than −1.96, the next most extreme but acceptable value in the same condition was found and replaced the extreme value that needed to be winsorized. This procedure eliminated all outliers and extreme skewness and kurtosis values. Parametric analyses were then performed, with descriptive results reported in Table 2 (note that results were similar if the data is not corrected for outliers).

Table 2. Means and standard deviations of dependent variables in each experimental condition for the three scenarios.

Measure and Scenario	Condition			
	IM-Exp/VR-Exp		VR-Exp/IM-Exp	
	M	*(SD)*	*M*	*(SD)*
STAI-Y1				
Neutral environment	39.67	(10.83)	41.92	(13.12)
Exposure scenario 1	50.20	(12.81)	46.00	(12.91)
Exposure scenario 2	47.00	(12.66)	51.00	(14.74)
PANAS_NA				
Neutral environment	15.47	(5.14)	15.08	(4.25)
Exposure scenario 1	18.33	(6.23)	17.23	(5.12)
Exposure scenario 2	15.67	(3.60)	19.46	(8.61)

Note: IM-Exp = exposure to a personalized scenario in imagination, VR-Exp = exposure to a standardized scenario in virtual reality.

Following data screening, variables were analyzed with repeated measures ANOVAs, followed by a priori orthogonal within-subjects contrasts. Contrasts focused on the impact of the neutral scenario and first exposure and of the first and second exposures on the cognitive exposure group compared to the virtual exposure group. All Mauchly's (sphericity) values were non-significant, therefore the non-corrected values were used. To control for Type-I error rate, Bonferroni corrections were applied. Controlling with ANCOVAs for the use of three standardized scenarios did not change the interpretation of the results. When results were not significant, the expected number of participants required to detect a significant difference at alpha = 0.05 with a power of 0.80 is reported based on Cohen [41] to illustrate the magnitude of the differences.

Descriptive information and results for all dependent variables following the ANOVAs are reported in Tables 2 and 3 respectively. For the main effect of Time, a repeated measures ANOVA showed a significant increase in anxiety as measured with the STAI-Y1, when comparing exposure to the neutral VE and exposure to either a catastrophic scenario (traditional personalized scenario or VR scenario, see Figure 1 for illustration). The interaction was non-significant, indicating that exposure to the traditional personalized scenario over time did not elicit more anxiety than exposure to the virtual scenario. The first contrast revealed that the first exposure to either the traditional personalized scenario or the virtual scenario was significantly more anxiety provoking than exposure to the neutral scenario [$t(26) = 3.82$, $p < 0.001$, eta-squared = 0.22, effect size = large, power = 0.96]. The interaction contrast was non-significant [$t(26) = -0.58$, $p > 0.05$, eta-squared = 0.006, effect-size = very small, power = 0.10, expected N to detect a significant difference with a power of 0.80 > 2000], showing that both scenarios induced anxiety. The contrast from the first exposure to the second exposure was non-significant [$t(26) = 0.48$, $p > 0.05$. eta-squared −0.004, effect-size = very small, power = 0.07, expected N to detect a significant difference with a power of 0.80 > 2000], suggesting that the first exposure was not more anxiety provoking than the second exposure, regardless of the scenario. However, the interaction contrast was significant [$t(26) = 2.20$, $p < 0.05$, partial eta-squared = 0.09, effect-size = medium, power = 0.65], indicating that the traditional personalized scenario elicited more anxiety than the VR scenario. The interaction did not remain significant when applying the Bonferroni correction.

Results on the negative affect scale of the PANAS were somewhat different (see Figure 2 for illustration). In the group first exposed to traditional cognitive exposure, negative affect decreased in the second exposure whereas the second group, first exposed to VR, shows an increase in negative affect when exposed to the traditional personalized scenario. The results for the main effect of Time from the ANOVA revealed non-significant increase in negative affect overall. The first a priori contrast indicated that negative affect did significantly increase from the neutral scenario to the first exposure in both scenarios [$t(26) = 2.59$, $p < 0.05$, eta-squared = 0.11, effect-size = medium, power = 0.78], although the increase did not remain significant when applying the Bonferroni correction. The interaction contrast was non-significant [$t(26) = 0.94$, $p > 0.05$, eta-squared = 0.02, effect-size = small, power = 0.20, expected N to detect a significant difference with a power of 0.80 = 344], revealing a similar and only slight increase in negative affect. The second a priori interaction contrast was non-significant [$t(26) = 2.03$, $p > 0.05$ eta-squared = 0.07, effect-size = medium, power = 0.60, expected N to detect a significant difference with a power of 0.80 = 120], although the effect size was close to significance.

Table 3. Results of main effects of repeated measures ANOVAs for the comparative effect of cognitive exposure generalized anxiety disorder (GAD) scenarios presented in imagination and in virtual reality.

Effect	*MS*	*df*	*F*	*p*	ηp^2
STAI-Y1					
Time	564.10	2	9.03	< 0.001	0.258
Time × Condition	129.96	2	2.08	0.135	0.074
Condition	4.06	1	0.01	0.92	0.000
PANAS_NA					
Time	53.87	2	2.97	0.60	0.102
Time × Condition	48.75	2	2.69	0.078	0.094
Condition	56.38	1	0.61	0.44	0.023

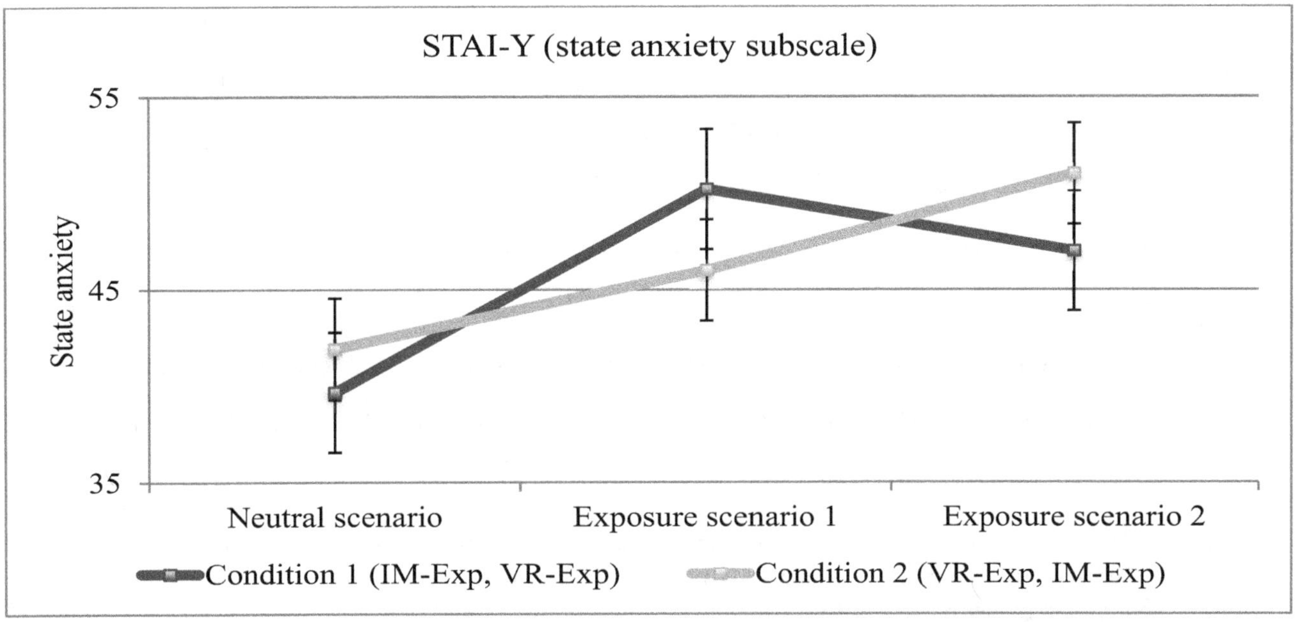

Figure 1. Illustration of the differential impact of exposure to a neutral scenario in virtual reality, a personalized scenario in imagination (IM-Exp) and a standardized scenario in virtual reality (VR-Exp) on the self-report measure of anxiety.

Further exploratory analyses were conducted to study predictors of the impact of the exposure to the standardized catastrophic scenarios in VR. To respect a subject-to-variable ratio that minimizes parameter inflation and maximizes replicability, only three predictors were selected: two variables related to GAD (intolerance of uncertainty—IUS, and beliefs about worry—WW-II) and one related to VR (immersive tendencies - ITQ). Prior to performing the analyses, data were screened for linearity (by examining a scatterplot), multicollinearity (by verifying the tolerance and VIF values), autocorrelation among the residuals (by verifying the Durbin-Watson values and examining a scatterplot), multivariate normality (by examining a histogram), and homoscedasticity (by examining a scatterplot). All assumptions were met.

In the exploratory predictor analyses of state anxiety during exposure to the standardized scenario in VR, the main regression was significant [adj$R^2 = 0.44$, $F_{(3, 24)} = 7.29$, $p < 0.01$]. Two predictors were significant, the usefulness of worrying (WW-II; $t = 2.99$, partial $r = 0.46$, $p < 0.01$) and the immersive tendency (ITQ; $t = 4.14$, partial $r = 0.63$, $p < 0.001$). Intolerance of uncertainty was not a significant predictor (IUS; $t = -0.9$, partial $r = -0.15$, $p = 0.35$ ns). The exploratory predictor analyses of negative affect was significant [adj$R^2 = 0.32$, $F_{(3, 24)} = 4.79$, $p < 0.05$], with only the immersive tendency standing out as a significant predictor (ITQ; $t = 3.54$, partial $r = 0.6$, $p < 0.01$). Regression parameters were not significant for the WW-II ($t = 1.62$, partial $r = 0.27$, $p = 0.12$ ns) and the IUS ($t = -0.22$, partial $r = -0.04$, $p = 0.83$ ns). The scaterplots in Figure 3 illustrate the tendecy, and individial differences, for higher predispositions to feel present in VR to be associated with more anxiety and negative affect.

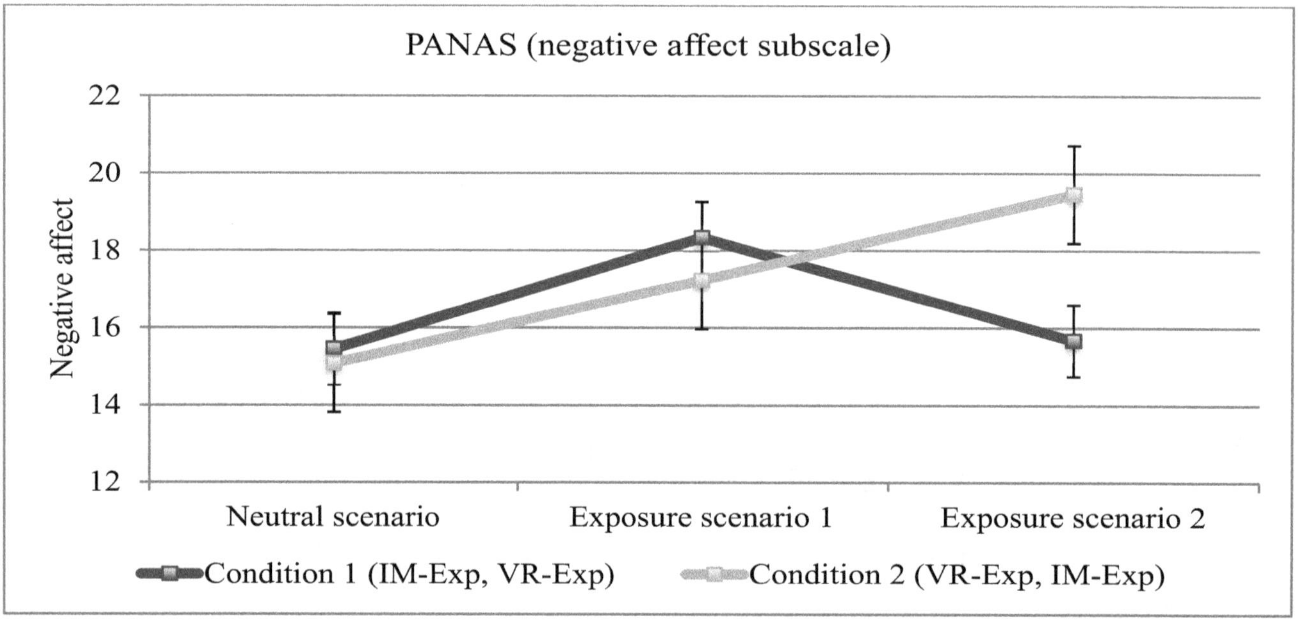

Figure 2. Illustration of the differential impact of exposure to a neutral scenario in virtual reality, a personalized scenario in imagination (IM-Exp) and a standardized scenario in virtual reality (VR-Exp) on the self-report measure of negative affect.

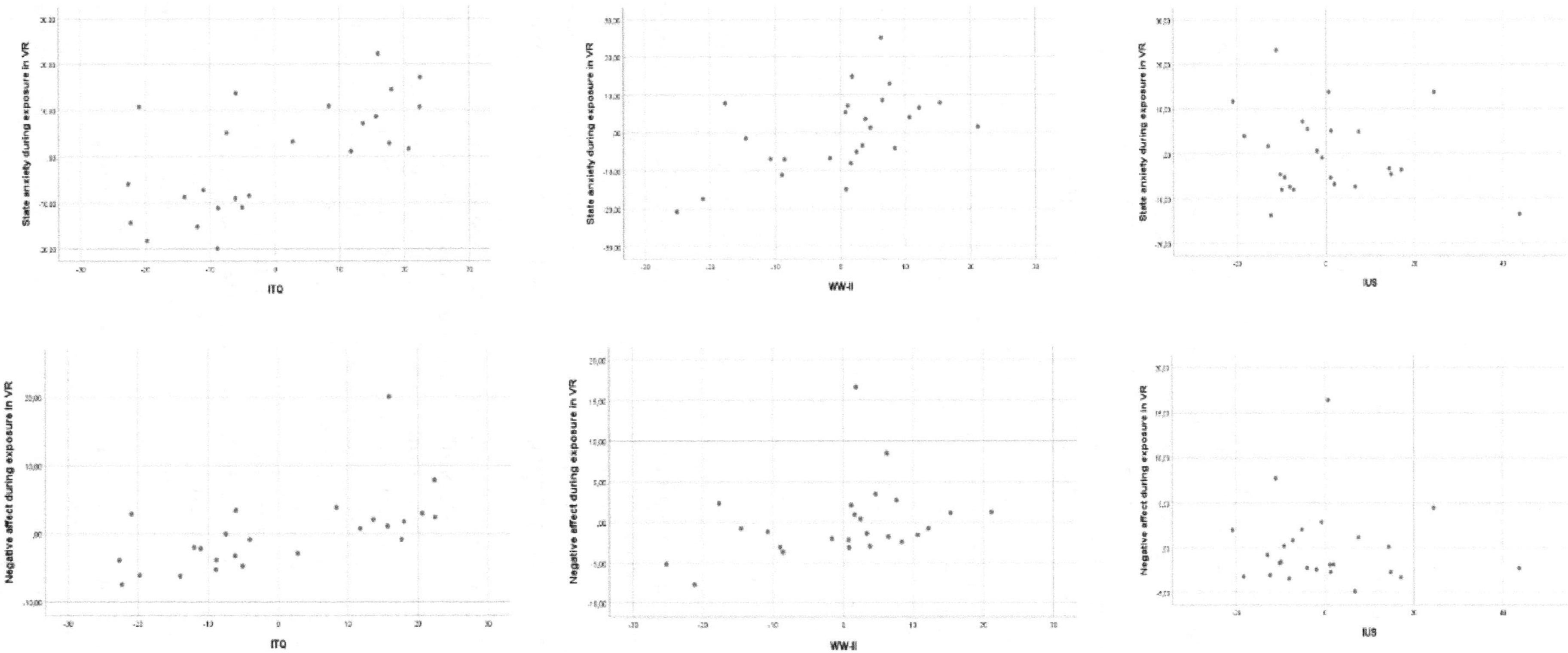

Figure 3. Scatterplots for the three predictors of state anxiety (**top** three) and negative affect (**bottom** three): immersive tendency (ITQ, **left** plot), positive beliefs about worry (WW-II, **center** plot), and intolerance of uncertainty (IUS, **right** plot).

4. Discussion

The goal of the current study was to assess the potential of VR scenarios to elicit anxiety in GAD patients, with the long-term research goal of facilitating cognitive exposure in CBT. The current study compared a standardized scenario in VR and a traditional personalized scenario. More precisely, we compared traditional exposure in imagination using a personalized catastrophic scenario to exposure in VR to a standardized scenario. Exposure to a neutral scenario was used as a baseline for comparisons. We hypothesized that exposure in VR to the standardized scenario would be significantly more anxiety provoking than the neutral scenario. No specific hypothesis was formulated for the comparison between the modalities of exposure.

Our first hypothesis was supported. The state anxiety scores during exposure in VR and in imagination were significantly higher than the baseline. Results were also in the same range than in the Guitard et al. [25] study, where participants had to imagine the scenarios instead of being exposed to them in VR, and to studies using VR for other anxiety disorders (e.g., [6,7]). The actual difference between exposure to standardized scenarios in VR and personalized scenarios in imagination was significant only when the sequence of exposure sessions was counterbalanced and it did not remain significant after controlling for the number of comparisons. The effect size and statistical power of the comparisons between the two exposure modalities deserve attention. When compared to the neutral scenario, the increase in anxiety experience in the personalized scenario in imagination versus the standardized scenario in VR is associated with a small effect size and more than 2 000 participants would be required to detect a significant difference in the two exposure modalities. This is supporting the potential of VR with GAD patients. However, the direct comparison of the two modalities with each other (i.e., the interaction contrast between the exposure scenarios) is associated with a medium effect size and a lack of power explains why the difference does not remain significant after controlling for the number of comparisons. Overall, this suggests that personalized scenarios may be more anxiety provoking. Based on the multiple regression analysis, we can speculate this may be especially relevant for people who have a strong susceptibility to be immersed in VR. Nevertheless, the potential of using standardized scenarios in VR remains promising because it did elicit anxiety in GAD patients.

The findings are even more interesting because they were observed on the anxiety measure, but not on the less specific measure of negative affect. To be more precise, the impact of the exposure sessions mirror those of the anxiety measure on the a priori contrasts, but the differences do not remain statistically significant after controlling for the number of comparisons. Readers relying more on effect sizes than probability levels, or on power analyses, would consider the finding meaningful, consistent with Guitard et al. [25] and actually revealing more specificity to fear and anxiety than to diffuse negative emotions.

A pilot and independent clinical trial based on our results support our interest in the use of VR with GAD patients. Labbé, Thibault, Côté, and Gosselin [42] assessed the effectiveness of conducting only exposure to one standardized scenario (the emergency waiting room) in VR with people diagnosed with GAD. Participants were exposed three times to the scenario. Results showed a significant improvement on all measures related to GAD post-treatment, including the tendency to worry, symptoms of GAD, and anxiety. Treatment gains were maintained at the two-month follow-up. In addition, the changes were specific to health-related worries, which is consistent with the content of the scenario used for exposure. Results from Labbé et al. [42] are in line with the pioneering paper from Repetto et al. [43] on GAD, although they are the first to address the core fear of GAD.

Some limitations of the current study must be pointed out and discussed. First, the sample is relatively small. The provision of effect sizes should help gauge the magnitude of the experimental manipulations and plan larger studies. The effect of repeated exposure to standardized versus personalized scenarios should also be documented. The sociodemographic and clinical characteristics of the sample are typical of a study sample of GAD patients, with the exception of slightly more women than what is found in the general population, where women are usually three times more likely than men to have GAD [44]. A larger proportion of males would allow comparing the potential impact of gender differences. Documenting sex, economic, marital, and educational status in research articles is important for clinicians and researchers in order to appraise the sample and generalize the results. Reviews have been conducted on the power of immersions in VR to induce anxiety responses (e.g., [45]), but the impact of these variables has not yet been examined. Because these variables are frequently associated with anxiety disorders, their impact on the effect of VR deserve to be explored. The addition of physiological measures of anxiety would have documented and complemented our findings with objective measures [25]. However, heart rate or skin conductance would have been biased and unreliable given implicit differences in the exposure sessions. Participants were seated in the session of exposure in imagination. But in VR, participants were standing up and were physically moving when exploring the virtual environment. The intensity of the anxiety response also deserves attention. The research protocol was not designed to show how much an experience in VR could be frightening to GAD patients, but to show the potential of scenarios with a feeling of uncertainty to elicit anxiety in a population that is known to perceive uncertainty as threatening [18]. Finally, to increase generalization of the results to the psychotherapy contexts, it would have been interesting to conduct the study while patients are already in therapy and ready to proceed with exposure. Such a study comes with methodological challenges and it was considered better to first show that scenarios that are not individualized and presented in VR bear some potential.

Furthermore, the choice of three different VEs instead of only one could be argued as another limitation. However, the drawback of using only one scenario would be not targeting the main worry themes of the participants. This would be far more detrimental than comparing only three slightly different generic scenarios to 28 totally different and individualized ones. A replication study with a sample selected on the basis of the main worry theme would allow a more direct comparison of the exposure modalities with similar themes, or a larger sample would allow comparisons between virtual scenarios. Comparisons with people suffering from other anxiety disorders and with non-anxious participants would help document the specificity of the reactions to GAD.

The results from the exploratory analyses revealed that immersive tendencies, or individual predispositions to feel present, significantly predicted the increase in emotional reactions of participants. The predictive importance of the ITQ was significant when predicting anxiety and negative affect during exposure *in virtuo*. Perceived usefulness of worrying was another significant predictor of state anxiety in VR, but not intolerance of uncertainty. Presenting the neutral immersion in VR to all participants at the beginning of the experiment may have protected against the elements of novelty in the task [25], leaving room for other variables to stand out, such as the severity of dysfunctional thoughts about the usefulness of worry in predicting state anxiety. Future research should document with a larger sample, more predictors, better control for the different VR scenarios and planned hypotheses, and predictors of emotional reactions of patients in VR.

5. Conclusions

Because uncertainty is the core fear underlying GAD [18,19], the current study examined if immersion in virtual standardized scenarios that were developed based on the feeling of uncertainty and typical GAD worry themes may be relevant to be used in CBT. The increase in anxiety during immersion support the potential of VR for exposure, even in the case where feared stimuli are not as specific as in phobias and other anxiety disorders. This paves the way for the development of psychotherapy protocols that would integrate *in virtuo* exposure to test in randomized control trials.

Author Contributions: Conceptualization, T.G., S.B., and C.B.; methodology, T.G., S.B., and C.B.; software, S.B.; validation, S.B. and C.B.; formal analysis, S.B. and M.B.; investigation, T.G.; resources, S.B.; data curation, T.G.; writing—original draft preparation, T.G. and M.B.; writing—review and editing, T.G., S.B., C.B., and M.B.; visualization, T.G., S.B., C.B., and M.B.; supervision, S.B. and C.B.; project administration, T.G.; funding acquisition, S.B.

References

1. Marshall, W.L. Exposure. In *Dictionary of Behavior Therapy Techniques*; Bellack, A.S., Herson, M., Eds.; Pergamon Press: New York, NY, USA, 1986; pp. 121–124.
2. Craske, M.G.; Treanor, M.; Conway, C.C.; Zbozinek, T.; Vervliet, B. Maximizing exposure therapy: An inhibitory learning approach. *Behav. Res. Ther.* **2014**, *58*, 10–23. [CrossRef] [PubMed]
3. Richard, D.C.S.; Lauterbach, D.; Gloster, A.T. Description, mechanisms of action, and assessment. In *Handbook of Exposure Therapies*; Richard, D.C.S., Lauterbach, D., Eds.; Academic Press: Cambridge, MA, USA, 2007; pp. 1–28.
4. Bouchard, S.; Robillard, G.; Larouche, S.; Loranger, C. Description of a treatment manual for *in virtuo* exposure with specific phobia. In *Virtual Reality in Psychological, Medical and Pedagogical Applications*; Eichenberg, C., Ed.; InTech: Rijeka, Croatia, 2012; pp. 82–108.
5. Robillard, G.; Bouchard, S.; Fournier, T.; Renaud, P. Anxiety and presence during VR immersion: A comparative study of the reactions of phobic and non-phobic participants in therapeutic virtual environments derived from computer games. *Cyberpsychol. Behav.* **2003**, *6*, 467–476. [CrossRef] [PubMed]
6. Laforest, M.; Bouchard, S.; Crétu, A.-M.; Mesly, O. Inducing an anxiety response using a contaminated virtual environment: Validation of a therapeutic tool for obsessive-compulsive disorder. *Front. ICT* **2016**, *3*, 18. [CrossRef]
7. Kim, K.; Roh, D.; Kim, C.H.; Cha, K.R.; Rosenthal, M.Z.; Kim, S.I. Comparison of checking behavior in adults with or without checking symptoms of obsessive-compulsive disorder using a novel computer-based measure. *Comput. Methods Programs Biomed.* **2012**, *108*, 434–441. [CrossRef] [PubMed]
8. McCann, R.A.; Armstrong, C.M.; Skopp, N.A.; Edwards-Stewart, A.; Smolenski, D.J.; June, J.D.; Metzger-Abamukong, M.; Reger, G.M. Virtual reality exposure therapy for the treatment of anxiety disorders: An evaluation of research quality. *J. Anxiety Disord.* **2014**, *28*, 625–631. [CrossRef] [PubMed]
9. Chesham, R.K.; Malouff, J.M.; Schutte, N.S. Meta-analysis of the efficacy of virtual reality exposure therapy for social anxiety. *Behav. Chang.* **2018**, *35*, 1–15. [CrossRef]
10. Fernández-Alvarez, J.; Rozental, A.; Carlbring, P.; Colombo, D.; Riva, G.; Anderson, P.L.; Baños, R.M.; Benbow, A.A.; Bouchard, S.; Bretón López, J.M.; et al. Deterioration rates in virtual reality exposure therapy: An individual patient data level meta-analysis. *J. Anxiety Disord.* **2018**, in press. [CrossRef]
11. Morina, N.; Ijntema, H.; Meyerbroker, K.; Emmelkamp, P.M.G. Can virtual reality exposure therapy gains be generalized to real-life? A meta-analysis of studies applying behavioral assessments. *Behav. Res. Ther.* **2015**, *74*, 18–24. [CrossRef] [PubMed]
12. Tisseau, J. In vivo, in vitro, in silico, in virtuo. In Proceedings of the 1st Workshop on SMA in Biology at Meso or Macroscopic Scales, Paris, France, 2 July 2008; pp. 1–17.
13. Fuchs, P.; Moreau, G.; Guitton, P. *Virtual Reality: Concepts and Technologies*; CRC Press: New York, NY, USA, 2011.
14. Wiederhold, B. Virtual Reality in the 1990s: What Did We Learn? *Cyberpsychol. Behav.* **2004**, *3*, 311–314. [CrossRef]
15. Blade, R.A.; Padgett, M.L. Virtual Environments Standards and Terminology. In *Handbook of Virtual Environments: Design, Implementation, and Applications*; Stanney, K., Ed.; Lawrence Erlbaum Associates Publishers: Mahwah, NJ, USA, 2002; pp. 21–33.
16. Hirai, M.; Vernon, L.L.; Cochran, H. Exposure for phobias. In *Handbook of Exposure Therapies*; Richard, D.C.S., Lauterbach, D., Eds.; Academic Press: San Diego, CA, USA, 2007; pp. 247–270.
17. Garcia-Palacios, A.; Hoffman, H.G.; Kwon See, S.; Tsai, A.; Botella, C. Redefining therapeutic success with VR exposure therapy. *Cyberpsychol. Behav.* **2001**, *4*, 341–348. [CrossRef] [PubMed]
18. Dugas, M.J.; Gagnon, F.; Ladouceur, R.; Freeston, M.H. Generalized anxiety disorder: A preliminary test of a conceptual model. *Behav. Res. Ther.* **1998**, *36*, 215–226. [CrossRef]
19. Dugas, M.; Ladouceur, R. Treatment of GAD. Targeting intolerance of uncertainty in two types of worry. *Bheav. Modif.* **2000**, *24*, 635–657. [CrossRef] [PubMed]
20. Freeston, M.H.; Rhéaume, J.; Letarte, H.; Dugas, M.J.; Ladouceur, R. Why do people worry? *Personal. Individ. Differ.* **1994**, *17*, 791–802. [CrossRef]
21. Dugas, M.J.; Robichaud, M. *Cognitive-Behavioral Treatment for Generalized Anxiety Disorder*; Routledge: New York, NY, USA, 2007.

22. Goldman, N.; Dugas, M.J.; Sexton, K.A.; Gervais, N.J. The impact of written exposure on worry. *Behav. Modif.* **2007**, *31*, 512–538. [CrossRef] [PubMed]
23. Bouchard, S.; Côté, S.; Richard, D.C.S. Virtual reality applications for exposure. In *Handbook of Exposure Therapies*; Richard, D.C.S., Lauterbach, D., Eds.; Academic Press: Cambridge, MA, USA, 2007; pp. 347–388.
24. Dallaire, L.; Bouchard, S. Identification des thèmes récurrents d'exposition dans le cadre du traitement cognitif du TAG. Unpublished Manuscript. 2007.
25. Guitard, T.; Bouchard, S.; Bélanger, C. Exposure to standardized catastrophic scenarios with patients suffering from GAD. Presented at the 45th Annual Convention of the Association for Behavioral and Cognitive Therapy (ABCT), Toronto, ON, Canada, 10–13 November 2011.
26. Brown, T.A.; DiNardo, P.A.; Barlow, D.H. *Anxiety Disorders Interview Schedule for DSM-IV (ADIS-IV)*; Psychological Corporation: San Antonio, TX, USA, 1994.
27. Meyer, T.J.; Miller, M.L.; Metzger, R.L.; Borkovec, T.D. Development and validation of the Penn State Worry Questionnaire. *Behav. Res. Ther.* **1990**, *28*, 487–495. [CrossRef]
28. Ladouceur, R.; Freeston, M.H.; Dumont, J.; Letarte, H.; Rhéaume, J.; Gagnon, F.; Thibodeau, N. Penn State Worry Questionnaire: Validity and reliability of a French translation. *Can. Psychol.* **1992**, *33*, 236.
29. Molina, S.; Borkovec, T.D. The Penn State Worry Questionnaire: Psychometric properties and associated characteristics. In *Worrying: Perspectives on Theory, Assessment and Treatment*; Davey, G.C.L., Tallis, F., Eds.; John Wiley & Sons: New York, NY, USA, 1994; pp. 265–283.
30. Gosselin, P.; Langlois, F.; Freeston, M.H.; Ladouceur, R.; Dugas, M.J.; Pelletier, O. Le questionnaire d'évitement cognitif: Développement et validation auprès d'adultes et d'adolescents. *Journal de thérapie comportementale et cognitive* **2002**, *12*, 24–37.
31. Gosselin, P.; Dugas, M.J.; Ladouceur, R.; Freeston, M.H. Évaluation des inquiétudes: Validation d'une traduction française du Penn State Worry Questionnaire. *L'Encéphale* **2001**, *27*, 475–484. [PubMed]
32. Robillard, G.; Bouchard, S.; Renaud, P.; Cournoyer, L.G. Validation canadienne-française de deux mesures importantes en réalité virtuelle: l'Immersive Tendencies Questionnaire et le Presence Questionnaire. In Proceedings of the 25ième congrès de la Société Québécoise pour la Recherche en Psychologie (SQRP), Trois-Rivières, QC, Canada, 1–3 November 2002.
33. Witmer, B.G.; Singer, M.J. Measuring presence in virtual environments: A presence questionnaire. *Presence* **1998**, *7*, 225–240. [CrossRef]
34. Bouchard, S.; Robillard, G.; Renaud, P. Revising the factor structure of the Simulator Sickness Questionnaire. *Annu. Rev. Cyberther. Telemed.* **2007**, *5*, 117–122.
35. Kennedy, R.S.; Lane, N.E.; Berbaum, K.S.; Lilienthal, M.G. Simulator sickness questionnaire: An enhanced method for quantifying simulator sickness. *Int. J. Aviat. Psychol.* **1993**, *3*, 203–220. [CrossRef]
36. Gauthier, J.; Bouchard, S. Adaptation canadienne-française de la forme révisée du State-Trait Anxiety Inventory de Spielberger. *Revue Canadienne des Sciences du Comportement* **1993**, *25*, 559–578. [CrossRef]
37. Spielberger, C.D.; Gorsuch, R.L.; Lushene, R.; Vagg, P.R.; Jacobs, G.A. *Manual for the State-Trait Anxiety Inventory*; Consulting Psychologists Press: Palo Alto, CA, USA, 1983.
38. Gaudreau, P.; Sanchez, X.; Blondin, J.P. Positive and negative affective states in a performance-related setting: Testing the factorial structure of the PANAS across two samples of French-Canadian participants. *Eur. J. Psychol. Assess.* **2006**, *22*, 240–249. [CrossRef]
39. Watson, D.; Clark, L.; Tellegen, A. Development and validation of brief measures of positive and negative affect: The PANAS scales. *J. Personal. Soc. Psychol.* **1988**, *54*, 1063–1070. [CrossRef]
40. Bouvard, M. *Questionnaires et échelles d'évaluation de la personnalité*, 3rd ed.; Elsevier Masson: Paris, France, 2009.
41. Cohen, J. *Statistical Power Analysis for the Behavioral Sciences*; Lawrence Erlbaum Associates: London, UK, 1988.
42. Labbé Thibault, P.; Côté, G.; Gosselin, P. Effet de l'exposition en réalité virtuelle sur les symptômes du trouble d'anxiété généralisée. Ph.D. Thesis, Université de Sherbrooke, Sherbrooke, QC, Canada, 2017.
43. Repetto, C.; Gaggioli, A.; Pallavicini, F.; Cipresso, P.; Raspelli, S.; Riva, G. Virtual reality and mobile phones in the treatment of generalized anxiety disorders: A phase-2 clinical trial. *Pers. Ubiquitous Comput.* **2013**, *17*, 253–260. [CrossRef]
44. Katzman, M.; Bleau, P.; Blier, P.; Chokka, P.; Kjernisted, K.; Van Ameringen, M.; Antony, M.; Bouchard, S.; Brunet, A.; Flament, M.; et al. Canadian clinical practice guidelines for the management of anxiety, posttraumatic stress and obsessive-compulsive disorders. *BMC Psychiatry* **2014**, *14* (Suppl. 1), S1. [CrossRef] [PubMed]

2

Can we Predict the Evolution of Depressive Symptoms, Adjustment and Perceived Social Support of Pregnant Women from their Personality Characteristics? A Technology-Supported Longitudinal Study

Laura Andreu-Pejó [1,2], Verónica Martínez-Borba [1,2], Carlos Suso-Ribera [1] and Jorge Osma [2,3,*]

[1] Nursing Department, Universitat Jaume I de Castelló, Castelló de la Plana, 12071 Valencia, Spain; pejo@uji.es (L.A.-P.); borba@uji.es (V.M.-B.); susor@uji.es (C.S.-R.)
[2] Instituto de Investigación Sanitaria de Aragón, 50009 Zaragoza, Spain
[3] Departmento de Psicología y Sociología, Universidad de Zaragoza, 44003 Teruel, Spain
* Correspondence: osma@unizar.es

Abstract: *Background*: Research exploring the relationship between personality and important pregnancy outcomes (i.e., depressive symptoms, adjustment, and perceived social support) tends to be cross-sectional, arguably due to the difficulties of conducting longitudinal and mental health research in this population. The objective of this study is to use a web-based solution to longitudinally explore how personality traits are associated, not only with the co-occurrence of these outcomes but also with their evolution during pregnancy. Stability and change of these outcomes will also be investigated. *Methods*: The sample included 85 pregnant women attending several medical centers in Spain. The web-based assessment included sociodemographic and obstetric variables (ad hoc) and personality (at the second trimester only), and outcomes at both the second and the third trimester (i.e., depressive symptoms, adjustment, and perceived social support). *Results*: The results showed that adjustment worsened from the second to the third trimester of pregnancy. Neuroticism (N), low extraversion (E), and psychoticism (P) were cross-sectionally and longitudinally associated with outcomes. In addition, N and, to a lesser extent P, uniquely contributed to the evolution of these outcomes in the multivariate analyses, including autoregressions. *Conclusion*: Personality and especially N and P should be evaluated early during pregnancy mental health screening. The use of a web page appears to be a useful tool for that purpose. Technologies might also help disseminate mental health prevention programs for these women, which would be especially recommended for those with a personality profile characterized by high N and P and, to a lesser extent, low E.

Keywords: information and communication technologies; pregnancy; personality; depression; adjustment; social support

---

1. Introduction

Pregnancy is a period of great changes and demands for women and often challenges their ability to adapt to important physiological, social, and psychological changes and to continue to perform despite these difficulties [1]. Additionally, there is a large body of research suggesting that pregnant women may be particularly vulnerable to the detrimental effects of environmental stressors on their mental health [2], which altogether would explain the existence of high emotional distress and stress in this period of the woman's life [3]. For example, it is estimated that prenatal depression (PD) can affect up to 25%–38% of women worldwide [4]. In Spain, studies on the prevalence of

PD are scarce, although the available data indicates that at least 14.8% of women would experience moderate-to-severe symptoms of depression during pregnancy [5]. In addition, in Spain, the healthcare services provided to the perinatal women are mainly focused on the physical aspects related to pregnancy and postpartum, living aside the mental health aspects [6]. Thus, the study of mental well-being during the perinatal period and its predictors is relevant in this country if routine practices are to be changed. The clinical practice guidelines developed by the most prominent organizations in the field of perinatal mental health agree in emphasizing the importance of developing screening strategies that facilitate the detection of women who present risk factors for emotional problems throughout the perinatal period [7–10]. The risk factors for PD that are most frequently included in these clinical guidelines are current anxious and depressive symptoms, previous history of psychiatric problems, history of sexual abuse or child maltreatment, history of gender violence, adjustment problems with the partner, the experience of a traumatic birth, and the death of the baby during childbirth. In addition to these factors, there is evidence to suggest that certain normal personality traits, especially high neuroticism (N), high psychoticism (P), and low extraversion (E), are related to greater psychopathology in this population [11–13]. However, these guidelines do not yet support the need for the evaluation of these personality traits in pregnant women, which suggests that further research is needed in this field.

Regarding N, this is a personality trait characterized by the tendency to experience frequent and intense negative emotions in response to a stressful situation (e.g., pregnancy or childbirth). Furthermore, N is associated with a perception of ineffective coping. Thus, when N is high and persistent, processes such as worry, rumination, or emotional avoidance are likely to appear [14]. Interest in this personality trait, which is considered a widespread biological vulnerability factor for the etiology and maintenance of emotional disorders, including depression, has increased in recent years [15]. For example, Bunevicius et al. [16] found that high scores in N were, together with an unplanned and unwanted pregnancy, independent determinants of prenatal depressive disorders throughout pregnancy. In this same line, several authors have concluded that, of all personality dimensions, N could be considered the most important predictive risk factors for depression both in pregnancy and in the postpartum [13,17]. Additionally and linked with this tendency to experience negative emotions, N has been associated with low perceived social support [18] and poor adjustment to childbirth stressors [19].

Different to N, E refers to the tendency to experience positive emotions such as happiness, optimism, or enthusiasm and attitudes of security, activation, and interest for social interaction [20,21] and is associated with reduced vulnerability to affective disorders [22], increased social support [18], and successful adjustment to childbirth stressors [19]. In this sense, recent studies argue that low E, also known as introversion, would be a key personality trait associated with the onset of emotional disorders and poor adjustment during the perinatal period [23].

Finally, P is a personality trait that includes severe psychopathological conditions, such as deception or interpersonal alienation, to more frequent human expressions such as hostility, anger, and social isolation [24]. The literature exploring the role of P in pregnant women is scarce, but research so far supports the idea that high P poses a risk for perinatal women of PD [25]. The relationship between P and adjustment and social support during pregnancy remains unexplored. However, because P is inversely related to agreeableness [26], a key factor associated with perceived availability of social support [18] and effective coping use and adaptation during pregnancy [27], a negative impact of P on these outcomes would be expected.

To date, the relationship between personality and outcomes in perinatal research (i.e., depressive symptomatology and adaptation to the challenges associated with the perinatal period) has been predominantly explored using cross-sectional designs [13,16,17,25]. Consequently, little is actually known about the influence of normal personality traits (N, E, and P) in the evolution of depressive symptoms and adjustment of women during the perinatal period. Additionally, while it has been argued that poor social support, which is known to negatively impact mood and adjustment during the perinatal period [28,29], might be partly influenced by the personality profile of the mothers (i.e., high N, low E, and high P would arguably represent the high-risk profile) [13,17,20], this also remains unexplored during pregnancy. Note that social support and adjustment are key factors associated with well-being in the mother. Social support (i.e., perceived support from family, partners, and peers) is important both during pregnancy and at the postpartum, and low perceived support appears to add to the mental burden associated with the perinatal period (i.e., depression) [29]. Regarding maladjustment, this measure of poor emotional adaptation to the challenges that can occur during the perinatal period has been associated not only with suffering in the mother but also with internalizing problems in the baby [30]. In the light of the previous, the goal of the present investigation is to investigate whether the personality profile of prenatal women indeed predicts the evolution of depressive symptoms, adjustment to pregnancy, and social support perceived by these women using a longitudinal design.

As noted in the previous lines, there is an evident lack of longitudinal and prospective studies that try to clarify the role of personality traits and other psychosocial variables with respect to important perinatal outcomes, such as depressive symptoms and adjustment [31]. It is possible that this lack of longitudinal research is due to its high cost, especially in terms of time, because longitudinal research implies carrying out repeated evaluations during pregnancy. This might indeed problematic for public health systems since the time available for consultations is limited and estimated (i.e., 10–15 min per patient globally) [32]. Furthermore, reluctance to face-to-face psychological evaluations by women in the perinatal stage are frequent as a consequence of the stigma associated with mental illness [33].

The use of information and communication technologies (ICTs) might help overcome some of these limitations of traditional paper-and-pencil, face-to-face evaluations in the perinatal period. Briefly stated, repeated assessment using ICTs imposes less burden on healthcare professional and users, facilitates data collection since evaluations are carried out in the real context of women and traveling to the clinic for assessments is no longer needed, and minimizes stigmatization as they are perceived as being more anonymous and private [34]. Additionally, it is important to note that the use of ICTs in the general population has grown considerably in the past years. In 2008, 61% of homes in the European Union had access to the Internet. Now, in 2019, this has risen to 87% of homes [35]. Most importantly, in our field, 57% of pregnant women download health-related apps to seek information associated with pregnancy, which suggests that the use of ICTs in this field is growing significantly [36]. For this reason, the use of ICT in the field of mental health problems and maladjustment prevention [37], and specifically in the screening of depressive symptoms [38], is becoming increasingly popular and more feasible than ever. Particularly in Spain, where the public health system is very frequently used by the population, the implementation of such ICT solutions would be particularly useful to reduce the current burden associated with face-to-face assessments and interventions [36].

However, despite these promising benefits of ICT use in perinatal settings, most of the screening studies are cross-sectional and do not include the evaluation of risk factors for mental distress and poor adjustment to pregnancy [39]. From this need arises (Mamáfeliz (MMF; HappyMom)), a project that studies the risk factors for the development of perinatal emotional disorders longitudinally through the Internet (i.e., a web page). Thus, the main objective of this study is to explore how certain personality traits are associated, not only with the co-occurrence of depressive symptoms, maladjustment, and poor social support but also with their evolution during pregnancy. Importantly, a web application will be used for the longitudinal assessment of study variables. In addition to exploring the predictive role of personality on outcomes, we will also investigate the stability and change of depressive symptoms, adjustment, and social support during pregnancy. Stability and change will be investigated both at the order level (what is called "differential continuity") and at the group mean level (what is called "mean-level change"). We hypothesize scoring high in N and P will present a deterioration of depressive symptoms, adjustment, and perceived social support. By contrast, we anticipate that women scoring high in E will report an improvement in outcomes (i.e., reduction in depression and maladjustment and increase in social support). With respect to changes in outcomes, these will be investigated in an exploratory manner due to the limited literature in this regard.

2. Materials and Methods

2.1. Participants

The study sample consisted of 85 pregnant women who voluntarily agreed to participate in the project MMF and to be evaluated with a website throughout pregnancy. Women responded to two evaluations during pregnancy (completers), that is, between weeks 16–24 (Time 1) and weeks 30–36 of gestation (Time 2).

The mean age of the participants was 33.54 years (SD = 4.06; range 25–42). Of these, 94.1% were Spanish, 81.2% had a partner with whom they lived in the home, 94.1% had higher education, and 67.1% were working at the time of the first assessment. The sociodemographic characteristics of the participants are shown in Table 1.

Table 1. Sociodemographic characteristics of the sample (N = 85).

	Total
Nationality	
Spanish	94.1%
Latin American	2.4%
Western Europe	3.5%
Marital Status	
With a living partner	81.2%
Without a living partner	18.8%
Educational level	
≤12 years of education	5.9%
>12 years of education	94.1%
Employment situation	
Working	67.1%
Unemployment	20%
Sick leave	12.9%

2.2. Method

The study dissemination was made by the midwives of the collaborating centers. Study participation was offered to all pregnant women treated at the collaborating centers, which belong to the public or the private health network of MMF. The eligibility criteria were being a pregnant woman over 18 years of age, being fluent in Spanish, and having Internet access.

The collaborating healthcare personnel delivered the study information in writing along with a unique code for each participant to register into the program MMF. Thus, the entire study was conducted online. Once the participants accessed the application with their code, they had to read and accept the data protection and confidentiality documents and accept the informed consent form.

When the registration was completed, and the sociodemographic, obstetric, and medical data were filled, the evaluation of the main study variables began. Finally, the participants received a thank-you message, and they were informed that they would receive an email to complete the following evaluation in the following trimester.

The approval of the Ethics and Clinical Research Committees of all the collaborating centers was obtained.

2.3. Instruments

Sociodemographic, obstetric, and personality variables were assessed at Time 1 only (during the second trimester). Study outcomes (depressive symptoms, maladjustment, and social support) were evaluated longitudinally twice (during the second trimester and in the third trimester, to explore changes). Personality was only evaluated once to reduce the burden of assessment, because personality characteristics are relatively stable dispositions [40], and because the study focus was not on evaluating changes in personality but on predicting changes in outcomes based on baseline personality profiles.

Assessment of sociodemographic and obstetric variables (ad hoc items): Participants answered questions about their marital status, educational level, employment status, and economic level. They also responded to questions of an obstetric nature, such as the period of gestation, the history of abortion, pregnancy planning, and the level of pregnancy risk.

Revised Eysenck Personality Questionnaire (EPQ-RS) [41,42]: The EPQ-RS was administered to assess the three dimensions of normal personality from the Big Three's Eysenck model, namely neuroticism, extraversion, and psychoticism. This short version consists of 12 items per dimension in which every item evaluates a series of usual behaviors or ways of thinking or feeling. The questionnaire response format is "Yes" =1 or "No" = 0, where higher scores represent a greater presence of the trait that it evaluates. Regarding their psychometric properties of the EPQ-RS, the three scales have an acceptable internal consistency in women, that is, a Cronbach's alpha of 0.82 for N, 0.79 for E, and 0.67 for P [42]. Similar results were found in our sample for N ($\alpha = 0.82$), E ($\alpha = 0.77$), and P ($\alpha = 0.60$).

Edinburgh Postnatal Depression Scale (EPDS) [43,44]: The EPDS consists of 10 items that evaluate the depressive symptoms experienced during the last seven days. Each item has four response options with a unique value that varies from 0 to 3. Items 1 and 2 are scored from 0 = "As much as always" to 3 = "Not at all", and items 3–10 are valued inversely, from 3 = "Yes, most of the time" to 0 = "No, never". The total score is obtained by summing the scores of all 10 items. Higher scores should be interpreted as indicating more severe depressive symptoms. The maximum total score is 30 points. The Spanish adaptation of the scale has obtained very good internal consistency estimates in pregnant women ($0.81 \leq \alpha \leq 0.85$, according to trimester during pregnancy) [43]. In our sample, good internal consistency was found both in the second ($\alpha = 0.86$) and the third ($\alpha = 0.85$) trimester of pregnancy.

Maladjustment Scale (MS) [45]. This scale consists of 5 items that evaluate to what extent the psychological distress experienced by the person affects different areas of daily life, that is work or studies, social activities, free time, family life, and relationship with their partner. In addition, the scale global item that refers to the overall degree of maladjustment. Each item is rated on a 6-point scale (0 = "None" to 5 = "Very Serious"). Higher scores represent higher maladjustment. Cronbach's alpha coefficient of the Spanish validation of the scale was 0.94 [45]. In our sample, good internal consistency was found both in the second ($\alpha = 0.85$) and the third ($\alpha = 0.82$) trimester of pregnancy.

Multidimensional scale of perceived social support (MSPSS) [46,47]. The MSPSS consists of 12 items evaluated on a 7-point Likert-type scale (1 = "Strongly disagree" to 7 = "Strongly agree"). The 12 items were designed to measure the perception of support in three areas: family (items 3, 4, 8, and 11), friends (items 6, 7, 9, and 12) and other significant persons (items 1, 2, 5, and 10). High scores indicate a greater perception of support received in each of the areas. In our study, we selected the family and friends scales to reduce the number of statistical analyses and to minimize the risk of multicollinearity problems. The use of the total score of the scale was discarded due to the interest in differentiating the support of the family from that of other agents, such as friends. The alpha coefficients of the family and friends scales were 0.89 and 0.92, respectively [47]. In our sample, good internal consistency was found both in the second ($\alpha = 0.94$) and the third ($\alpha = 0.94$) trimester in the family-scale. Similar results were found in the friends-scale both in the second ($\alpha = 0.97$) and the third ($\alpha = 0.95$) trimester.

2.4. Data Analysis

First, a descriptive analysis was made. Next, the change in the study variables was explored. Two different procedures were used to investigate the evolution of the study outcomes (i.e., depressive symptoms, adjustment, and social support) during pregnancy. On the one hand, the Student *t*-test for related samples was used to assess the change in mean scores (mean-level change). Additionally, Pearson's correlations were calculated to explore order changes between the two measurement times (differential continuity).

In order to explore the cross-sectional and prospective associations between baseline personality and outcomes, we first conducted a series of Pearson's correlations.

Finally, multivariate regression was carried out to explore to what extent the changes in study outcomes (i.e., depressive symptoms, adjustment, and perceived social support) at Time 2 (third trimester of pregnancy) were explained by personality factors, after controlling for important covariates (i.e., age the corresponding outcome at Time 1, that is during the second trimester of pregnancy). Age was included as a covariate because it has been related to psychosocial adjustment during the perinatal period in the literature [48]. A Holm–Bonferroni correction was used for all statistical analyses, which resulted in a p-value of 0.0125.

3. Results

3.1. Retention of the Participants Into the Online Assessment Program MMF

Regarding the participation of women in the online program MMF, 4500 women received codes to enroll in the program. Of these, 62.2% (n = 2797) effectively registered into the web, but only 5.9% (n = 266) participated at some point in the prenatal evaluation of the program. Finally, only 85 women completed both evaluations during the second and the third trimester during pregnancy. Figure 1 describes the flow diagram of study participation.

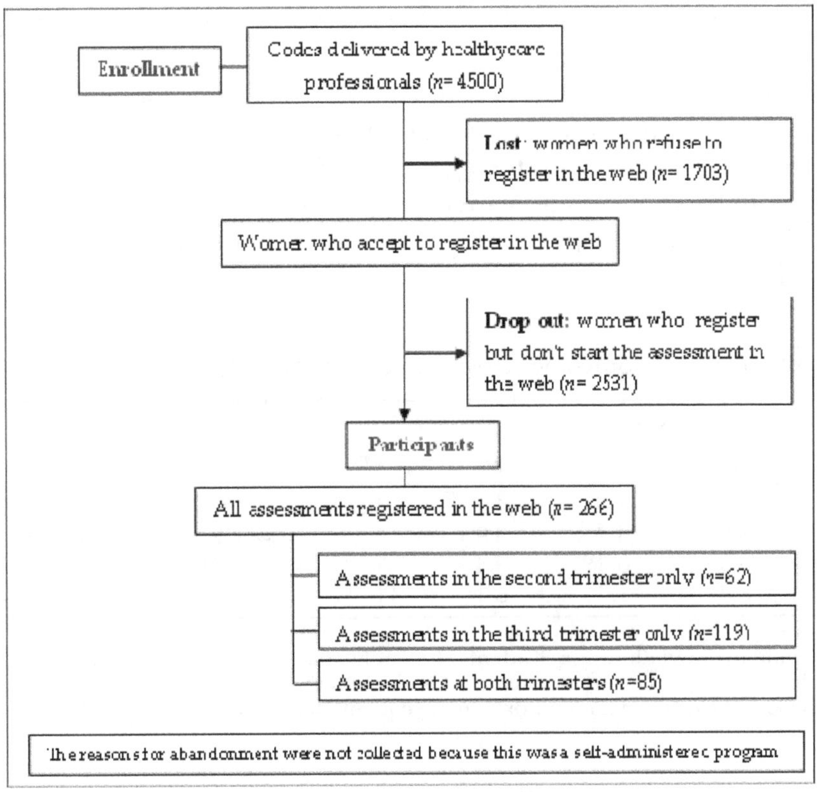

Figure 1. Flow chart of the participants in the study.

3.2. Descriptive Results of the Study Variables

Table 2 shows the means and standard deviations of the women's scores in the study variables, as well as a comparison with population normative scores. Overall, the women in our study showed a personality profile characterized by low N ($t = 7.17$, $p < 0.001$), average E ($t = 1.50$, $p = 0.135$), and low P ($t = 6.04$, $p < 0.001$). The levels of depressive symptoms during pregnancy in our sample were comparable to those of normative populations (all $p > 0.0125$). Perceived social support by family ($t = 3.59$, $p < 0.001$) and friends ($t = 4.55$, $p < 0.001$) was higher in our sample. Maladjustment scores could not be compared because normative scores do not exist for women.

Table 2. Descriptive statistics of study variables and comparison with normative scores.

Variables	N	Pregnant Women M (*SD*)	N	Reference Female Population M (*SD*)	*t*	*p*	*d*
Personality	85		583				
EPQ-RS (N)		3.8 *(3.1)*		6.6 *(3.4)*	7.169	<0.001	0.86
EPQ-RS (E)		8.7 *(2.7)*		8.2 *(2.9)*	1.498	0.135	0.18
EPQ-RS (P)		2.1 *(1.8)*		3.8 *(2.5)*	6.043	<0.001	0.78
Depressive symptoms	85		569				
EPDS (2nd T)		5.2 *(4.6)*		5.7 *(3.9)*	1.076	0.282	0.12
EPDS (3rd T)		4.7 *(4.3)*		5.7 *(4.3)*	1.999	0.046	0.23
Maladjustment	85						
MS		6.2 *(5.3)*		-	-	-	-
Social support	85		265				
MSPSS (Family)		6.5 *(0.8)*		6.0 *(1.2)*	3.592	<0.001	0.49
MSPSS (Friends)		6.3 *(1.0)*		5.6 *(1.3)*	4.549	<0.001	0.60

EPQ-RS = Eysenck Personality Questionnaire (N: neuroticism; E: extraversion; P: psychoticism); EPDS = Edinburgh Postnatal Depression Scale; T = trimester; MS = maladjustment scale; MSPSS = Multidimensional Scale of Perceived Social Support.

3.3. Evolution of Outcomes (Depressive Symptoms, Adjustment, and Perceived Social Support) During Pregnancy

Table 3 presents the means and standard deviations of study outcomes, as well as the analyses of change at the mean level and at the rank order level. Regarding mean values, only a significant increase in maladjustment was observed during pregnancy ($t = 4.83$, $p < 0.001$). Taking changes at the order level, the moderate-to-strong significant correlations should be interpreted as indicating some stability at the order level. Social support variables were the ones that remained more stable in terms of order (strong correlation).

Table 3. Evolution of study outcomes from the second (Time 1) to the third trimester (Time 2).

	Time 1		Time 2		*t*	95% CI	*r*
	M	***SD***	**M**	***SD***			
EPDS	5.2	4.6	4.7	4.3	−1.024	−1.42,0.46	0.53 **
MS	6.2	5.3	8.9	5.4	4.832 **	1.59, 3.80	0.54 **
MSPSS (F)	6.5	0.8	6.4	1.0	−0.744	−0.15, 0.07	0.85 **
MSPSS (Fr)	6.3	1.0	6.1	1.0	−1.493	−0.29, 0.04	0.71 **

M = mean; SD = standard deviation; t = Student's t ; r = Pearson's correlation; EPDS = Edinburgh Postnatal Depression Scale; T = trimester; MS = maladjustment scale; MSPSS = Multidimensional Scale of Perceived Social Support; F = family; Fr = friends. * p (Holm Bonferroni sequential correction) < 0.0125; ** $p < 0.001$.

3.4. Bivariate Associations Between Personality Variables, Depressive Symptoms, Adjustment, and Perceived Social Support

Table 4 shows the bivariate associations between the main study variables. The results of the correlations between the variables evaluated at Time 1 (second trimester) showed that N was associated with greater depressive symptoms ($r = 0.61$, $p < 0.001$), greater maladjustment ($r = 0.29$, $p = 0.007$), and poorer perceived family ($r = -0.31$, $p = 0.004$) and friends support ($r = -0.34$, $p = 0.002$). Conversely, high levels in E were associated with a decreased depressive symptoms ($r = -0.43$, $p < 0.001$), reduced maladjustment ($r = -0.30$, $p = 0.006$), and increased perceived support by the family ($r = 0.34$, $p < 0.001$) and friends ($r = 0.34$, $p = 0.002$).

Table 4. Correlations between personality, age, and outcomes (i.e., depressive symptoms, adjustment, and social support).

	2	3	4	5	6	7	8	9	10	11	12
Second trimester											
1. Neuroticism	−0.36 **	0.19	−0.31 *	−0.34 *	0.61 **	0.29 *	0.10	−0.29 *	−0.48 **	0.54 **	0.46 **
2. Extraversion		−0.09	0.34 **	0.34 *	−0.43 **	−0.30 *	−0.12	0.28 *	0.38 **	−0.29 *	−0.36 **
3. Psychoticism			−0.34 *	−0.19	0.11	0.03	−0.09	−0.29 *	−0.34 *	0.33 *	0.08
4. Family support				0.65 **	−0.23	−0.20	−0.05	**0.85 ****	0.67 **	−0.33 *	−0.29 *
5. Friends support					−0.27	−0.18	0.04	0.60 **	**0.71 ****	−0.31 *	−0.16
6. Depression						0.67 **	0.13	−0.18	−0.28 *	**0.53 ****	0.48 **
7. Maladjustment							0.11	−0.13	−0.22	0.27	**0.54 ****
8. Age (third trimester)								−0.10	−0.04	0.18	0.15
9. Family support									0.71 **	−0.38 **	−0.27
10. Friends support										−0.47 **	−0.34 *
11. Depression											0.44 **
12. Maladjustment											

In bold, the intercorrelations between variables at the second trimester and their corresponding variable at the third trimester. * p (Holm Bonferroni sequential correction) < 0.0125; ** $p < 0.001$.

The cross-sectional associations between study variables evaluated in Time 2 (third trimester) showed family support ($r = -0.38$, $p < 0.001$) and friends support ($r = -0.47$, $p < 0.001$) were associated with decreased depressive symptoms. Support from friends ($r = -0.34$, $p = 0.001$) and depressive symptoms ($r = 0.44$, $p < 0.001$) were inversely associated with maladjustment.

Finally, the results of the longitudinal correlations showed that N at Time 1 was prospectively related to more severe depressive symptomatology ($r = 0.54$, $p < 0.001$), maladjustment ($r = 0.46$, $p < 0.001$), and poorer support from family ($r = -0.29$, $p = 0.008$) and friends ($r = -0.48$, $p < 0.001$) at Time 2. Similarly, P at Time 1 was related to greater depressive symptomatology ($r = 0.33$, p = 0.002) and less support from family members ($r = -0.29$, $p = 0.007$) and friends ($r = -0.34$, $p = 0.002$) at Time 2. Conversely, E at Time 1 was associated with less intense depressive symptoms ($r = -0.29$, $p = 0.008$) and maladjustment ($r = -0.36$, $p < 0.001$), as well as with increased support from the family ($r = 0.28$, $p = 0.010$) and friends ($r = 0.38$, $p < 0.001$) at Time 2.

Different to personality, age was not cross-sectionally or longitudinally related to outcomes (all $p > 0.050$).

3.5. Personality Factors as Predictors of Depressive Symptoms, Maladjustment, and Perceived Social Support Evolution During Pregnancy: Multivariate Analysis)

Table 5 presents the results of the multivariate regression analyzes. In order to decide whether potential covariates should be included in the regressions, we investigated the bivariate associations between economic level, abortion history, pregnancy risk, and history of childbirth. None of the correlations were significant and they were all very small in size (all $r < 0.20$, all $p > 0.05$), which might have been influenced by the low heterogeneity of responses (approximately 75% of women had moderately high economic levels, did not have previous abortions, and had very a low risk pregnancy and over 65% of them were primiparous). Thus, there was no evidence to support their inclusion in the multivariate regression and doing so would only increase the risk of multicollinearity.

Across personality variables, both N ($\beta = 0.40$, $t = 2.62$, $p < 0.001$, 95% CI = 0.10, 0.71) and P ($\beta = 0.58$, $t = 2.62$, $p < 0.001$, 95% IC = 0.10, 0.71) uniquely and significantly contributed to the prediction of depressive symptoms at a prospective level after controlling for the effect of baseline depressive symptoms. In relation to maladjustment, the only personality factor to prospectively and significantly contribute to this outcome above and beyond baseline maladjustment levels was N ($\beta = 0.50$, $t = 2.99$, $p < 0.0125$, 95% CI = 0.17, 0.84). Finally, and similar to depressive symptomatology, N ($\beta = -0.07$, $t = -2.65$, $p < 0.0125$, 95% CI = −0.12, −0.02) and P ($\beta = -0.10$, $t = -2.58$, $p < 0.0125$, 95% CI = −0.18, 0.02) were the personality dimensions to significantly and uniquely contribute to the prediction of perceived social support from friends at a prospective level and after controlling for baseline perceived friends support. Regarding perceived family support, the results did not indicate that personality variables contributed to the evolution of this outcome.

Table 5. Multivariate regression predicting study outcomes.

DV		Beta	t	95% CI	R^2 Change	F Change
	Depression (T2)					
Block 1: depression (T1)		0.28	2.70 **	0.07, 0.50	0 .279	32.15 **
Block 2: age (T1)		0.14	1.56	−0.04, 0.33	0.013	1.55
Block 3: personality (T1)					0.133	6.08 **
Neuroticism		0.40	2.62 **	0.10, 0.71		
Extraversion		−0.02	−0.16	−0.33, 0.28		
Psychoticism		0.58	2.84 **	0.17, 0.99		
	Maladjustment (T2)					
Block 1: maladjustment (T1)		0.42	4.44 **	0.23, 0.60	0.291	34.09 **
Block 2: age (T1)		0.09	0.74	−0.15, 0.32	0.009	1.09
Block 3: personality (T1)					0.112	5.04 *
Neuroticism		0.50	2.99 *	0.17, 0.84		
Extraversion		−0.26	−1.35	−0.64, 0.12		
Psychoticism		0.03	0.12	−0.48, 0.55		
	Family support (T2)					
Block 1: family support (T1)		0.95	12.48 **	0.80, 1.10	0.719	212.81 **
Block 2: age (T1)		−0.02	−1.03	−0.04, 0.01	0.004	1.08
Block 3: personality (T1)					0.001	0.06
Neuroticism		−0.06	−0.31	−0.05, 0.03		
Extraversion		−0.07	−0.31	−0.05, 0.04		
Psychoticism		−0.04	−0.12	−0.07, 0.06		
	Social support friends (T2)					
Block 1: friends support (T1)		0.56	7.39 **	0.41, 0.71	0.506	84.95 **
Block 2 : age (T1)		−0.01	−0.68	−0.05, 0.02	0.005	0.82
Block 3: personality (T1)					0.100	6.73 **
Neuroticism		−0.07	−2.65 *	−0.12, −0.02		
Extraversion		0.03	1.15	−0.03, 0.09		
Psychoticism		−0.10	−2.58 *	−0.18, 0.02		

T1 = second trimester; T2 = third trimester. * p (Holm Bonferroni sequential correction) < 0.0125; ** $p < 0.001$.

4. Discussion

The present study aims at providing further evidence into the role of personality (N, E, and P) and important pregnancy outcomes, namely, depressive symptoms, adjustment to pregnancy challenges, and perceived social support. In order to achieve this goal and in order to address some limitations observed in the literature, this investigation included two major improvements compared to previous studies, namely, the implementation of a longitudinal design and the use of ICTs for assessment. Overall, the results indicated an important contribution of N and, to a lesser extent, P on the evolution of study outcomes, but failed to reveal a significant prospective association between E and outcomes when controlling for the remaining personality factors and baseline outcome scores. Additionally, while the inclusion of ICTs for technology made the longitudinal evaluation more feasible for healthcare professionals, response rates by participants were very poor, which will be discussed in more detail in the following lines.

Indeed, one of the strengths of the present study was the longitudinal investigation of the evolution of important perinatal outcomes. In this sense, the results showed that significant mean-level changes only occurred in maladjustment, so that women reported a poorer adaptation when comparing the second and the third trimester of pregnancy. As evidenced in past research, pregnancy imposes major changes in the lifestyles of women and requires important psychological resources for an adequate adaptation to these changes [1], which means that pregnancy can become a stressful period for women [49]. An interesting finding was that, according to our results, it is at the last stage during pregnancy when women experience greater limitations in their life areas (e.g., work activity, leisure, or social life). Based on our data, these increased difficulties in adaptation did not result in a proportional depressed mood, which suggests that a deterioration of adjustment with time might have been expected by the participants or was well tolerated at an emotional level. While acknowledging the aforementioned increase in adjustment challenges in the third trimester due to biological reasons, it is also true that preventive interventions focused on offering information about changes during pregnancy and guidelines to better adjust to such changes, such as maintaining social and leisure activities and physical activity, could help mitigate the degree of maladjustment in this period of pregnancy. As stated in previous research, ICTs can help to provide information-based interventions, physical exercise, or behavioral activation in perinatal women at reduced costs and high disseminability [37,50,51].

As noted in the previous lines, depressive symptomatology did not change during pregnancy in the present study, which contrasts with some past research [16]. These differences could be explained by several reasons, such as the sample sizes used in previous investigations, the country of origin of women participating in the studies, or their educational level, which was very high in the present study and this is known to be a protective factor for depression [52]. In addition, it is also possible that our participants have present protective factors for depression, such as an adequate evolution of pregnancy, an overall good health status, or adequate coping strategies.

Similar to depression, no changes were observed in perceived social support, which was high at both assessment times. This is an important finding considering that social support seems to have a buffering effect on women's health during the perinatal stage and, as some authors affirm, social support could contribute to reducing the impact of stress and depressive symptomatology [48]. Related to this, the fact that in the present study baseline support from family and friends was prospectively associated with reduced depressive symptomatology is consistent with the idea that social support facilitates the journey to motherhood [53].

Regarding the relationships between personality and outcomes, our results showed significant associations both at the cross-sectional and longitudinal level between personality traits and outcomes. Consistent with the literature, N and E showed the strongest associations with outcomes, and P was mostly associated with the social variables included in the study (i.e., social support) [16,17]. As expected, women who presented high N and low E scores reported more depressive symptoms, poorer adjustment, and less social support cross-sectionally. This adds to the existing literature showing that N is a risk factor for well-being and adaptation to challenges, such as those experienced during pregnancy, while E would be a protective factor in such situations [11,17,25].

Interestingly and one of the key contributions of the present study was the finding that the aforementioned contribution of personality, particularly in the case of N and P, was preserved in the multivariate analyses, including prospective data and controlling for the auto-regressions. This design allowed us to confirm that personality is not only associated with prenatal outcomes in a cross-sectional manner, but that N and P might be risk factors for the deterioration of many of these outcomes. It is important to note that personality explained an important percentage of the variance of prospective outcomes (13.3% for depressive symptoms, 11.2% for adjustment, and 10% for perceived social support), considering baseline scores in the outcomes were controlled for. While cross-sectional associations are indeed important and informative, the prospective relationships evidenced in the present investigation add to past research in suggesting that, if prevention or intervention programs are not provided to populations at risk (i.e., high N and P), they are likely to continue to worsen in the mental symptomatology, adaptation, and social satisfaction during pregnancy, which puts them at risk for their own well-being and that of the newborns [54].

Note that one of the present study goals was to investigate whether personality characteristics were indeed associated with social support during pregnancy. Our results support past research in showing that E is associated with satisfaction with social life, and N and P are inversely associated with this outcome [40]. Because social support was inversely associated with depressive symptoms and maladjustment, these results support the idea that intervention programs should be addressed to women at risk for poor perceived social support (i.e., those with a low E and high N and P profile). Again, ICT solutions might be useful tools to provide social support to women during pregnancy [55].

Contrary to our expectations, age did not show significant associations with any of the study variables. The literature is ambiguous when establishing a relationship between age and the risk of depression during pregnancy [11]. While some studies suggest that younger women are at greater risk of developing depressive symptoms [56], inconsistent findings have also been reported [57]. These discrepancies are probably due to differences in the mean age of women from the different studies. However, a review by Biaggi et al. [11] indicated no association between age and perinatal outcomes, which is consistent with our findings and suggests that older age might not be a key protective factor for well-being and adjustment in pregnant women.

A final contribution of the present study was the implementation of a web-based application for data collection. From our experience, the use of a web page for the longitudinal evaluation of risk factors and associated psychological variables during pregnancy has represented a simple, inexpensive, and confidential alternative that we believe helped overcome some of the current barriers for the longitudinal assessment of mental health problems in perinatal care, most notably the insufficient consultation time [34,58]. Additionally, research suggests that the application of ICT facilitates perinatal mental health screening due to the reduced stigma associated with non-face-to-face evaluations, the flexibility with which assessments can be completed (anywhere and anytime), and the reduced costs in terms of professional time [50,59].

While acknowledging the benefits of ICT for mental health screening, as noted by our low participation and retention rates, the implementation of online longitudinal assessments with very limited professional involvement is still challenging. One of the main barriers for participation, as informally reported by some of the participants, was associated with the time required to complete the evaluation protocol, which was perceived as being too extensive. As indicated by recent research conducting longitudinal and ecological momentary assessments, a reduction of items (e.g., validation of individual item measures against full traditional scales) and the selection of key questionnaires only is fundamental in design with technology and longitudinal designs [60]. The use of apps, which are more accessible and acceptable for perinatal women, might help as well in this direction [39]. Finally, the inclusion of gamification or treatment elements (i.e., tips to be used during pregnancy) might also facilitate engagement with longitudinal studies [61].

Limitations

This study has some limitations that should be taken into account. First, note that the sample is composed of a group of women with very similar sociodemographic characteristics, which limits the generalization of our findings. The small sample size (N = 85) also represents a problem. In this sense, it is important to consider the main obstacle associated with using the Internet in self-applied screening, prevention, or treatment programs, which is low adherence. In our case, as noted in the previous lines, the fact that this was a longitudinal study with a significant load in terms of the number of questionnaires to be completed might have negatively impacted on sample participation and retention. Note, however, that this is a frequent finding in the perinatal research using technology, even when treatment is provided [62]. As noted earlier, there are a number of initiatives that could be implemented to minimize this problem when conducting longitudinal assessments. Another limitation refers to the reliance on self-report measures only, which might have led to interpretation bias or social desirability. However, and in relation to social desirability, the anonymous and online nature of the evaluations should have encouraged honesty [63].

5. Conclusions

In sum, our results support the idea that certain personality characteristics (high N and P) might pose a risk to women for a deterioration of important well-being outcomes. This is important for prevention purposes and would suggest that women characterized by high N or high P should be monitored more frequently during pregnancy (e.g., using ICTs). Additionally, in order to promote changes in personality tendencies, self-applied programs, again using ICTs, could be the first solution in a stepped manner of care, which is more feasible than offering face-to-face individual treatments for all, considering the limited existing resources in public health settings in Spain [64].

It is important to note that an intervention program specifically aimed at reducing N and the negative consequences derived from this vulnerability factor currently exists [14]. This intervention, called the Unified Protocol, allows individuals to acquire a set of emotional regulation strategies that facilitate tolerance to discomfort derived from intense emotions, such as sadness or anxiety [65]. Future studies should test if the Unified Protocol effectively reduces N levels in a sample of pregnant women and whether, consequently, an improvement in outcomes (e.g., depressive symptoms, adaptation to pregnancy, and perceived social support) occurs. Again, and according to previous similar research, ICTs could be used to conduct and easily disseminate these interventions in women in the perinatal stage [60]. This opens fascinating avenues for future research in the field.

Author Contributions: Conceptualization J.O., C.S.-R., L.A.-P., and V.M.-B.; methodology, J.O. and C.S.-R.; formal analysis, C.S.-R.; investigation, L.A.-P.; resources, J.O., C.S.-R., L.A.-P., and V.M.-B.; data curation, J.O. and C.S.-R.; writing—original draft preparation, L.A.-P.; writing—review and editing, J.O., C.S.-R., and V.M.-B.; supervision, J.O.; project administration, J.O.; funding acquisition J.O. and V.M.-B. All authors have read and agreed to the published version of the manuscript.

Acknowledgments: The authors thank all the women who voluntarily participate in this study and all collaborating centers for their support in the dissemination campaigns.

References

1. Glazier, R.H.; Elgar, F.J.; Goel, V.; Holzapfel, S. Stress, social support, and emotional distress in a community sample of pregnant women. *J. Psychosom. Obstet. Gynecol.* **2005**, *25*, 247–255. [CrossRef] [PubMed]
2. Rubertsson, C.; Hellström, J.; Cross, M.; Sydsjö, G. Anxiety in early pregnancy: Prevalence and contributing factors. *Arch. Women's Ment. Heal.* **2014**, *17*, 221–228. [CrossRef] [PubMed]
3. Rallis, S.; Skouteris, H.; McCabe, M.P.; Milgrom, J. A prospective examination of depression, anxiety and stress throughout pregnancy. *Women Birth* **2014**, *27*, e36–e42. [CrossRef] [PubMed]
4. Accortt, E.E.; Cheadle, A.C.D.; Schetter, C.D. Prenatal depression and adverse birth outcomes: An updated systematic review. *Matern. Child Heal. J.* **2015**, *19*, 1306–1337. [CrossRef]
5. Rodriguez, M.D.L.F.; Le, H.-N.; La Cruz, I.V.-D.; Crespo, M.E.O.; Méndez, N.I. Feasibility of screening and prevalence of prenatal depression in an obstetric setting in Spain. *Eur. J. Obstet. Gynecol. Reprod. Boil.* **2017**, *215*, 101–105. [CrossRef]
6. Clinical Practice Guideline for Care in Pregnancy and Puerperium. Available online: https://portal.guiasalud.es/wp-content/uploads/2018/12/GPC_533_Embarazo_AETSA_compl_en.pdf (accessed on 6 May 2020).
7. The American College os Obstetricians and Gynecologist. ACOG Screening for perinatal depression. *Obstet. Gynecol.* **2018**, *132*, e208–e212. [CrossRef]
8. Antenatal and Postnatal Mental Health: Clinical Management and Service Guidance. Available online: https://www.nice.org.uk/guidance/cg192 (accessed on 6 May 2020).
9. Guia De Practica Clinica de atención en el embarazo y puerperio. Available online: https://portal.guiasalud.es/wp-content/uploads/2018/12/GPC_533_Embarazo_AETSA_compl.pdf (accessed on 6 May 2020).
10. Force, U.P.S.T.; Curry, S.J.; Krist, A.H.; Owens, U.K.; Barry, M.J.; Caughey, A.B.; Davidson, K.W.; Doubeni, C.A.; Epling, J.W.; Grossman, D.C.; et al. Interventions to Prevent Perinatal Depression: US Preventive Services Task Force Recommendation Statement. *JAMA* **2019**, *321*, 580–587. [CrossRef]
11. Biaggi, A.; Conroy, S.; Pawlby, S.; Pariante, C.M. Identifying the women at risk of antenatal anxiety and depression: A systematic review. *J. Affect. Disord.* **2015**, *191*, 62–77. [CrossRef]
12. Lancaster, C.A.; Gold, K.J.; Flynn, H.A.; Yoo, H.; Marcus, S.M.; Davis, M.M. Risk factors for depressive symptoms during pregnancy: A systematic review. *Am. J. Obstet. Gynecol.* **2010**, *202*, 5–14. [CrossRef]
13. Dennis, C.-L.; Boyce, P. Further psychometric testing of a brief personality scale to measure vulnerability to postpartum depression. *J. Psychosom. Obstet. Gynecol.* **2005**, *25*, 305–311. [CrossRef]
14. Barlow, D.H.; Sauer-Zavala, S.; Carl, J.R.; Bullis, J.R.; Ellard, K.K. The Nature, Diagnosis, and Treatment of Neuroticism. *Clin. Psychol. Sci.* **2013**, *2*, 344–365. [CrossRef]
15. Barlow, D.; Ellard, K.K.; Sauer-Zavala, S.; Bullis, J.R.; Carl, J.R. The Origins of Neuroticism. *Perspect. Psychol. Sci.* **2014**, *9*, 481–496. [CrossRef] [PubMed]

16. Bunevicius, R.; Kusminskas, L.; Bunevicius, A.; Nadisauskiene, R.J.; Jureniene, K.; Pop, V.J. Psychosocial risk factors for depression during pregnancy. *Acta Obstet. et Gynecol. Scand.* **2009**, *88*, 599–605. [CrossRef] [PubMed]

17. Podolska, M.Z.; Bidzan, M.; Majkowicz, M.; Podolski, J.; Sipak-Szmigiel, O.; Ronin-Walknowska, E. Personality traits assessed by the NEO Five-Factor Inventory (NEO-FFI) as part of the perinatal depression screening program. *Med Sci. Monit.* **2010**, *16*, 77–81.

18. Swickert, R. Personality and social support processes. In *The Cambridge Handbook of Personality Psychology*; Cambridge University Press: New York, NY, USA, 2012; pp. 524–540.

19. Johnston, R.; Brown, A. Maternal trait personality and childbirth: The role of extraversion and neuroticism. *Midwifery* **2013**, *29*, 1244–1250. [CrossRef]

20. Watson, D.; Clark, L.A. Extraversion and Its Positive Emotional Core. In *Handbook of Personality Psychology*, 1st ed.; Hogan, R., Johnson, J., Briggs, S., Eds.; Academic Press: Amsterdam, The Netherlands, 1997; pp. 767–793.

21. Yang, S.K.; Ha, Y. Predicting Posttraumatic Growth among Firefighters: The Role of Deliberate Rumination and Problem-Focused Coping. *Int. J. Environ. Res. Public Heal.* **2019**, *16*, 3879. [CrossRef]

22. Kotov, R.; Gamez, W.; Schmidt, F.; Watson, D. Linking "big" personality traits to anxiety, depressive, and substance use disorders: A meta-analysis. *Psychol. Bull.* **2010**, *136*, 768–821. [CrossRef]

23. Peñacoba-Puente, C.; Marín-Morales, D.; Carmona-Monge, F.J.; Furlong, L.V. Post-Partum Depression, Personality, and Cognitive-Emotional Factors: A Longitudinal Study on Spanish Pregnant Women. *Heal. Care Women Int.* **2015**, *37*, 1–21. [CrossRef]

24. Eysenck, H. The definition and measurement of psychoticism. *Pers. Individ. Differ.* **1992**, *13*, 757–785. [CrossRef]

25. Zeng, Y.; Cui, Y.; Li, J. Prevalence and predictors of antenatal depressive symptoms among Chinese women in their third trimester: A cross-sectional survey. *BMC Psychiatry* **2015**, *15*, 66. [CrossRef]

26. McCrae, R.R.; Costa, P.T., Jr. Comparison of EPI and psychoticism scales with measures of the five-factor model of personality. *Pers. Individ. Differ.* **1985**, *6*, 587–597. [CrossRef]

27. Peñacoba, C.; Rodriguez, L.; Carmona, J.; Marin, D. Agreeableness and pregnancy: Relations with coping and psychiatric symptoms, a longitudinal study on Spanish pregnant women. *Women Heal.* **2017**, *58*, 204–220. [CrossRef] [PubMed]

28. Martini, J.; Petzoldt, J.; Einsle, F.; Beesdo-Baum, K.; Höfler, M.; Wittchen, H.-U. Risk factors and course patterns of anxiety and depressive disorders during pregnancy and after delivery: A prospective-longitudinal study. *J. Affect. Disord.* **2015**, *175*, 385–395. [CrossRef] [PubMed]

29. Milgrom, J.; Hirshler, Y.; Reece, J.; Holt, C.; Gemmill, A.W. Social Support-A Protective Factor for Depressed Perinatal Women? *Int. J. Environ. Res. Public Heal.* **2019**, *16*, 1426. [CrossRef]

30. Bouvette-Turcot, A.-A.; Bernier, A.; Leblanc, E. Maternal Psychosocial Maladjustment and Child Internalizing Symptoms: Investigating the Modulating Role of Maternal Sensitivity. *J. Abnorm. Child Psychol.* **2016**, *45*, 157–170. [CrossRef]

31. Field, T. Prenatal depression effects on early development: A review. *Infant Behav. Dev.* **2011**, *34*, 1–14. [CrossRef]

32. Outomuro, D.; Actis, A. Estimación del tiempo de consulta ambulatoria en clínica médica. *Revista médica de Chile* **2013**, *141*, 361–366. [CrossRef]

33. McLoughlin, J. Stigma associated with postnatal depression: A literature review. *Br. J. Midwifery* **2013**, *21*, 784–791. [CrossRef]

34. Kingston, D.; Austin, M.-P.; Heaman, M.; McDonald, S.; Lasiuk, G.; Sword, W.A.; Giallo, R.; Hegadoren, K.; Vermeyden, L.; Van Zanten, S.V.; et al. Barriers and facilitators of mental health screening in pregnancy. *J. Affect. Disord.* **2015**, *186*, 350–357. [CrossRef]

35. Internet Use by Individuals. Available online: https://ec.europa.eu/eurostat/databrowser/view/tin00028/default/table?lang=en (accessed on 15 April 2020).

36. Osma, J.; Barrera, A.Z.; Ramphos, E. Are Pregnant and Postpartum Women Interested in Health-Related Apps? Implications for the Prevention of Perinatal Depression. *Cyberpsychol. Behav. Soc. Netw.* **2016**, *19*, 412–415. [CrossRef]

37. Lewis, B.A.; Gjerdingen, D.K.; Avery, M.D.; Guo, H.; Sirard, J.R.; Bonikowske, A.R.; Marcus, B.H. Examination of a telephone-based exercise intervention for the prevention of postpartum depression: Design, methodology, and baseline data from The Healthy Mom study. *Contemp. Clin. Trials* **2012**, *33*, 1150–1158. [CrossRef] [PubMed]
38. Belisario, J.M.; Gupta, A.K.; O'Donoghue, J.; Ramchandani, P.; Morrison, C.; Car, J. Implementation of depression screening in antenatal clinics through tablet computers: Results of a feasibility study. *BMC Med Inform. Decis. Mak.* **2017**, *17*, 59. [CrossRef]
39. Martínez-Borba, V.; Suso-Ribera, C.; Osma, J. The Use of Information and Communication Technologies in Perinatal Depression Screening: A Systematic Review. *Cyberpsychol. Behav. Soc. Netw.* **2018**, *21*, 741–752. [CrossRef] [PubMed]
40. Ozer, D.; Benet-Martinez, V. Personality and the Prediction of Consequential Outcomes. *Annu. Rev. Psychol.* **2006**, *57*, 401–421. [CrossRef] [PubMed]
41. Eysenck, S.; Eysenck, H.; Barrett, P. A revised version of the psychoticism scale. *Pers. Individ. Differ.* **1985**, *6*, 21–29. [CrossRef]
42. Eysenck, H.J.; Eysenck, S.B.G. *EPQ-R: Cuestionario Revisado de Personalidad de Eysenck: Versiones Completa (EPQ-R) y Abreviada (EPQ-RS): Manual*, 2nd ed.; Hodder & Stoughton: London, UK, 2001.
43. Vázquez, M.B.; Míguez, M.D.C. Validation of the Edinburgh postnatal depression scale as a screening tool for depression in Spanish pregnant women. *J. Affect. Disord.* **2019**, *246*, 515–521. [CrossRef]
44. Cox, J.L.; Holden, J.M.; Sagovsky, R. Detection of postnatal depression. Development of the 10-item Edinburgh Postnatal Depression Scale. *Br. J. Psychiatry* **1987**, *150*, 782–786. [CrossRef]
45. Echeburúa, E.; de Corral, P.; Fernandez-Montalvo, J. Escala de inadaptación (EI): Propiedades psicométricas en contextos clínicos. *Análisis y Modificación de Conducta* **2000**, *26*, 325–340.
46. Zimet, G.D.; Dahlem, N.W.; Zimet, S.G.; Farley, G.K. The Multidimensional Scale of Perceived Social Support. *J. Pers. Assess.* **1988**, *52*, 30–41. [CrossRef]
47. Landeta, O.; Calvete, E. Adaptación y validación de la escala multidimensional de apoyo social percibido. *Ansiedad y estrés* **2002**, *8*, 173–182.
48. Guedes, M.; Canavarro, M.C. Personal competencies, social resources, and psychosocial adjustment of primiparous women of advanced maternal age and their partners. *Child Adolesc. Soc. Work. J.* **2015**, *36*, 506–521. [CrossRef] [PubMed]
49. Rodriguez, A.; Bohlin, G.; Lindmark, G. Symptoms across pregnancy in relation to psychosocial and biomedical factors. *Acta Obstet. et Gynecol. Scand.* **2001**, *80*, 213–223. [CrossRef] [PubMed]
50. O'Mahen, H.; A Richards, D.; Woodford, J.; Wilkinson, E.; McGinley, J.; Taylor, R.S.; Warren, F.C. Netmums: A phase II randomized controlled trial of a guided Internet behavioural activation treatment for postpartum depression. *Psychol. Med.* **2013**, *44*, 1675–1689. [CrossRef] [PubMed]
51. Salonen, A.; Pridham, K.F.; Brown, R.L.; Kaunonen, M. Impact of an internet-based intervention on Finnish mothers' perceptions of parenting satisfaction, infant centrality and depressive symptoms during the postpartum year. *Midwifery* **2014**, *30*, 112–122. [CrossRef]
52. Bjelland, I.; Krokstad, S.; Mykletun, A.; Dahl, A.A.; Tell, G.S.; Tambs, K. Does a higher educational level protect against anxiety and depression? The HUNT study. *Soc. Sci. Med.* **2008**, *66*, 1334–1345. [CrossRef]
53. Warren, P.L. First-time mothers: Social support and confidence in infant care. *J. Adv. Nurs.* **2005**, *50*, 479–488. [CrossRef]
54. Gavin, N.I.; Gaynes, B.; Lohr, K.; Meltzer-Brody, S.; Gartlehner, G.; Swinson, T. Perinatal Depression: A Systematic Review of Prevalence and Incidence. *Obstet. Gynecol.* **2005**, *106*, 1071–1083. [CrossRef]
55. Caramlau, I.; Barlow, J.; Sembi, S.; McKenzie-McHarg, K.; McCabe, C. Mums 4 Mums: Structured telephone peer-support for women experiencing postnatal depression. Pilot and exploratory RCT of its clinical and cost effectiveness. *Trials* **2011**, *12*, 88. [CrossRef]
56. Siegel, R.S.; Brandon, A.R. Adolescents, Pregnancy, and Mental Health. *J. Pediatr. Adolesc. Gynecol.* **2014**, *27*, 138–150. [CrossRef]
57. Fellenzer, J.L.; Cibula, D.A. Intendedness of Pregnancy and Other Predictive Factors for Symptoms of Prenatal Depression in a Population-Based Study. *Matern. Child Heal. J.* **2014**, *18*, 2426–2436. [CrossRef]
58. Goodman, J.H. Women's Attitudes, Preferences, and Perceived Barriers to Treatment for Perinatal Depression. *Birth* **2009**, *36*, 60–69. [CrossRef] [PubMed]

59. Danaher, B.G.; Milgrom, J.; Seeley, J.R.; Stuart, S.; Schembri, C.; Tyler, M.S.; Ericksen, J.; Lester, W.; Gemmill, A.W.; Lewinsohn, P.; et al. Web-based Intervention for Postpartum Depression: Formative Research and Design of the MomMoodBooster Program. *JMIR Res. Protoc.* **2012**, *1*, e18. [CrossRef] [PubMed]
60. Suso-Ribera, C.; Castilla, D.; Zaragozá, I.; Ribera-Canudas, M.V.; Arbona, C.B.; Palacios, A.G. Validity, Reliability, Feasibility, and Usefulness of Pain Monitor, a Multidimensional Smartphone App for Daily Monitoring of Adults with Heterogeneous Chronic Pain. *Clin. J. Pain* **2018**, *34*, 900–908. [CrossRef] [PubMed]
61. Sardi, L.; Idri, A.; Fernández-Alemán, J.L. A systematic review of gamification in e-Health. *J. Biomed. Inform.* **2017**, *71*, 31–48. [CrossRef]
62. Barrera, A.Z.; Kelman, A.R.; Muñoz, R.F.; Donker, T.; Danaher, B. Keywords to Recruit Spanish- and English-Speaking Participants: Evidence From an Online Postpartum Depression Randomized Controlled Trial. *J. Med Internet Res.* **2014**, *16*, e6. [CrossRef]
63. Kingston, D.; Biringer, A.; Toosi, A.; Heaman, M.; Lasiuk, G.C.; McDonald, S.; Kingston, J.; Sword, W.A.; Jarema, K.; Austin, M.-P. Disclosure during prenatal mental health screening. *J. Affect. Disord.* **2015**, *186*, 90–94. [CrossRef]
64. Commissioning Stepped Care for People with Common Mental Health Disorders. Available online: http://www.swscn.org.uk/wp/wp-content/uploads/2015/03/non-guidance-commissioning-stepped-care-for-people-with-common-mental-health-disorders-pdf.pdf (accessed on 6 May 2020).
65. Barlow, D.; Farchione, T.J.; Bullis, J.R.; Gallagher, M.W.; Murray-Latin, H.; Sauer-Zavala, S.; Bentley, K.H.; Thompson-Hollands, J.; Conklin, L.R.; Boswell, J.F.; et al. The Unified Protocol for Transdiagnostic Treatment of Emotional Disorders Compared With Diagnosis-Specific Protocols for Anxiety Disorders: A Randomized Clinical Trial. *JAMA Psychiatry* **2017**, *74*, 875–884. [CrossRef]

3

Non-Immersive Virtual Reality for Rehabilitation of the Older People: A Systematic Review into Efficacy and Effectiveness

Roberta Bevilacqua [1], Elvira Maranesi [1,*], Giovanni Renato Riccardi [2], Valentina Di Donna [2], Paolo Pelliccioni [3], Riccardo Luzi [4], Fabrizia Lattanzio [1] and Giuseppe Pelliccioni [5]

1 Scientific Direction, IRCCS INRCA, 60129 Ancona, Italy; r.bevilacqua@inrca.it (R.B.); f.lattanzio@inrca.it (F.L.)
2 Clinical Unit of Physical Rehabilitation, IRCCS INRCA, 60100 Ancona, Italy; g.riccardi@inrca.it (G.R.R.); v.didonna@inrca.it (V.D.D.)
3 Eye Clinic, Polytechnic University of Marche, 60100 Ancona, Italy; paopel@hotmail.it
4 Medical Direction, IRCCS INRCA, 60100 Ancona, Italy; r.luzi@inrca.it
5 Neurology Unit, IRCCS INRCA, 60100 Ancona, Italy; g.pelliccioni@inrca.it
* Correspondence: e.maranesi@inrca.it

Abstract: Objective: the objective of this review is to analyze the advances in the field of rehabilitation through virtual reality, while taking into account non-immersive systems, as evidence have them shown to be highly accepted by older people, due to the lowest "cibersikness" symptomatology. Data sources: a systematic review of the literature was conducted in June 2019. The data were collected from Cochrane, Embase, Scopus, and PubMed databases, analyzing manuscripts and articles of the last 10 years. Study selection: we only included randomized controlled trials written in English aimed to study the use of the virtual reality in rehabilitation. We selected 10 studies, which were characterized by clinical heterogeneity. Data extraction: quality evaluation was performed based on the Physioterapy Evidence Database (PEDro) scale, suggested for evidence based review of stroke rehabilitation. Of 10 studies considered, eight were randomized controlled trials and the PEDro score ranged from four to a maximum of nine. Data synthesis: VR (Virtual Reality) creates artificial environments with the possibility of a patient interaction. This kind of experience leads to the development of cognitive and motor abilities, which usually positively affect the emotional state of the patient, increasing collaboration and compliance. Some recent studies have suggested that rehabilitation treatment interventions might be useful and effective in treating motor and cognitive symptoms in different neurological disorders, including traumatic brain injury, multiple sclerosis, and progressive supranuclear palsy. Conclusions: as it is shown by the numerous studies in the field, the application of VR has a positive impact on the rehabilitation of the most predominant geriatric syndromes. The level of realism of the virtual stimuli seems to have a crucial role in the training of cognitive abilities. Future research needs to improve study design by including larger samples, longitudinal designs, long term follow-ups, and different outcome measures, including functional and quality of life indexes, to better evaluate the clinical impact of this promising technology in healthy old subjects and in neurological patients.

Keywords: virtual reality; cognitive and physical rehabilitation; oldest old person

1. Introduction

Virtual reality (VR) is a trending, widely accessible, contemporary technology of increasing utility to biomedical and health applications [1]. VR is the technological experience that allows for a full immersion in virtual spaces with which you can interact via specific wearable or using only your hand.

A key feature of all VR applications is interaction. Virtual environments (VE) are created and allow for the user to interact with not only the VE, but also with virtual objects within the environment. In some systems, the interaction might be achieved via a pointer operated by a mouse or joystick button. In other systems, a representation of the user's hand (or other body part) might be created within the environment where the virtual hand movement is generated [2].

VR ranges from non-immersive to fully immersive, depending on the degree to which the user is isolated from the physical surroundings when interacting with the virtual environment. Non-immersive virtual reality allows for interacting with the environment through mouse or joystick; immersive virtual reality, instead, uses tools that are connected to the human body in order to perform the same motor task [3,4]. Non-immersive VR systems have been studied as a therapeutic tool for improving symptoms in neurological disorders and have shown potential to promote cognitive and motor improvements even in advanced stages of different neurological diseases (e.g., stroke, Alzheimer and Parkinson disease (AD, PD), multiple sclerosis (MS), and traumatic brain injury) because of these characteristics [5–9].

The use of VR technology in rehabilitation derives from research in computational neuroscience involving motor learning mechanisms [10]. VR provides real-time visual feedback for movements, thereby increasing engagement in enjoyable rehabilitation tasks [11].

VR provides alternative rehabilitation programs with new and effective therapeutic tools that can improve the functional abilities in a wide variety of rehabilitation patients in a neurological setting, offering several features, such as goal-oriented tasks and repetition. The use of VR environments for virtual augmented exercise has recently been proposed as having the potential to increase exercise behavior in older adults [12] and it also has the potential to influence cognitive abilities in this population segment [13]. Therefore, VR represents a real opportunity for the cognitive rehabilitation of neurological patients with different neuropsychological symptoms, especially in attention, memory, problem-solving and executive dysfunction, and in behavioral impairments [7–9].

Moreover, VR training has been mostly described for the upper limb [14,15], but also for the lower limb [16], balance and walking [17,18], as well as for perceptual/cognitive skills [19].

To our knowledge, systematic reviews or meta-analyses have been undertaken to review the utility of VR technologies in a single arm of rehabilitation (i.e., motor or cognitive rehabilitation, upper or lower limb rehabilitation), focusing on a specific pathology (stroke, PD, AD, MS) [6,7,9].

Despite the growing evidence of the positive effects of VR in rehabilitation of functional and cognitive abilities, some systems still raised concerns regarding their acceptability with complex clinical populations, as, for example, the older people. In particular, during trials with immersive systems, few adverse events have been described by participants, including headache and dizziness [20]. Finally, little is known about the perceived effect of the exposure at multisensory input during a complex activity, such as treadmill walking with VR in patients during post-stroke rehabilitation to improve balance and gait ability [6,21].

The objective of this review is to analyze the advances in the field of rehabilitation through VR, while taking non-immersive systems into account, as evidence have shown to be highly accepted by older people, due to the lowest "cibersikness" symptomatology [20]. For this purpose, Randomized Controlled Trials (RCTs) were analyzed in order to investigate the effects of rehabilitation programs integrated with innovative non-immersive VR systems and suggest future clinical applications.

2. Methods

2.1. Literature Search and Study Selection

The methodology of this systematic review was based on the Preferred Reporting Items for Systematic Reviews and Meta-Analyses (PRISMA) guidelines, as the main aim of this work is mapping all the available literature in the rehabilitation with non-immersive virtual reality. A systematic review of the literature was conducted in June 2019. The data were collected from Cochrane, Embase, Scopus,

PubMed, and Science Direct databases, analyzing manuscripts and articles of the last 10 years (from June 2009 to June 2019), in order to obtain the latest evidence in the field.

Based on consultation with the multidisciplinary team, non-immersive VR studies and applications related to rehabilitation intervention were searched while using the following search terms, and the combination thereof: non-immersive, virtual reality, virtual game, rehabilitation, motor impairment, and cognitive impairment.

After the preliminary search, 26 articles resulted from PubMed, 19 from Scopus, 283 from Science Direct, 10 from Embase, and 11 from Cochrane.

The findings were analyzed and screened by four experts of the team, a bioengineer, a clinical neuropsychologist, a statistician, and a neurologist. In particular, three review authors independently reviewed titles and abstracts that were retrieved from the search in order to determine whether they met the predefined inclusion criteria. A fourth review author (a statistician) moderate any disagreement. The full text articles were subsequently analyzed.

The first screening was based on the analysis of the title and of the abstract, as well as deduplication of the findings. Another researcher confirmed the accuracy of the papers selection and screened for any possible omission. After the first step, 11 articles resulted from PubMed, two from Scopus, and 0 from Science Direct, Embase, and Cochrane.

2.2. Study Selection

We included RCTs and reviews written in English that aimed to study the use of non-immersive virtual reality in rehabilitation. Thus, we selected studies meeting the following criteria:

1. Studies conducted on adult patients aged ≥65 years
2. Studies devoted to use a non-immersive virtual reality in rehabilitation
3. Studies including upper limb rehabilitation, lower limb rehabilitation, or cognitive rehabilitation
4. Randomized clinical trials, with control group that received conventional rehabilitation therapy
5. Before-after comparison of a single group
6. Review articles

On the contrary, we excluded studies that met the following criteria:

1. Conference proceedings
2. Studies for which the full text was not found
3. Studies written in languages other than English
4. Technical papers
5. Qualitative studies

All case-report studies and case-control studies were excluded for a lack of sustainability of results, as well as works concerning the development of new technologies.

2.3. Data Collection

After the screening based on the inclusion/exclusion criteria, conducted on the full text articles, the studies were selected as follows: 0 from Scopus, 10 from PubMed, and no one from Cochrane, Science Direct and Embase, and one from other sources. The countries of the selected studies are: Spain (2), France (2), Italy (2), Israel (1), United State of America (1), Canada (2), and Brazil (1). The fact that the studies have been performed in different countries shows that the topic is of general interest. Figure 1 shows the flowchart search strategy applied.

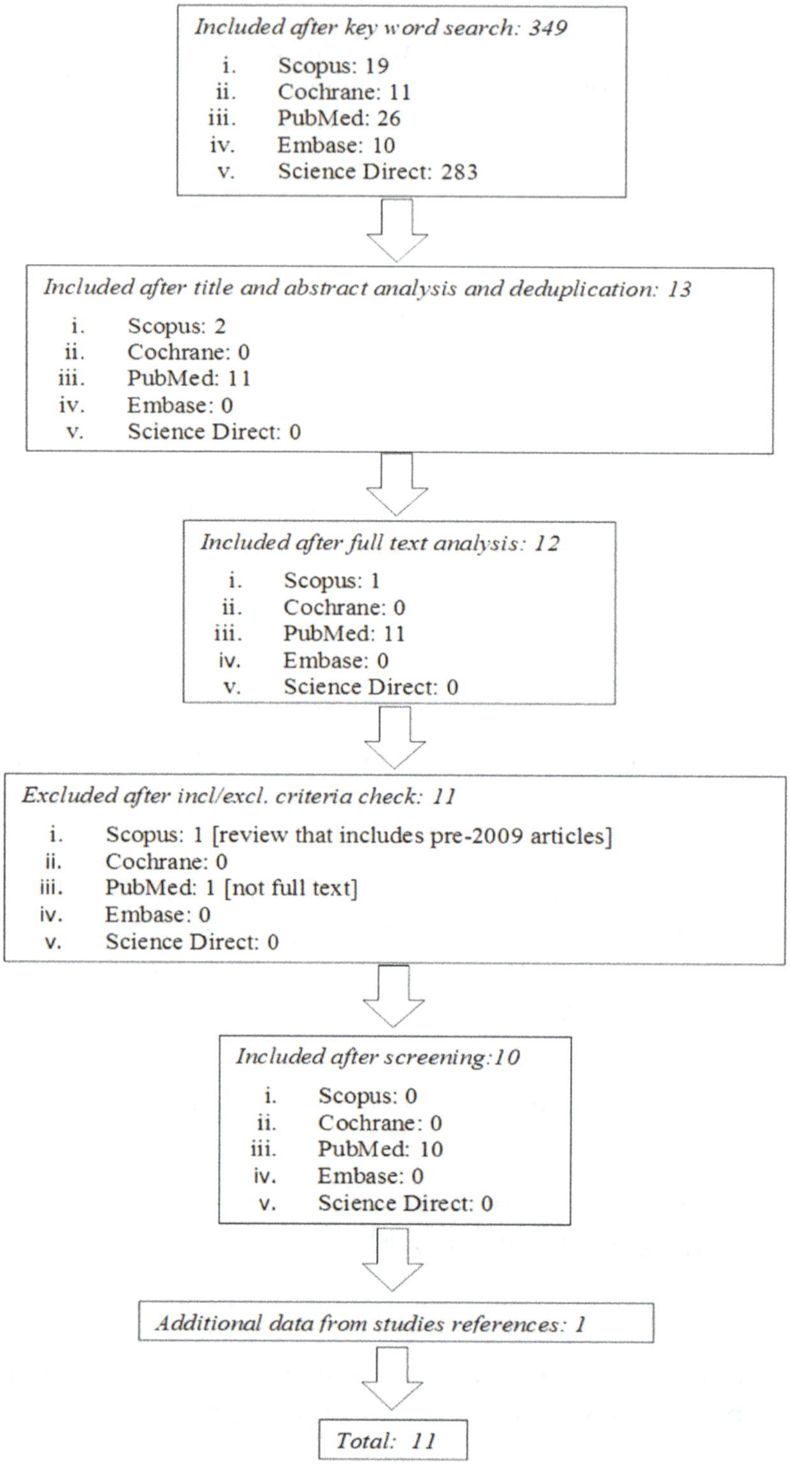

Figure 1. Flow diagram of the study selection process.

3. Results

A total of 10 papers were included. Studies are both reviews [22,23] and clinical papers [24–31].

3.1. *Study Quality Evaluation*

Quality evaluation was performed based on the PEDro scale and on the Cochrane's Risk of Bias (RoB) tool, suggested for evidence based review of rehabilitation while using non-immersive virtual reality [32,33]. The final score was settled when three authors reached agreement after repeated review and analysis. Of eight studies considered, five were randomized controlled trials and the PEDro score ranged from four to a maximum of nine, and the RoB score ranges from one to five (Table 1).

3.2. *General Characteristics of the Study Population*

All of the studies were focused on older people with a mean age of 65.2 (±9.4) years for the experimental group and 69.2 (±9.4) years in the control group. The number of participants that were involved in all the studies is 1008 ranged from 6 to 376.

To our knowledge, of the older people involved in the trials, 586 were males and 392 females.

The majority of the patients suffered from stroke ($n = 593$), followed by older people at high risk of falls, with more than two falls in six months ($n = 182$), patients with amyotrophic lateral sclerosis ($n = 30$), AD ($n = 24$), or PD ($n = 24$).

3.3. *Descriptive Analysis and Outcome Measures*

Table 2 shows the characteristics of the studies. The outcome could not be pooled into meta-analysis due to the following reasons. Clinical heterogeneity (Table 2) can be clearly observed from the participant, intervention, exercise mode, and outcome measures of the included studies. Diversity is seen in patient conditions and pathology, frequency, and duration of VR intervention, whether the impairment concerns the upper or the lower limb, whether the experiment conducted was pure VR (only VR) or VR mixed with traditional physical therapy or with exercise therapy, and whether the outcome measure contains follow-up.

Table 1. Scores of methodological quality assessment of the included studies.

PEDro [32]	**Walker et al., 2010 [24] RCT**	**Turolla et al., 2013 [25] RCT**	**Allain et al., 2014 [26] RCT**	**Saposnik et al., 2016 [27] RCT**	**Mirelman et al., 2016 [28] RCT**	**Seguera-Ortì et al., 2018 [29] RCT**	**Trevizan et al., 2018 [30] RCT**	**Pelosin et al., 2019 [31] RCT**
Eligibility	Y	Y	Y	Y	Y	Y	Y	Y
Randomized allocation	N	N	N	Y	Y	Y	Y	Y
Concealed allocation	N	N	N	Y	Y	Y	Y	Y
Baseline comparability	Y	Y	N	Y	N	N	N	N
Blinded subject	N	N	N	N	N	N	N	N
Blinded therapists	N	N	N	N	N	N	N	N
Blinded raters	N	N	N	Y	Y	Y	Y	Y
Key outcomes	Y	Y	Y	Y	Y	Y	Y	Y
Intention to treat	N	N	N	Y	Y	Y	Y	N
Comparison between groups	N	Y	Y	Y	Y	Y	Y	Y
Precision and variability	Y	Y	Y	Y	Y	Y	Y	Y
	4/11	5/11	4/11	9/11	8/11	8/11	8/11	7/11
Cochrane's Risk of bias tool [33]								
Sequence generation	N	N	N	Y	Y	Y	Y	Y
Allocation concealment	N	N	N	Y	Y	Y	Y	Y
Blinding of participants, personnel and outcome assessors.	N N N	N N N	N N N	N N Y	N N Y	N N Y	N N Y	N N Y
Incomplete outcome data.	N	N	N	N	N	N	N	N
Selective outcome reporting	Y	Y	Y	Y	Y	Y	Y	Y
Other sources of bias	N	Y	Y	Y	Y	N	N	Y
	1/8	2/8	2/8	5/8	5/8	4/8	4/8	5/8

Y: yes; N: no.

Table 2. Descriptive analysis of the included clinical studies.

	Population		**Technological Devices**	**Intervention**		**Comparison Control Group**	**Outcome**
	Partecipants in Experimental Group	**Partecipants in Control Group**		**Training Frequency**	**Intervention Group**		
Walker et al., 2010 [24]	6 adults within 1-year post-stroke $N = 6$, 3 F/3 M Age: 54.3 years (range 41–70 years)	-	A partial body weight-support treadmill in conjunction with a television mounted on a stand in front of the treadmill to display the VR walkthrough environment.	2 or 3 training sessions per week with partial body weight-supported tredmill with virtual reality system (total 12 training sessions). Initial training duration is 10 minutes; duration was progressed as tolerated.	-		(1) FGA scores increased by 30% (2) BBS scores improved by 10% (3) Overground walking speed increased by 38%

Table 2. *Cont.*

	Population		Technological Devices	Intervention		Comparison Control Group	Outcome
	Partecipants in Experimental Group	Partecipants in Control Group		Training Frequency	Intervention Group		
Turolla et al., 2013 [25]	n = 263 post-stroke patients, 105 F/158 M Age: 60.2 ± 14.3 years	n = 113 post-stroke patients, 41 F/72 M Age: 65.4 ±12.5	The Virtual Reality Rehabilitation System (Khymeia group. Noventa padovana, Italy) includes a pc workstation connected to 3D motion-tracking system and a high-resolution LCD projector displaying the virtual scenarios on a large wall screen.	40 sessions of daily therapy provided 5 days per week, for 4 weeks.	40 sessions of daily therapy provided 5 days per week, for 4 weeks. 1 hour of conventional therapy and 1 hour of VR therapy	2 hours of conventional treatment.	Within groups: F-M UE score improved by 4% in control group, and 10% in experimental group. Between groups: significantly greater motor improvement in experimental group. Within groups: FIM scores improved in both groups. Between groups: FIM scores improved by 5% in experimental group than in control group.
Allain et al., 2014 [26]	n = 24 AD patients, 14 F/10 M Age: 76.96 ± 6.05 years	n = 32 healthy older patients, 25 F/7 M Age: 74.13 ± 5.93	The virtual environment simulated a fully texture, medium-size kitchen. In the foreground, there was a work plane with all the objects needed to prepare a cup of coffee with milk and sugar. Patients controlled the 2D cursor using a computer mouse.	1. Virtual reality: 3 sessions: 2 of training and one test session to prepare a cup of coffee in virtual condition 2. Reality: to prepare a cup of coffee	Each training sessions lasts 15 minutes	Each training sessions lasts 15 minutes	Within groups: time to complete the virtual task and MMSE score are correlated in both groups
Saposnik et al., 2016 [27]	n = 71 stroke patients, 25 F/46 M Age: 62 ± 13 years	n = 70 stroke patients, 22 F/48 M Age: 62 ± 12 years	The Nintendo Wii gaming system or recreational activities (playing cards, bingo, jenga or ball game).	10 sessions, 60 minutes each, over a 2 week period.	30 minutes of traditional rehabilitation of the upper extremity + 30 minutes of virtual reality training	60 minutes of traditional rehabilitation of the upper extremity	1. Within groups: WMFT performance time improves from baseline to the end of treatment in both groups. 2. Between groups: no differences in WMFT at the end and at 4-weeks post-intervention 3. Between groups: better performance in BBT in control group at the end of treatment.
Mirelman et al., 2016 [28]	n = 146 older people at high risk of falls (more than 2 falls in 6 months), 48 F/98 M Age: 74.2 ± 6.9 years	n = 136 older people at high risk of falls (more than 2 falls in 6 months), 52 F/84 M Age: 73.3 ± 6.4 years	The treadmill plus VR intervention included a camera for motion capture and a computer generated simulation. The virtual environments included real-life challenges with obstacles, multiple pathway and distracters.	3 times per week for 6 weeks, with each session lasting about 45 minutes	45 minutes of treadmill training with virtual reality	45 minutes of traditional treadmill training	In the 6 months after training, the incident rate was significantly lower in the treadmill training plus VR group.

Table 2. *Cont.*

	Population		Technological Devices	Intervention		Comparison Control Group	Outcome
	Partecipants in Experimental Group	Partecipants in Control Group		Training Frequency	Intervention Group		
Seguera-Orti et al., 2018 [29]	$n = 9$ patients on hemodialysis, 4 F/5 M Age: 61.8 ± 13.0	$n = 9$ patients on hemodialysis, 3 F/6 M Age: 68.3 ± 15.6	The system is an adapted version of ACT (A la Caza del Tesoro), in which the subject tries to catch a series of targets by moving their leg.	16 weeks of intra-dialysis exercise program. The program lasted 4 additional weeks.	5 minutes warm-up; 30 minutes of virtual reality training.	5 minutes warm-up and strengthening exercises; 30 minute of aerobic training; 5 minutes of stretching.	1. Between groups: no significant differences in STS-60 2. Between groups: significant differences in gait speed 3. Within groups: significant improvements for STS-10, gait speed, 6 minute walking test between baseline-16 and 20 weeks, and 16–20 weeks.
Trevizan et al., 2018 [30]	$n = 30$ people with ALS, 12 F/18 M Age: 59 years (range 44–74 years)	$n = 30$ healthy people, equally matched for age and gender with experimental group	The VR environment is a 3D game in which the goal was to reach as many bubbles displayed on the computer monitor. The game was controlled by three different device system: motion tracking, finger motion and touch-screen.	Participants were randomly divided in 3 groups: motion tracking, finger motion control, touchscreen, to perform 3 task phases (acquisition, retention, transfer)			Both experimental and control group showed better performance whn using the touchscreen device in the transfer phase.
Pelosi net al., 2019 [31]	$n = 10$ PD + 7 OA 11 F/6 M Age: 73.2 ± 3.6	$n = 14$ PD + 8 OA 15 F/7 M Age: 71.9 ± 4.1	Treadmill with a non-immersive virtual reality that reacts to a virtual environment that included real-life challenges	45 minutes/session, 3 times a week for 6 weeks	To walk on a treadmill with virtual reality that included obstacles, distracters.	To walk on a treadmill without virtual reality.	Experimental group increased SAI, reduced the number of falls, improved obstacle negotiation performance.

FGA: Functional Gait Assessment. BBS: Berg Balance Scale. VR: Virtual Reality. F-M UE: Fugl-Meyer upper extremity. FIM: Functional Independence Measure. AD: Alzheimer's disease. MMSE: Mini Mental State Examination. WMFT: Wolf Motor Function Test. BBT: Box and Block Test. STS-60: sit-to-stand tests 60. ARAT: Action Research Arm Test. MMAS: Modified Modified Ashworth Scale. MAL: Motor Activity Log. FSS-7: Fatigue Severity Scale seven-item. SIPSO: Subjective Index of Physical and Social Outcome 10-item. VAS: Visual Analogue Scale. ALS: Amyotrophic Lateral Sclerosis. PD: Parkinson Disease. OA: older adults. SAI: Short-latency afferent inhibition.

3.4. *Intervention Effects*

Eight papers report the results of clinical trials involving a group of patients that performed a training with VR system versus a control group that performed a traditional physiotherapy training [25–29,31], or a comparison within the same group performing a VR training while using different exercise control modalities [30].

The period of VR training ranged from four to six weeks, each day of the week or three training sessions per week, while the duration of each single session with VR system ranged from 15 to 60 minutes. Only in one study [27] the duration of intervention was two weeks. Generally, all the experimental groups (EGs) in the studies have received both therapies with VR and traditional physiotherapy, while the control groups (CGs) have only received traditional physiotherapy. Two studies have a follow up after eight and 12 weeks [29] or six months [28].

The study of Walker et al. [24] reported the lowest number of subjects ($n = 6$) within one-year post-stroke. It is a before-after study and all the subjects performed training with a treadmill equipped with a VR system. All the participants made significant improvements in their ability to walk, increasing the over ground walking speed and the Berg Balance Scale (BBS) scores.

The study of Turolla et al. [25] involves 376 post-stroke patients randomized into two groups, receiving combined VR and upper limb conventional therapy or traditional therapy alone. VR rehabilitation seems more effective than conventional interventions in restoring upper limb motor impairments and motor related functional abilities.

The study of Allain et al. [26] involves 24 Alzheimer's disease patients as compared with 32 healthy elderly controls on a task designed to assess their ability to prepare a virtual cup of coffee, comparing the performance with an identical daily living task. Significant relations are found between virtual and real coffee-making scores, and between virtual score and Instrumental activities of daily living (IADL) scale, which supports the validity of the virtual reality training.

In a study of Saposnik et al. [27], 141 post-stroke patients were randomized into two groups: the first received the VR therapy and the second received recreational therapy. The results show that within each group the performance time improves from baseline to the end of treatment, whereas no differences are found between groups.

The objective of Mirelman et al. [28] was to verify whether an intervention combining treadmill training with non-immersive virtual reality (to target both cognitive aspects and mobility) would lead to fewer falls than treadmill training alone would. To do this, the authors recruited 282 older people at high risk of falls and randomized them into two groups to receive treadmill training plus VR or treadmill training alone. In the six months after training, the incident rate was significantly lower in the experimental group.

The study of Segura-Ortì et al. [29] involves 18 patients on hemodialysis: nine performed 30 minutes of non-immersive virtual reality training and nine performed 30 minutes of aerobic training. Both interventions improved physical function, such as gait speed and no significant differences, were found between groups.

In the study of Trevizan et al. [30], the performance on a computer task in patients with amyotrophic lateral sclerosis while using three (motion tracking, finger motion control, or touch screen) different commonly used non-immersive devices was evaluated. The control and experimental group both showed better performance on the computer task when using the touch screen device.

Pelosin et al. [31] analyzed 39 patients with Parkinson's disease, assigned to treadmill training group or treadmill training with non-immersive virtual reality intervention group to assess cholinergic activity. The results showed that the experimental group improved obstacle negotiation performance, and reduced the number of falls as compared with control group.

4. Discussion

A review of the evidence on VR efficacy in patients affected by a neurological disease is mandatory due to the rapid development of VR programs in the last years and the increasing literature on VR application in neurological conditions, in order to enable clinicians to have an up-to-date understanding of the potential clinical beneficial effects of these techniques.

Therefore, the aim of this paper was to systematically evaluate the evidence of the effectiveness of VR compared to conventional therapies. It must be stressed that few studies summarize the current best evidence on the effectiveness, user compliance, feasibility, and safety of VR interventions for rehabilitation treatment in neurological disorders.

VR creates artificial environments with the possibility of a patient interaction. This kind of experience leads to the development of cognitive and motor abilities, which usually positively affect the emotional state of the patient, increasing collaboration and compliance.

Moreover, the VR rehabilitative treatment might be personalized according to the specific abilities and needs of the subject.

Parkinson disease is one of the most common age-related brain disorders with both dopamine-related motor symptoms and nonmotor symptoms due to other neurotransmitter circuits involvement, such as the cholinergic, noradrenergic, and serotonergic pathways.

The cognitive decline is among the most common and relevant nonmotor symptoms in PD and it affects different cognitive domains, in particular attentional, visuospatial and executive domains, and also memory. VR in the cognitive PD treatment could be useful in improving, in particular, the visuospatial and executive abilities, which represent the most compromised aspects of cognitive decline in PD patients [7].

Moreover, falls are frequent in ageing and PD patients, due to an impairment in the cholinergic-mediated gait pathway. A rehabilitation approach using treadmill training combined with non-immersive VR seems to induce changes in cortical cholinergic activity, which enables functional gait improvements and reduces the fall rate in comparison to a traditional rehabilitation method [31].

A reduction in static and dynamic balance is a major risk factor for falls also in stroke survivors [34]. In fact, the majority of the individuals with stroke who have fallen usually develop fear of falling again (88%). Fear of falling is related to balance and gait deficits [35], and it often leads to reduced physical activity and deconditioning. In fact, 44% of stroke fallers report restriction of activity after the fall. Given the very low physical activity and cardiovascular fitness levels already near the lower limit of those required for basic ADL, further activity reduction and deconditioning due to the fear of falling can easily lead to a loss of independence in individuals with stroke.

A recent review on post-stroke rehabilitation therapy [6] provided evidence for a moderate beneficial effect in balance improvement of VR combined with conventional therapy, as compared to conventional therapy alone.

More promising effects seem to be evident in the case of upper limb motor impairments in stroke rehabilitation [25], but further studies are needed on this subject. In fact, the trial described in [27] found that non-immersive VR as an add-on therapy to conventional rehabilitation was not superior to a recreational activity intervention in improving motor function, which suggested that the added intensity of training only induces early motor recovery of the upper limb, and that this can be achieved with VR or with other simple and inexpensive arm activities.

VR technology has considerable potential for detecting functional limitations in IADL performance in AD patients, beyond that of current neuropsychological measures, as shown by Allain et al. [26]. Moreover, studies were carried out to assess the effectiveness of a VR cognitive training program on cognition in mild cognitive impairment (MCI) and AD patients [36].

VR cognitive training for individuals with MCI and dementia has proven to result in improvements in the cognitive domains of attention, executive function, and visual and verbal memory. Moreover, significant reductions in depressive symptoms and anxiety were evident, with a delay in the progression of cognitive impairment [37].

Additionally, the VR format might help in training adherence, as individuals with MCI and dementia patients seem to prefer the VR format of a task over the paper version, as confirmed by a feasibility study with image-based rendered VR in patients with mild cognitive impairment and dementia [38].

Some recent studies have suggested that rehabilitation treatment interventions might be useful and effective in treating motor and cognitive symptoms in different neurological disorders, including traumatic brain injury [8], multiple sclerosis [9], and progressive supranuclear palsy [39].

Finally, VR represents an effective tool that could improve the traditional cognitive and motor rehabilitation in patients that are affected by a neurological disease. Moreover, home-based VR might offer a promising addition or alternative to existing rehabilitation programs, and a chance to provide and/or prolong the required therapy after discharge in a more accessible setting, potentially improving clinical outcomes.

Future research needs to improve the study design by including larger samples, longitudinal designs, long term follow-ups, and different outcome measures, including functional and quality of life indexes, to better evaluate the clinical impact of this promising technology in healthy old subjects and in neurological patients. In particular, the next challenge for the research on VR and rehabilitation can be summarized in the following questions:

1. Does an innovative intervention enriched with VR provide a significant improvement in mobility, compared to traditional physiotherapy?
2. Is the intervention cost-effective for the health management systems?

To answer to these questions, it is crucial to understand how to improve the rehabilitation path of older people, through multidisciplinary multicomponent and person-centered intervention, integrated with VR.

The evidence reported in the paper are in line with the aims that were expressed by the National Plan for Health Research, whose priorities are defined in accordance with the indications contained in the regulation of the European Parliament and of the Council on the establishment of the "Health for growth" program, which pursues as a goal the achievement of a strong potential for economic growth thanks to the improvement of the state of health, through the facilitation of innovation in health care, the improvement of skills and information on specific diseases, and the identification of good practices for effective prevention [40]. In line with what has been expressed, the role of health technology assessment is of crucial importance. In this perspective, the available services must necessarily be enriched with adequate equipment of proven efficacy, as the promising sector of VR, to be able to advance at both the methodological and assistance level.

5. Conclusions

As it is shown by the numerous studies in the field, the application of VR has a positive impact on the rehabilitation of the most predominant geriatric syndromes. The level of realism of the virtual stimuli seems to have a crucial role in the training of the cognitive abilities. Nevertheless, semi-immersive or non-immersive VR systems have the advantage of being more accepted by the users, as they experienced less cybersickness after the training. Moreover, the integration of these devices in the health management systems are still lacking despite the evidence and the peculiarity of VR technologies with different level of immersivity. A tentative explanation can be found, not only in the cost of technology that seems to be more affordable in the recent years, but, most of all, in the absence of a standardized protocol and procedure, to harmonize traditional rehabilitation therapies and innovative VR systems. For this reason, it will be necessary to improve the research in the field, adopting RCTs study design as well as indicators of health technology assessment, to understand the effectiveness and efficacy also in terms of optimization of the clinical pathways. In addition, as VR systems can be easily adopted at home, it can be considered to be useful for the continuity of care.

Author Contributions: Study concept and design: E.M., R.B.; Acquisition of data (Literature search and Study Selection): E.M., R.B.; Analysis and interpretation of data (literature): E.M., R.B.; Drafting of the manuscript: E.M., R.B., V.D.D., G.R.R., G.P.; Critical revision of the manuscript for important intellectual content: F.L., L.R., P.P.

Abbreviations

VR	Virtual Reality
AD	Alzheimer disease
PD	Parkinson disease
MS	Multiple sclerosis
RCTs	Randomized Controlled Trials
EGs	experimental groups
CGs	control groups
BBS	Berg Balance Scale
IADL	Instrumental activities of daily living
MCI	Mild cognitive impairment

References

1. Torner, J.; Skouras, S.; Molinuevo, J.L.; Gispert, J.D.; Alpiste, F.; Molinuevo, J.L. Multipurpose Virtual Reality Environment for Biomedical and Health Applications. *IEEE Trans. Neural Syst. Rehabil. Eng.* **2019**, *27*, 1511–1520. [CrossRef] [PubMed]
2. Sveistrup, H. Motor rehabilitation using virtual reality. *J. Neuroeng. Rehabil.* **2004**, *1*, 1–10. [CrossRef] [PubMed]
3. Henderson, A.; Korner-Bitensky, N.; Levin, M. Virtual reality in stroke rehabilitation: A systematic review of its effectiveness for upper limb motor recovery. *Top. Stroke Rehabil.* **2007**, *14*, 52–61. [CrossRef] [PubMed]
4. Piron, L.; Turolla, A.; Agostini, M.; Zucconi, C.S.; Ventura, L.; Tonin, P.; Dam, M. Motor Learning Principles for Rehabilitation: A Pilot Randomized Controlled Study in Poststroke Patients. *Neurorehabil. Neural Repair* **2010**, *6*, 501–508. [CrossRef] [PubMed]
5. Perrochon, A.; Borel, B.; Istrate, D.; Compagnat, M.; Daviet, J.C. Exercise-based games interventions at home in individuals with a neurological disease: A systematic review and meta-analysis. *Ann. Phys. Rehabil. Med.* **2019**, *62*, 366–378. [CrossRef] [PubMed]
6. Mohammadi, R.; Semnani, A.V.; Mirmohammadkhani, M.; Grampurohit, N. Effects of Virtual Reality Compared to Conventional Therapy on Balance Poststroke: A Systematic Review and Meta-Analysis. *J. Stroke Cerebrovasc. Dis.* **2019**, *28*, 1787–1798. [CrossRef] [PubMed]
7. Maggio, M.G.; De Cola, M.C.; Latella, D.; Maresca, G.; Finocchiaro, C.; La Rosa, G.; Cimino, V.; Sorbera, C.; Bramanti, P.; De Luca, R.; et al. What about the Role of Virtual Reality in Parkinson Disease's Cognitive Rehabilitation? Preliminary Findings from a Randomized Clinical Trial. *J. Geriatr. Psychiatry Neurol.* **2018**, *31*, 312–318. [CrossRef]
8. Alashram, A.R.; Annino, G.; Padua, E.; Romagnoli, C.; Mercuri, N.B. Cognitive rehabilitation post traumatic brain injury: A systematic review for emerging use of virtual reality technology. *J. Clin. Neurosci.* **2019**, *66*, 209–219. [CrossRef]
9. Maggio, M.G.; Russo, M.; Cuzzola, M.F.; Destro, M.; La Rosa, G.; Molonia, F.; Bramanti, P.; Lombardo, G.; De Luca, R.; Calabrò, R.S. Virtual reality in multiple sclerosis rehabilitation: A review on cognitive and motor outcomes. *J. Clin. Neurosci.* **2019**, *65*, 106–111. [CrossRef]
10. Freeman, D.; Reeve, S.; Robinson, A.; Ehlers, A.; Clark, D.; Spanlang, B.; Slater, M. Virtual reality in the assessment, understanding, and treatment of mental health disorders. *Psychol. Med.* **2017**, *47*, 2393–2400. [CrossRef]
11. Ahn, S.; Hwang, S. Virtual rehabilitation of upper extremity function and independence for stoke: A meta-analysis. *J. Exerc. Rehabil.* **2019**, *15*, 358–369. [CrossRef] [PubMed]
12. Van Schaik, P.; Blake, J.; Pernet, F.; Spears, I.; Fencott, C. Virtual augmented exercise gaming for older adults. *Cyberpsychol. Behav.* **2008**, *11*, 103–106. [CrossRef] [PubMed]
13. Zelinski, E.M.; Reyes, R. Cognitive benefits of computer games for older adults. *Gerontechnology* **2009**, *8*, 220–235. [CrossRef] [PubMed]
14. Patel, J.; Fluet, G.; Qiu, Q.; Yarossi, M.; Merians, A.; Tunik, E.; Adamovich, S. Intensive virtual reality and robotic based upper limb training compared to usual care, and associated cortical reorganization, in the acute and early sub-acute periods post-stroke: A feasibility study. *J. Neuroeng. Rehabil.* **2019**, *16*, 92. [CrossRef]

15. Lee, S.H.; Jung, H.Y.; Yun, S.J.; Oh, B.M.; Seo, H.G. Upper Extremity Rehabilitation Using Fully Immersive Virtual Reality Games with a Head Mount Display: A Feasibility Study. *PM R.* **2019**. [CrossRef]
16. Dos Santos, L.F.; Christ, O.; Mate, K.; Schmidt, H.; Krüger, J.; Dohle, C. Movement visualisation in virtual reality rehabilitation of the lower limb: A systematic review. *Biomed. Eng. Online* **2016**, *15* (Suppl. 3), 144.
17. Ku, J.; Kim, Y.J.; Cho, S.; Lim, T.; Lee, H.S.; Kang, Y.J. Three-Dimensional Augmented Reality System for Balance and Mobility Rehabilitation in the Elderly: A Randomized Controlled Trial. *Cyberpsychol. Behav. Soc. Netw.* **2019**, *22*, 132–141. [CrossRef]
18. Vogt, S.; Skjæret-Maroni, N.; Neuhaus, D.; Baumeister, J. Virtual reality interventions for balance prevention and rehabilitation after musculoskeletal lower limb impairments in young up to middle-aged adults: A comprehensive review on used technology, balance outcome measures and observed effects. *Int. J. Med. Inform.* **2019**, *126*, 46–58. [CrossRef]
19. Törnbom, K.; Danielsson, A. Experiences of treadmill walking with non-immersive virtual reality after stroke or acquired brain injury—A qualitative study. *PLoS ONE* **2018**, *13*, e0209214. [CrossRef]
20. An, C.M.; Park, Y.H. The effects of semi-immersive virtual reality therapy on standing balance and upright mobility function in individuals with chronic incomplete spinal cord injury: A preliminary study. *J. Spinal. Cord Med.* **2018**, *41*, 223–229. [CrossRef]
21. Darekar, A.; McFadyen, B.J.; Lamontagne, A.; Fung, J. Efficacy of virtual reality-based intervention on balance and mobility disorders post-stroke: A scoping review. *J. Neuroeng. Rehabil.* **2015**, *12*, 46. [CrossRef] [PubMed]
22. García-Betances, R.I.; Arredondo Waldmeyer, M.T.; Fico, G.; Cabrera-Umpiérrez, M.F. A succinct overview of virtual reality technology use in Alzheimer's disease. *Front. Aging Neurosci.* **2015**, *7*, 80. [PubMed]
23. Palacios-Navarro, G.; Albiol-Pérez, S.; García-Magariño García, I. Effects of sensory cueing in virtual motor rehabilitation. A review. *J. Biomed. Inform.* **2016**, *60*, 49–57. [CrossRef]
24. Walker, M.L.; Ringleb, S.I.; Maihafer, G.C.; Walker, R.; Crouch, J.R.; Van Lunen, B.; Morrison, S. Virtual Reality–Enhanced Partial Body Weight–Supported Treadmill Training Poststroke: Feasibility and Effectiveness in 6 Subjects. *Arch. Phys. Med. Rehabil.* **2010**, *91*, 115–122. [CrossRef] [PubMed]
25. Turolla, A.; Dam, M.; Ventura, L.; Tonin, P.; Agostini, M.; Zucconi, C.; Kiper, P.; Cagnin, A.; Piron, L. Virtual reality for the rehabilitation of the upper limb motor function after stroke: A prospective controlled trial. *J. Neuroeng. Rehabil.* **2013**, *10*, 85. [CrossRef]
26. Allain, P.; Foloppe, D.A.; Besnard, J.; Yamaguchi, T.; Etcharry-Bouyx, F.; Le Gall, D.; Nolin, P.; Richard, P. Detecting everyday action deficits in Alzheimer's disease using a nonimmersive virtual reality kitchen. *J. Int. Neuropsychol. Soc.* **2014**, *20*, 468–477. [CrossRef]
27. Saposnik, G.; Cohen, L.G.; Mamdani, M.; Pooyania, S.; Ploughman, M.; Cheung, D.; Shaw, J.; Hall, J.; Nord, P.; Dukelow, S.; et al. Efficacy and safety of non-immersive virtual reality exercising in stroke rehabilitation (EVREST): A randomised, multicentre, single-blind, controlled trial. *Lancet Neurol.* **2016**, *15*, 1019–1027. [CrossRef]
28. Mirelman, A.; Rochester, L.; Maidan, I.; Del Din, S.; Alcock, L.; Nieuwhof, F.; Rikkert, M.O.; Bloem, B.R.; Pelosin, E.; Avanzino, L.; et al. Addition of a non-immersive virtual reality component to treadmill training to reduce fall risk in older adults (V-TIME): A randomised controlled trial. *Lancet* **2016**, *388*, 1170–1182. [CrossRef]
29. Segura-Ortí, E.; Pérez-Domínguez, B.; Ortega-Pérez de Villar, L.; Meléndez-Oliva, E.; Martínez-Gramage, J.; García-Maset, R.; Gil-Gómez, J.A. Virtual reality exercise intradialysis to improve physical function: A feasibility randomized trial. *Scand. J. Med. Sci. Sports* **2019**, *29*, 89–94. [CrossRef]
30. Trevizan, I.L.; Silva, T.D.; Dawes, H.; Massetti, T.; Crocetta, T.B.; Favero, F.M.; Oliveira, A.S.B.; de Araújo, L.V.; Santos, A.C.C.; de Abreu, L.C.; et al. Efficacy of different interaction devices using non-immersive virtual tasks in individuals with Amyotrophic Lateral Sclerosis: A cross-sectional randomized trial. *BMC Neurol.* **2018**, *18*, 209. [CrossRef]
31. Pelosin, E.; Cerulli, C.; Ogliastro, C.; Lagravinese, G.; Mori, L.; Bonassi, G.; Mirelman, A.; Hausdorff, J.M.; Abbruzzese, G.; Marchese, R.; et al. A multimodal training modulates short-afferent inhibition and improves complex walking in a cohort of faller older adults with an increased prevalence of Parkinson's disease. *J. Gerontol. A Biol. Sci. Med. Sci.* **2019**. [CrossRef] [PubMed]
32. Maher, C.G.; Sherrington, C.; Herbert, R.D.; Moseley, A.M.; Elkins, M. Reliability of the PEDro scale for rating quality of randomized controlled trials. *Phys. Ther.* **2003**, *83*, 713–721. [PubMed]

33. Doniger, G.M.; Beeri, M.S.; Bahar-Fuchs, A.; Gottlieb, A.; Tkachov, A.; Kenan, H.; Livny, A.; Bahat, Y.; Sharon, H.; Ben-Gal, O.; et al. Virtual reality-based cognitive-motor training for middle-aged adults at high Alzheimer's disease risk: A randomized controlled trial. *Alzh. Dement. (N. Y.)* **2018**, *4*, 118–129. [CrossRef] [PubMed]
34. Savović, J.; Weeks, L.; Sterne, J.A.C.; Turner, L.; Altman, D.G.; Moher, D.; Higgins, J.P.T. Evaluation of the Cochrane Collaboration's tool for assessing the risk of bias in randomized trials: Focus groups, online survey, proposed recommendations and their implementation. *Syst. Rev.* **2014**, *3*, 37. [CrossRef] [PubMed]
35. Weerdesteyn, V.; de Niet, M.; van Duijnhoven, H.J.R.; Geurts, A.C.H. Falls in individuals with stroke. *JRRD* **2008**, *45*, 1195–1214. [CrossRef]
36. Botner, E.M.; Miller, W.C.; Eng, J.J. Measurement properties of the Activities-specific Balance Confidence Scale among individuals with stroke. *Disabil. Rehabil.* **2005**, *27*, 156–163. [CrossRef]
37. Coyle, H.; Traynor, V.; Solowij, N. Computerized and virtual reality cognitive training for individuals at high risk of cognitive decline: Systematic review of the literature. *Am. J. Geriatr. Psychiatry* **2015**, *23*, 335–359. [CrossRef]
38. Manera, V.; Chapoulie, E.; Bourgeois, J.; Guerchouche, R.; David, R.; Ondrej, J.; Drettakis, G.; Robert, P. A feasibility study with image-based rendered virtual reality in patients with mild cognitive impairment and dementia. *PLoS ONE* **2016**, *11*, e0151487. [CrossRef]
39. Maggio, M.G.; Maresca, G.; Scarcella, I.; Latella, D.; De Domenico, C.; Destro, M.; De Luca, R.; Calabro, R.S. Virtual reality-based cognitive rehabilitation in progressive supranuclear palsy. *Psychogeriatr. Soc.* **2019**. [CrossRef]
40. Regulation (EU) No 282/2014 of the European Parliament and of the Councilof 11 March 2014 on the Establishment of a Third Programme for the Union's Action in the Field of Health (2014–2020) and Repealing Decision No 1350/2007/EC. Available online: https://eur-lex.europa.eu/legal-content/EN/TXT/PDF/?uri=CELEX:32014R0282&from=EN (accessed on 23 October 2019).

4

Randomized Clinical Trial of an Internet-Based Adolescent Depression Prevention Intervention in Primary Care: Internalizing Symptom Outcomes

Tracy Gladstone [1,*], Katherine R. Buchholz [1], Marian Fitzgibbon [2,3,4], Linda Schiffer [3], Miae Lee [2] and Benjamin W. Van Voorhees [2]

1 The Robert S. and Grace W. Stone Primary Prevention Initiatives, Wellesley Centers for Women, Wellesley College, Wellesley, MA 02481, USA; katherine.buchholz@wellesley.edu

2 Department of General Pediatrics, College of Medicine, University of Illinois at Chicago, Chicago, IL 60612, USA; mlf@uic.edu (M.F.); mlee9@uic.edu (M.L.); bvanvoor@uic.edu (B.W.V.V.)

3 Institute for Health Research and Policy, School of Public Health, University of Illinois at Chicago, Chicago, IL 60608, USA; lschiff@uic.edu

4 University of Illinois Cancer Center, University of Illinois at Chicago, Chicago, IL 60612, USA

* Correspondence: tgladsto@wellesley.edu

Abstract: Approximately 20% of people will experience a depressive episode by adulthood, making adolescence an important developmental target for prevention. CATCH-IT (Competent Adulthood Transition with Cognitive-behavioral, Humanistic, and Interpersonal Training), an online depression prevention intervention, has demonstrated efficacy in preventing depressive episodes among adolescents reporting elevated symptoms. Our study examines the effects of CATCH-IT compared to online health education (HE) on internalizing symptoms in adolescents at risk for depression. Participants, ages 13–18, were recruited across eight US health systems and were randomly assigned to CATCH-IT or HE. Assessments were completed at baseline, 2, 6, 12, 18, and 24 months. There were no significant differences between groups in change in depressive symptoms (b = −0.31 for CATCH-IT, b = −0.27 for HE, $p = 0.80$) or anxiety (b = −0.13 for CATCH-IT, b = −0.11 for HE, $p = 0.79$). Improvement in depressive symptoms was statistically significant ($p < 0.05$) for both groups ($p = 0.004$ for CATCH-IT, $p = 0.009$ for HE); improvement in anxiety was significant for CATCH-IT ($p = 0.04$) but not HE ($p = 0.07$). Parental depression and positive relationships with primary care physicians (PRPC) moderated the anxiety findings, and adolescents' externalizing symptoms and PRPC moderated the depression findings. This study demonstrates the long-term positive effects of both online programs on depressive symptoms and suggests that CATCH-IT demonstrates cross-over effects for anxiety as well.

Keywords: web-based interventions; internalizing symptoms; depressive symptoms; adolescents; prevention; primary care

1. Introduction

Depression is a significant public health concern for adolescents. It is estimated that as many as 20% of people will experience a depressive episode before adulthood [1]. Depression is associated with significant impairments in day-to-day functioning, and it can affect developmental trajectories in adolescence and early adulthood [2–4]. Episodic in its course, a single depressive episode increases the risk of future episodes that are often more severe [2,3]. Depressive symptoms, including subthreshold symptoms, are associated with an increased risk of depressive episodes, physical health problems, comorbid mental health concerns, and suicide [4–7]. The personal and societal cost of depression can be eased through depression prevention interventions [8,9].

A recent Cochrane review revealed that depression prevention programs for adolescents are associated with a moderate reduction in depressive episodes (risk difference = −0.03) across one-year follow-up [10], and a meta-analysis of 19 randomized preventive trials revealed that, for adolescents with elevated symptoms of depression, preventive interventions are associated with benefits across a two-year follow-up [11]. Several trials of specific depression prevention approaches for adolescents at risk for depression also have been found to be effective for certain subsets of teens [12–17]. The majority of these interventions involve in-person groups that rely on training therapists and recruiting participants who can attend regular sessions; these approaches are limited by lack of access due to barriers related to seeking in-person interventions [14–17]. Therefore, it can be difficult to provide these interventions cost-effectively to the large number of adolescents who may benefit from them. Given the high rate of depression among adolescents and the long-term consequences of depression, public health interventions that can reach a broad population of adolescents are needed.

Similar to depression, anxiety is a significant public health problem among adolescents. In fact, anxiety, frequently grouped with depression as an internalizing disorder, is the most common mental health concern among adolescents [18,19]. The lifetime prevalence of anxiety disorders in adolescents is just over 30% [18]. Developmentally, anxiety has an earlier age of onset than depression [18,20,21]. Some studies have found that anxiety starting in childhood precedes depression that begins in adolescence [22,23], while other studies report that there is a bidirectional relationship between anxiety and depression in children and adolescents [24,25]. Comorbid presentations result in poorer overall prognosis [26]. With both disorders, onset during childhood or adolescence is associated with chronic symptoms or functional impairment in adulthood [27,28]. Anxiety often co-occurs with depression [29–32], and adolescents with depression have been found to be at greater risk for also having an anxiety disorder compared to adolescents without depression [32,33]. Epidemiological studies suggest that 30–75% of children or adolescents with depression have comorbid anxiety [33]. Therefore, prevention and treatment of depression in adolescents must consider anxiety.

Given the high rates of co-occurring depression and anxiety, research has focused on identifying transdiagnostic factors that may represent shared etiological mechanisms or latent factors that underlie both disorders [34]. These transdiagnostic factors include negative affectivity or emotionality [35], cognitive or information processing biases [36], emotional awareness [37], and emotional regulation skills [38]. Given that comorbidity is more common than just anxiety or depression in clinical settings [26], researchers have recently developed transdiagnostic treatments to address the underlying factors associated with both depression and anxiety [39,40]. However, it has been suggested that treatments developed for depression or anxiety alone may also have cross-over effects on comorbid symptoms. In fact, clinical research confirms that many treatments developed for depression also result in decreased symptoms of anxiety. One meta-analysis [41] reviewing randomized clinical treatment or prevention trials found that crossover effects were present in both depression treatments and anxiety treatments, although the effects were stronger for the targeted symptoms. That is, depression treatments had a greater effect on depressive symptoms than anxiety symptoms, and anxiety treatments had a greater effect on anxiety symptoms than depressive symptoms. However, there were no significant cross-over effects of depression or anxiety prevention interventions.

To address the need for preventive interventions that may reduce a range of symptoms in adolescents, CATCH-IT (Competent Adulthood Transition with Cognitive-behavioral, Humanistic, and Interpersonal Training), an online prevention intervention, was developed as a low cost, universally available intervention. Disseminated through primary care settings, CATCH-IT uses a population-health based model (screening and outreach in settings where youth and their families usually receive care) [42]. CATCH-IT contains elements of CBT and interpersonal psychotherapy in a highly interactive interface, which is described in more detail in previous publications [42,43]. Early pilot studies demonstrated that participants who used CATCH-IT reported decreases in symptoms of depression at 6, 12, and 30 months, relative to baseline [13,44,45]. A more recent randomized clinical trial found CATCH-IT to be efficacious in preventing depressive episodes at six months, relative to an attention-control condition that combined usual care with monitoring and an online general health education program (HE) in adolescents who were experiencing elevated symptoms of depression, though not in the full intention to treat analysis [12]. These initial findings suggest that CATCH-IT may have great potential as a public health intervention for adolescents at risk of developing Major Depressive Disorder (MDD). As an online intervention, CATCH-IT is easy to access, cost-effective, decreases stigmatization through anonymity, and does not require highly trained professionals [46].

Even though no cross-over effects on anxiety were reported for depression prevention interventions, there is some indication that CATCH-IT may affect symptoms of anxiety as well as depression. A study of CATCH-IT adapted for Chinese adolescents found that participants in the CATCH-IT condition demonstrated a decrease in symptoms of both depression and anxiety at eight-months [47]. While CATCH-IT is specifically designed for depression prevention, many of the skills it teaches may affect transdiagnostic factors, and therefore, decrease symptoms of anxiety as well. For example, cognitive behaviorally-based A-B-C exercises presented in CATCH-IT may increase emotional awareness, and the cognitive restructuring taught in CATCH-IT may decrease negative cognitive biases as well as negative affectivity. These effects could positively impact symptoms of anxiety in addition to depression. Given the accessibility, reach, and potential public health impact of the CATCH-IT intervention, it is important to investigate and understand the potential cross-over effects that CATCH-IT may offer.

The current study uses data from the randomized clinical trial comparing CATCH-IT to HE, an online program providing general health education, in a sample that was composed of adolescents with an intermediate to high risk of depression recruited from primary care settings [43]. As mentioned above, at six months, CATCH-IT, compared to HE, prevented depressive episodes in high-risk adolescents with significant subthreshold depressive symptoms at baseline [12], and additionally, depressive symptoms significantly decreased in both conditions. Moreover, preventive effects for CATCH-IT were found for up to 24 months for those with low levels of hopelessness or adequate levels of paternal monitoring [48]. The current study expands these initial findings to examine the possibility that the CATCH-IT intervention has long-term preventive effects on symptoms of anxiety as well as on symptoms of depression, and also to examine moderators of intervention effects on symptoms of both disorders. We hypothesize that participants in the CATCH-IT condition will have experienced greater decreases in self-reported symptoms of anxiety and depression, relative to participants in the HE group. Secondary analyses will examine potential moderators that may affect findings across both groups.

2. Materials and Methods

2.1. Study Design and Setting

This study utilized a hybrid type I efficacy-implementation design to evaluate the effectiveness of CATCH-IT in a scalable setting [49]. The efficacy of CATCH-IT was evaluated while simultaneously gathering information on CATCH-IT's implementation to prepare for scaling up [12]. This trial was implemented in eight major US Health Systems (N = 31 primary care sites, 42,310 adolescents) in a population health approach (screen all youth, offer intervention, assessment, refer those in need of treatment) with over 1200 primary care staff consented and trained. This process has been previously described in further detail [43,50]. Data were collected from urban and suburban clinics located in Chicago, Illinois, and surrounding areas including northern Indiana, and Boston, Massachusetts and surrounding areas. The protocol, CONSORT statement, and a description of the implementation process have been described previously [43,50]. Institutional review board (IRB) approval was received from the University of Chicago IRB (protocol # 2011-0505), the IRB of record, on 15 December 2011, and also by local review boards. A data safety and monitoring board (DSMB) reviewed the trial and results twice per year.

2.2. Participants

The final sample included 369 adolescents, ages 13 to 18 years old, who were at risk for depression as indicated by elevated symptoms of depression (score of 8–17 on the 10-item or score of ≥16 on the 20-item Center for Epidemiologic Studies Depression scale (CES-D)) and/or a history of a major depressive episode or dysthymia. Exclusion criteria included a DSM-IV diagnosis of major depressive disorder (MDD), bipolar disorder, schizophrenia, psychosis, or current drug/alcohol abuse. Additionally, adolescents were excluded if they were in current treatment for MDD, had a significant developmental disability or reading impairment, were assessed to be at imminent risk of suicide, or were being treated for serious medical conditions [13,44].

2.3. Study Procedures

Participants were recruited from February 2012 to July 2016 through posted flyers, recruitment letters sent by primary care offices (sent to all families of adolescents in the targeted age range), and information given directly by the primary care physician (PCP) during clinic visits. Following verbal consent from a parent, the study staff administered a phone screen to assess adolescents for eligibility (Figure 1). Eligible adolescents and their parents attended an enrollment appointment at the office of their PCP. Informed consent was obtained before the completion of the baseline assessment. Depression risk was assessed by the KSADS, a clinician-administered, semi-structured interview. All baseline assessments were completed before informing the participants, their parents, or their PCPs of the intervention assignment. Follow-up assessments were conducted at 2, 6, 12, 18, and 24 months following baseline.

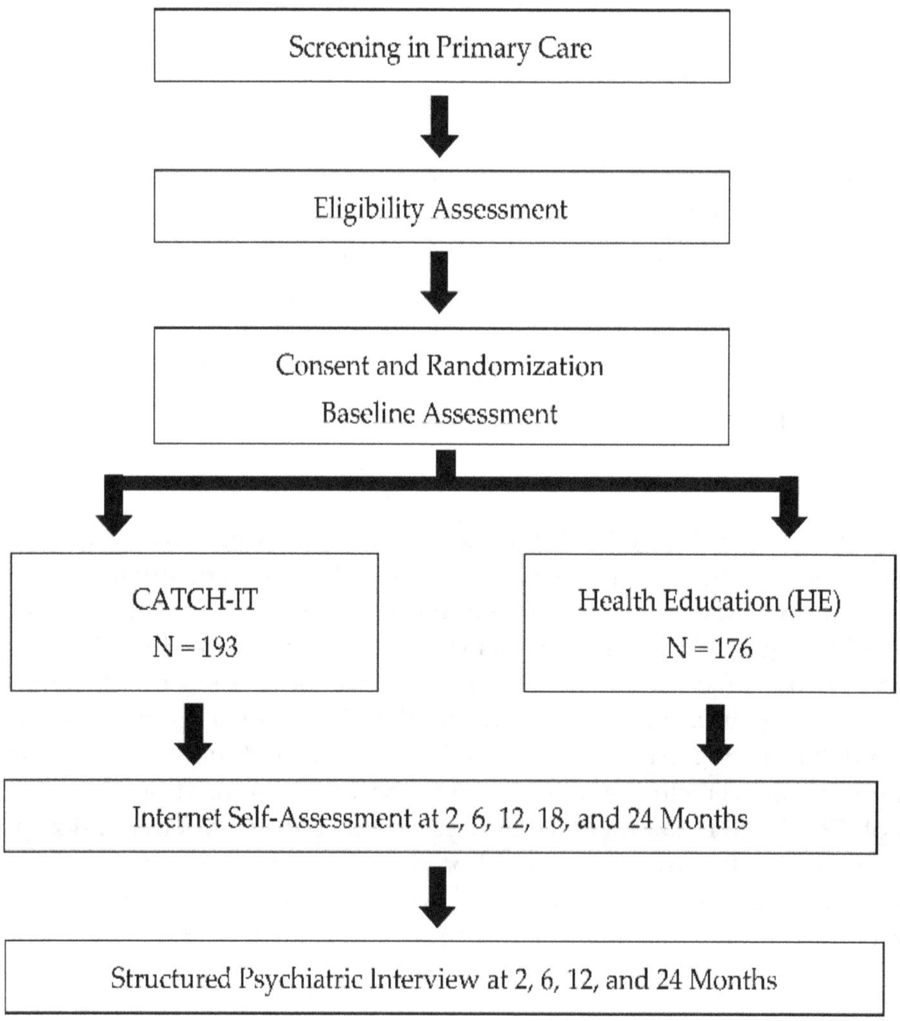

Figure 1. Study design.

2.4. Randomization and Blinding

A computer-generated sequence blocked by site and time of entry was used to randomly assign participants to CATCH-IT or HE. Participants were also stratified by age (13–14 years vs. 15–18 years), gender, and severity of their risk of a depressive episode (high risk: elevated score on the Center for Epidemiological Studies-Depression Scale (CES-D_{10}) and prior depressive episode; low risk: elevated CESD or prior depressive episode). The assignment of participants to HE versus CATCH-IT was 1:1. Assessors were blinded for the duration of the study, while investigators were blinded until all 12-month data were collected. PCPs were not blinded, since they provided motivational interviews to the adolescent participants in the CATCH-IT intervention.

2.5. Treatment Arms

2.5.1. The CATCH-IT Intervention

CATCH-IT consists of 14 online modules designed to help adolescents develop coping strategies to decrease symptoms related to depression and prevent depressive episodes, plus an additional, optional module to address symptoms of anxiety. CATCH-IT was adapted from the Coping with Depression Adolescent Course, a group cognitive-behavioral intervention. It also includes elements of behavioral activation strategies as well as Interpersonal Psychotherapy techniques [51–53]. The program was designed using the Instructional Design Theory to maximize learning and maintain the learner's attention [53]. In addition to the online modules, phone coaching by research staff (one to three calls) and a series of three motivational interviews conducted by the PCP (baseline, 2 months, and 12 months) were provided to support participants' use of CATCH-IT. Parents were also invited to complete four online modules to support their child's skills development, as well as an optional module for parents who worry they may themselves be depressed. Parent modules have been described in detail in previous publications [12,43,54].

2.5.2. The Health Education Intervention

The HE intervention consists of 14 online modules providing general health information, and it was used as the control intervention. The first 13 modules of the HE program provide general health information, while the final module focuses on identifying mood symptoms, the importance of treating mental health issues, and how mental health stigma may interfere with seeking treatment. In addition to the online modules, up to three check-in calls were provided to each HE participant to ensure that they had access to the website within three weeks of the study enrollment. Parents were also invited to complete four modules consisting of similar information to the adolescent modules.

2.6. Measures

Measures were chosen to capture the range of ways that internalizing symptoms are expressed by adolescents and possible mediators and moderators of intervention response. All measures were descriptive and were appropriate for adolescents ages 13–18.

Demographics. Demographic information including sex, race, ethnicity, and maternal education was collected from adolescents and their parents at baseline.

Kiddie Schedule for Affective Disorders and Schizophrenia (KSADS). The KSADS is a semi-structured, clinician-administered, clinical interview that was used to determine if participants met the criteria for depression and/or were experiencing suicidal thinking [55]. Additionally, the KSADS was used to assess global functioning (GAS score) at baseline. The GAS score can range from 1–100, with higher scores indicating higher functioning.

Center for Epidemiological Studies-Depression Scale (CES-D_{10}). The CES-D_{10} is a 10-item self-report or clinician-administered measure that assesses symptoms of depression over the past week. Scores can range from 0–30, with higher scores indicating higher levels of depressive symptoms. Adolescents and parents completed the CES-D_{10} at all time points [56]. Internal consistency of the CES-D in this sample was $\alpha = 0.71$ for youth report, and $\alpha = 0.84$ for parent report.

Screen for Child Anxiety Related Emotional Disorders (SCARED). The SCARED is a 41-item self-report measure that assesses symptoms of anxiety. Scores can range from 0–82, with higher scores indicating higher levels of anxiety symptoms [57]. The internal consistency of the SCARED in this sample was $\alpha = 0.91$ for youth report.

Disruptive Behaviors Disorder Scale (DBD). The DBD is a 41-item self-report measure that assesses behavioral concerns in adolescents. The Attention Deficit Disorder (ADHD) subscale, which includes both the Inattentive and Hyperactivity/Impulsivity domains, and the Oppositional Defiant Disorder/Conduct Disorder (ODD/CD) subscale of the DBD can range from 0–3, with a higher score indicating more externalizing behavior [58]. Internal consistency for youth report in this sample was $\alpha = 0.84$ for the ADHD subscale, and $\alpha = 0.87$ for the ODD/CD subscale.

Social Adjustment Scale (SAS-SR). The SAS-SR is a 36-item self-report measure that assesses social functioning over the past two weeks. Scores can range from 0–4 with a higher score indicating a lower level of functioning [59]. The internal consistency of the SAS-SR in this sample was $\alpha = 0.79$ for youth report.

Beck Hopelessness Scale (BHS). The BHS is a 21-item self-report measure that assesses pessimism about the future. Scores can range from 0–20, with a higher score indicating greater hopelessness [60]. The internal consistency of the BHS in this sample was $\alpha = 0.82$ for youth report.

Child Report of Parental Behavior Inventory (CRPBI). The CRPBI is a 15-item measure that assesses a child's relationship with their parents. Six subscales were used in this study: maternal and paternal acceptance (range = 10–30), psychological control (range = 8–24), and monitoring (range = 5–15). Higher scores indicate higher acceptance, control, and monitoring [61]. Internal consistency for youth report in this sample was $\alpha = 0.91$ for maternal acceptance, $\alpha = 0.78$ for maternal control, $\alpha = 0.80$ for maternal monitoring, $\alpha = 0.92$ for paternal acceptance, $\alpha = 0.82$ for paternal control, and $\alpha = 0.87$ for paternal monitoring.

Theory of Planned Behavior (TPB). The TPB Scale is a 19-item self-report measure that assesses attitude toward participating in a depression prevention intervention. Scores range from 1–5, with a higher score indicating a more positive attitude [62]. The internal consistency of the TPB in this sample was $\alpha = 0.87$ for youth report.

Trans-Theoretical Model. The Trans-Theoretical Model Scale is a 10-item self-report measure that asks the adolescent to rate the importance of preventing an episode of clinical depression, plus their ability and readiness to reduce their depression risk. Scores can range from 1–10, with a higher score indicating a higher overall intention to prevent future episodes [63]. The internal consistency of the Trans-Theoretical Model Scale in this sample was $\alpha = 0.86$ for youth report.

The Adolescent Life Events Questionnaire (ALEQ). The ALEQ is a retrospective self-report measure that asks about life events in the past 6 months. Scores can range from 0–51, with a higher score indicating more life events [64].

Engagement. Engagement in each of the interventions was assessed by the number of modules completed by parents and the number of modules completed by adolescents. A third variable was created to assess overall family engagement by summing the number of modules completed by an adolescent with the number of modules completed by the parent.

Positive Relationships in Primary Care (PRPC). The PRPC was administered at two months and asked the adolescent about their most recent interview with their primary care provider. For CATCH-IT participants, this may have been a motivational interview; for HE participants, it was their last PCP visit. The measure included both general questions ("I feel the primary care provider listened to me") and questions specific to the intervention ("It was helpful to focus on behaviors I would like to change.") Scores can range from 1–5, with higher scores indicating a more positive rating [44,65].

2.7. Statistical Analysis

Linear mixed-effect growth models with random intercept and slope were used to examine differences between groups in change over time in CES-D_{10} and SCARED scores. The CES-D_{10} analysis was conducted with and without a square root transformation of the time scale to improve linearity. All models were adjusted for sex, ethnicity (Hispanic, non-Hispanic), race (white, non-white), baseline age, and site, and the SCARED analysis was also adjusted for baseline teen CES-D_{10}. The p-value for the group*time interaction was used to test for a significant difference in slopes between CATCH-IT and HE. Within-group changes over time were estimated using simple slopes, and adjusted mean change over 24 months was calculated by multiplying the estimated slope by 24 (or the square root of 24 in the time-transformed model).

We also examined the moderating effects of theory-based covariates by including interaction terms in the models. The p-value of the group * time * moderator interaction was used to test for potential moderation of the effect of the intervention. For both the CES-D_{10} and SCARED outcomes, we examined the following potential moderators: demographics (sex, race, ethnicity, maternal education), site (Chicago or Boston), engagement (modules completed by teens, parents, teens + parents), PRPC scores at two months, and baseline scores for GAS, CRAFFT, DBD (ADHD, ODCD), SAS-SR, Theory of Planned Behavior, ALEQ, BHS, Trans-Theoretical Model, Parent CES-D_{10}, and the CRPBI (3 maternal and 3 paternal scales). We also tested SCARED as a potential moderator of the CES-D_{10} outcome and vice versa. In the moderator models with CES-D_{10} as the outcome variable, time was square-root transformed to improve linearity.

Completion or use of the supplementary CATCH-IT anxiety module was not included as a potential moderator in the analyses since only 18 (9.3%) teens completed the module, simply not a large enough percentage of the sample to allow us to test the effects of the module on anxiety and depressive symptoms. Additionally, our models included both CATCH-IT and HE participants to allow us to look for between-group differences. Therefore, we were unable to include variables that only applied to CATCH-IT as either covariates in the model or potential moderators.

Multivariable logistic regression models were used to test for differences between participants with and without CES-D_{10} or SCARED data at 12 and 24 months, including the following covariates: site, intervention group, age at baseline, gender, ethnicity, race, maternal education, parents' marital status, birth order (firstborn, other), past depressive episode at study entry, and high CES-D score at study entry. All analyses were conducted using SAS, version 9.4 (SAS Institute, Cary, NC, USA).

3. Results

3.1. Participants

One hundred ninety-three participants were randomized to CATCH-IT and 176 to HE. The mean age of the participants was 15.4 years (SD = 1.5), and 21% of the participants identified as Hispanic, 26% non-Hispanic black, 43% non-Hispanic white, 4% Asian, and 6% multiracial or other. Over half of the adolescents' parents reported having no more eduction than a high school diploma (60% of mothers and 53% of fathers), and 39.4% reported not being married. Clinically, 62% of participants reported a past sub-threshold or full depressive episode that had ended at least two months before study enrollment. Participants reported a mean score of 25.3 (SD = 12.3) on the SCARED, and a mean score of 9.4 (SD = 4.6) on the CES-D_{10} at baseline.

Site differences were found between the Chicago and Boston participants. Participants from Boston reported higher levels of parent education and a greater likelihood that parents were married. Additionally, the Boston sample was comprised of a lower percentage of ethnic minority participants, and a greater percentage of adolescents in Boston qualified for the study based on only a prior depressive episode. A complete description of the cohort data at baseline is provided in a prior publication [12].

Regarding attrition over the study period, at 24 months CESD scores were available for 182 participants (49.3%), and SCARED scores were available for 93 participants (25.2%). For the CES-D_{10}, missing scores at 24 months were associated with CATCH-IT assignment, the Chicago site, higher age at baseline, lower parent education, and elevated depressed mood at baseline (see Table S1); for the SCARED, missing scores at 24 months were associated with CATCH-IT assignment, the Chicago site, and lower maternal education (see Table S2).

3.2. *Symptoms of Anxiety and Depression*

There was not a significant difference between groups in change over time for either the SCARED ($p = 0.79$) or the CES-D_{10} ($p = 0.80$), see Table 1. Anxiety appeared to improve in both groups, though the change was only statistically significant in CATCH-IT. The estimated slope for SCARED scores was −0.13, SE = 0.06, $p = 0.04$ for CATCH-IT and −0.11, SE = 0.06, $p = 0.07$ for HE. The estimated mean change from baseline to 24 months was −3.1 (SE = 1.5) points in the CATCH-IT group and −2.6 (1.4) points in the HE group. Depressive symptoms improved significantly in both groups. The estimated slope for the CES-D_{10} scores with time square-root transformed was −0.31, $p = 0.004$ for CATCH-IT and −0.27, $p = 0.009$ for HE. The estimated mean change from baseline to 24 months was −1.5 (SE = 0.5) points for CATCH-IT and −1.3 (0.5) points for HE.

Table 1. Internalizing symptoms, baseline to 24 months.

	Unadjusted Means						Within-Group Slopes [1]							Btw Grp Diff
Outcome Variables	CATCH-IT (N = 193)			HE (N = 176)				CATCH-IT			HE			
	N	Mean	SD	N	Mean	SD	Time Variable	b	SE	p	b	SE	p	p
SCARED [2] total score (0–82)							Months	−0.13	(0.06)	0.04	−0.11	(0.06)	0.07	0.79
Baseline	171	25.5	(12.7)	141	25.2	(11.9)								
2 months	94	26.2	(13.1)	90	25.7	(14.3)								
6 months	74	25.1	(15.0)	92	24.0	(13.9)								
12 months	83	22.4	(13.0)	73	23.2	(13.6)								
18 months	64	25.6	(13.3)	81	23.2	(13.4)								
24 months	39	19.6	(12.2)	54	20.9	(13.7)								
CES-D_{10} (0–30)							Months	−0.06	(0.02)	0.01	−0.04	(0.02)	0.10	0.44
Baseline	190	9.5	(4.5)	172	9.4	(4.6)	Sqrt (months)	−0.31	(0.11)	0.004	−0.27	(0.10)	0.009	0.80
2 months	123	9.2	(4.2)	140	7.9	(5.2)								
6 months	116	8.2	(4.9)	133	7.9	(4.7)								
12 months	115	7.9	(5.3)	126	7.1	(4.7)								
18 months	67	7.9	(5.9)	81	7.5	(5.6)								
24 months	79	7.7	(5.8)	103	8.1	(5.6)								

[1] From linear mixed effect growth models with random intercept and slope, adjusted for sex, ethnicity (Hispanic, non-Hispanic), race (white, non-white), baseline age, site, and baseline teen CES-D_{10}. Within-group estimated slopes and p-values are from estimates of simple slopes. The p-value for the visit*time interaction is used to test for a significant difference between slopes. [2] Higher scores indicate greater anxiety.

3.3. Analyses of Potential Moderators

Symptoms of Anxiety. Two significant moderators of the effect of CATCH-IT and HE on change in SCARED scores across the 24-month study period were identified: parental CES-D10 scores at baseline (b = −0.05, p = 0.004) and positive relationships in primary care scores at 2 months (b = −0.41, p = 0.009) (Table 2). Anxiety appeared to decrease more in the HE group than in the CATCH-IT group when parental depressive symptoms at baseline were very low. When parental CES-D10 was set to 0 in the model, the estimated slope for HE was −0.25 (SE = 0.09), and the estimated slope for CATCH-IT was 0.04 (0.09), p = 0.03 (see Table S3). However, anxiety decreased more in the CATCH-IT group than the HE group when parental depressive symptoms at baseline were very high. When parental CES-D10 was set to 27, the maximum score in our sample, the estimated CATCH-IT slope was −0.62 (0.23), while the estimated HE slope was 0.36 (0.26), p = 0.005. At intermediate parental CES-D10 scores (25th percentile, median, 75th percentile), the model did not show significant differences between groups in anxiety change.

Table 2. Summary of moderator analyses for Screen for Child Anxiety Related Emotional Disorders (SCARED): Group*Visit*Moderator Interaction Term.

Moderator	N [1]	Beta	Standard Error	p [2]
Sex = male (reference = female)	362	0.16	0.19	0.41
Race = not white (reference = white) [3]	362	0.14	0.18	0.43
Ethnicity = Hispanic (reference = not Hispanic)	362	−0.17	0.25	0.50
Site = Boston (reference = Chicago)	362	0.29	0.17	0.09
Maternal education= college degree (reference = no college degree)	352	0.15	0.19	0.43
Teen GAS, baseline	360	0.00	0.01	0.66
Teen CES-D_{10}, baseline	362	0.02	0.02	0.17
Parent CES-D_{10}, baseline	332	−0.05	0.02	0.004
ADHD (DBD-A), baseline	196	0.12	0.26	0.64
ODCD (DBD-A), baseline	193	0.28	0.52	0.59
Social adjustment (SAS-SR), baseline	212	0.15	0.23	0.51
Hopelessness (BHS), baseline	270	−0.01	0.03	0.74
Maternal acceptance (CRPBI), baseline	196	−0.04	0.02	0.06
Maternal control (CRPBI), baseline	197	0.04	0.03	0.18
Maternal monitoring (CRPBI), baseline	187	−0.10	0.06	0.12
Paternal acceptance (CRPBI), baseline	176	−0.04	0.02	0.07
Paternal control (CRPBI), baseline	176	0.00	0.03	0.88
Paternal monitoring (CRPBI), baseline	170	−0.04	0.04	0.25
Positive relationships in primary care, 2 months	133	−0.41	0.16	0.009
Theory of planned behavior, baseline	164	−0.47	0.25	0.06
Stressful life events (LEQ), baseline	300	−0.02	0.02	0.24
Trans-theoretical model, baseline	191	−0.07	0.05	0.12
Teen modules completed	362	0.00	0.01	0.83
Parent modules completed	340	−0.03	0.04	0.45

[1] Number of participants included in the analysis. Participants with missing data for the moderator variable or baseline CESD (covariate) were excluded. [2] From linear mixed effect growth models with random intercept and slope and a group*visit*moderator interaction term, adjusted for sex, ethnicity (Hispanic, non-Hispanic), race (white, non-white), baseline age, site, and baseline teen CES-D_{10}. [3] No significant effects of race were detected when the race categorization was changed to Black or multi-racial vs. all others.

Similarly, anxiety appeared to show greater improvement in the HE group than the CATCH-IT group when adolescents gave a very low score to their most recent interaction with their primary care provider (see Table S4). When PRPC was set to 1.0 in the model, the estimated slope for HE was −1.05 (SE = 0.31), while the estimated slope for CATCH-IT was 0.20 (0.37), p = 0.01. However, when PRPC was set to the maximum score of 5.0, the estimated slope was 0.18 (0.14) for HE but −0.22 (0.14) for CATCH-IT, p = 0.050. The model did not predict significant differences in anxiety change between groups at intermediate PRPC scores.

Symptoms of Depression. Three significant moderators of the effect of CATCH-IT and HE on change in adolescent CES-D10 scores across the 24-month study period were identified: baseline DBD-ADHD subscale score (b = 1.42, p = 0.004), baseline DBD-ODD/CD subscale score (b = 2.37,

$p = 0.01$), and PRPC score at two months ($b = -0.60$, $p = 0.046$) (Table 3). In the ADHD moderator model, CATCH-IT appeared superior to HE in reducing CES-D10 scores when ADHD scores were low, but HE appeared superior when ADHD scores were high (see Table S5). When the ADHD score was set to 0 in the model, the estimated slope for CATCH-IT was −0.31 (SE = 0.28), while the estimated slope for HE was 0.89 (0.32), $p = 0.006$. CATCH-IT still appeared superior when ADHD was set to the approximate 25th percentile in our sample (0.5), though the difference between slopes was smaller: −0.25 (0.16) for CATCH-IT vs 0.24 (0.18) for HE, $p = 0.04$. However, when ADHD was set to the maximum value for our sample (2.0), the estimated CES-D10 slope was only −0.06 (0.43) for CATCH-IT but −1.70 (0.44) for HE, $p = 0.008$. For ADHD scores at the median and 75th percentiles for our sample, the model did not predict a significant difference between groups.

Table 3. Summary of moderator analyses for CESD: Group*Visit*Moderator Interaction Term.

Moderator	N[1]	Estimate	SE	p[2]
Sex = male (reference = female)	369	0.06	0.33	0.86
Race = not white (reference = white)	369	0.54	0.30	0.07
Ethnicity = Hispanic (reference = not Hispanic)	369	−0.09	0.38	0.81
Site = Boston (reference = Chicago)	369	0.01	0.31	0.98
Maternal education = college degree (reference = no college degree)	359	0.03	0.31	0.91
Teen GAS, baseline	367	0.00	0.02	0.93
Anxiety (SCARED), baseline	312	0.00	0.01	0.99
Parent CES-D_{10}, baseline	338	0.01	0.03	0.84
ADHD (DBD-A), baseline	196	1.42	0.48	0.004
ODCD (DBD-A), baseline	193	2.37	0.93	0.01
Social adjustment (SAS-SR), baseline	212	−0.22	0.45	0.64
Hopelessness (BHS), baseline	270	0.03	0.05	0.55
Maternal acceptance (CRPBI), baseline	196	−0.04	0.05	0.40
Maternal control (CRPBI), baseline	197	0.07	0.06	0.23
Maternal monitoring (CRPBI), baseline	187	0.02	0.10	0.86
Paternal acceptance (CRPBI), baseline	176	−0.05	0.04	0.21
Paternal control (CRPBI), baseline	176	0.06	0.06	0.35
Paternal monitoring (CRPBI), baseline	170	−0.07	0.07	0.29
Positive relationships in primary care, 2 months	134	−0.60	0.30	0.046
Theory of planned behavior, baseline	164	−0.91	0.50	0.07
Stressful life events (LEQ), baseline	302	0.05	0.03	0.10
Trans-theoretical model, baseline	191	0.08	0.10	0.42
Teen modules completed	369	0.00	0.03	0.88
Parent modules completed	346	−0.05	0.08	0.52

[1] Number of participants included in the analysis. Participants with missing data for the moderator variable were excluded. [2] From linear mixed effect growth models with random intercept and slope and a group*visit*moderator interaction term, adjusted for sex, ethnicity (Hispanic, non-Hispanic), race (white, non-white), baseline age, and site. Time square-root transformed to improve linearity.

Results were similar for the DBD-ODCD subscale (see Table S6). When ODCD was set to 0 in the model, the estimated improvement in depressive symptoms was greater in the CATCH-IT group: slope = −0.29 (0.19) for CATCH-IT and 0.38 (0.23) for HE, $p = 0.03$. When ODCD was set to the maximum score in our sample (still quite low at 1.25), the estimated slopes were 0.18 (0.71) for CATCH-IT and −2.11 (0.65) for HE, $p = 0.02$. The model did not predict significant differences between slopes at intermediate values of ODCD.

As was noted for anxiety, the HE group showed a greater estimated reduction in depressive symptoms than the CATCH-IT group when the PRPC rating was very low (see Table S7). With PRPC set to 1 (minimum score) in the model, the estimated CATCH-IT slope was 0.76 (0.70), but the HE slope was −1.22 (0.58), $p = 0.03$. However, the model did not show significant differences between groups at any other PRPC value tested, including the maximum score of 5.

4. Discussion

In a long-term follow-up investigation, the current study examined symptoms of anxiety and depression in at-risk adolescents who were recruited through primary care and were assigned randomly to the CATCH-IT prevention intervention or HE. Consistent with data from a 6-month follow-up of this sample [12], adolescents assigned to both the CATCH-IT intervention and the HE intervention experienced decreasing depressive symptoms over the course of 24 months. Moreover, differences in score trajectories were not found between the conditions, suggesting that both interventions had a positive effect on depressive symptoms. The multiple study contacts (i.e., screenings, assessments, safety calls) that accompanied both intervention approaches may have obscured group differences. In addition, while the content of the HE program focused on health behaviors and not on mental health, participants and parents may have received some sense of mastery and self-efficacy from completing the program, which may account for lower depression scores for HE participants.

The current study also provided evidence for cross-over effects in the CATCH-IT group. Although there was not an overall group difference in anxiety symptoms, teens at risk for depression who were assigned to CATCH-IT experienced a significant decrease in symptoms of anxiety across the 24 months, while there was no significant change in anxiety symptoms for teens assigned to HE. This finding is consistent with results from Ip et al. [47], who found that adolescents who used a Chinese adaptation of the CATCH-IT prevention intervention, Grasp the Opportunity, reported fewer symptoms of anxiety at 8 months, relative to adolescents assigned to a control (attention) intervention. Evidence of cross-over effects from CATCH-IT suggests that this prevention intervention, which was developed to address risk for depression only, may in fact target shared underlying mechanisms for both depression and anxiety. These results are counter to Garber et al. [41], who, in a meta-analysis exploring cross-over effects for depression and anxiety treatment and prevention interventions, reported no evidence of cross-over effects for depression prevention programs. It is possible that the recruitment process, intervention engagement, and motivational interviews that accompany the CATCH-IT intervention, all of which emphasize building resilience, managing stressors, and working toward goals in addition to preventing low mood and depression, may help teens to generalize depression prevention skills to other distressing symptoms such as anxiety. It is also true that the CATCH-IT intervention includes an optional anxiety module (Module #15), which addresses symptoms of anxiety more directly and provides instructions for exercises such as progressive muscle relaxation. Because so few adolescents ($N = 18$) in our sample completed the anxiety module, however, it is more likely that the observed improvement in anxiety symptoms is explained by participants' use of other skills taught in CATCH-IT, such as cognitive restructuring and behavioral activation, both of which are commonly used to treat symptoms of anxiety in adolescents [66–68].

Secondary analyses revealed that parental depression moderates the trajectory of anxiety symptoms in teens assigned to CATCH-IT compared to HE. Specifically, when parents had no or low-level symptoms of depression at baseline, their adolescents reported a greater improvement in anxiety when assigned to HE; when parents had high-level symptoms of depression at baseline, their adolescents reported a greater improvement in anxiety when assigned to CATCH-IT. This finding, that CATCH-IT is associated with better outcomes for teens when parents report high-level depressive symptoms, contrasts with prior research suggesting that parental depressive symptoms are associated with *poorer* intervention outcomes for children with internalizing symptoms [69,70]. Our findings are consistent, however, with research reporting better youth intervention outcomes when parents report symptoms of anxiety [71–73], and may reflect the additional motivation symptomatic parents feel to support their children's engagement in the CATCH-IT intervention. It is also possible that parents with depressive symptoms were more engaged in the CATCH-IT parent intervention, and that their use of the on-line parent modules, as well as the motivational interviews focusing on their goals for supporting their child in completing CATCH-IT, improved their child's long-term outcomes. In fact, Legerstee and colleagues [71] suggested that anxious mothers may have benefitted from the parent intervention that accompanied their adolescent's intervention, and therefore were able to support their teen's engagement in treatment, leading to better outcomes over time. Unfortunately, baseline parental anxiety was not measured in this trial, but adolescents with elevated symptoms of depression at baseline were found to benefit more from CATCH-IT than non-symptomatic adolescents [12].

Additionally, the adolescent's relationship with their primary care physician moderated the trajectory of anxiety symptoms in adolescents assigned to CATCH-IT relative to HE. Adolescents who reported a weak connection to their primary care physician experienced a greater improvement in anxiety when they were assigned to HE rather than CATCH-IT. The benefits adolescents received from the HE intervention are likely a function of the non-specific factors associated with study involvement (e.g., recruitment, assessments, check-in phone calls, sense of achievement from completing modules), and perhaps these non-specific factors were more motivating for adolescents in the absence of a close connection with their primary care physician.

Secondary analyses also revealed some interesting moderating effects of adolescents' externalizing behaviors on their depressive symptoms across the 24-month follow-up interval, such that, when adolescents reported more symptoms of attentional and oppositional behaviors, they experienced a greater improvement in depressive symptoms if they were assigned to the HE group. By extension, this finding suggests that the CATCH-IT intervention, relative to HE, may be less helpful to adolescents who are struggling with externalizing concerns, perhaps due to its high reading demand, and its demand for attention, homework completion, and compliance. Solanto [74] suggests that the self-management challenges for adolescents with ADHD may interfere with their response to cognitive-behavioral and self-directed interventions. Nevertheless, given the overall low mean score for this sample on the DBD, the measure of externalizing behaviors used in this trial, these moderating effects must be interpreted with caution. Similar to our findings on symptoms of anxiety, depressive symptoms decreased more across the 24 months for adolescents in HE than in CATCH-IT when they reported a weak connection to their primary care physician.

There are several limitations associated with this study. We experienced attrition in the sample over the 24-month study period, particularly among adolescents with fewer resources (e.g., Chicago site, higher depressed mood, lower parental education). It is noteworthy that, to our knowledge, this is the only Internet-based intervention trial for youth with a 2-year follow-up, and such attrition is to be expected when such a long interval follows an intervention with relatively minimal face-to-face interaction. It is also noteworthy that attrition was higher for adolescents assigned to CATCH-IT versus HE, despite the presence of physician contact through motivational interviews in the CATCH-IT condition only. It is difficult to account for this finding, but it is possible that adolescents who benefitted most from the CATCH-IT intervention were less likely to feel a need to remain connected with the study throughout the follow-up interval. To address attrition in our sample, we chose to use mixed effect models, which are thought to be robust to missing data. The use of a second, potentially active internet-based intervention as a control is another limitation to the study. While the content of HE was not focused on mental health (only a single module towards the end of the intervention addressed mental health concerns), the program did present information on other health behaviors. It is possible that teens assigned to the HE condition received benefit above what they would have in an inactive or waitlist control. In addition, the examination of very long-term intervention effects (24 months) is necessarily constrained by the possibility of intervening environmental factors (e.g., natural disasters, family disruption) that may limit the ability to draw conclusions regarding causality.

5. Conclusions

Despite these limitations, the current study demonstrates long-term reductions in symptoms of depression in both intervention groups (HE and CATCH-IT). Additionally, participants assigned to CATCH-IT were found to have cross-over effects as seen in a reduction of anxiety symptoms, demonstrating that it is possible to develop preventive interventions for adolescent depression that target transdiagnostic factors representing shared underlying mechanisms for both disorders. Similarly, moderation results of depression and anxiety symptoms reported here, in addition to earlier moderation results of depressive disorder outcomes [48], suggest that CATCH-IT is beneficial when certain conditions are present (i.e., no significant externalizing symptoms (depressed mood), no significant hopelessness (depressive episodes), a supportive relationship with a physician (anxiety and depressive symptoms), heightened parental symptoms (anxiety), and adequate paternal monitoring (depressive episodes)). That is, pre-conditions (current depressed mood), lack of substantial co-morbidity, and supportive environmental factors may be necessary for adolescents to benefit from this largely self-directed model. Given that comorbid presentations of depression and anxiety are common and are associated with poor long-term outcomes, the discovery of a single preventive intervention that targets both disorders has significant implications for youth mental health promotion. These findings, along with the ability to implement the program across multiple primary care clinics, demonstrates the value of CATCH-IT as a feasible, online, population-based depression prevention intervention for at-risk adolescents.

Supplementary Materials: Table S1: Predictors of missing 24-month SCARED, all participants, Table S2: Predictors of missing 24-month CES-D_{10}, all participants, Table S3: SCARED Moderator: Between-Group Comparisons: difference between CATCH-IT and HE simple slopes for time at selected levels of Parent CES-D[a], Table S4: SCARED Moderator: Between-Group Comparisons: difference between CATCH-IT and HE simple slopes for time at selected levels of PRPC, Table S5: CES-D_{10} Moderator: Between-Group Comparisons: difference between CATCH-IT and HE simple slopes for time at selected levels of ADHD, Table S6: CES-D_{10} Moderator: Between-Group Comparisons: difference between CATCH-IT and HE simple slopes for time at selected levels of ODCD, and Table S7: CES-D10 Moderator: Between-Group Comparisons: difference between CATCH-IT and HE simple slopes for time at selected levels of PRPC1.

Author Contributions: Conceptualization, T.G., K.R.B., L.S., M.L., and B.W.V.V.; methodology, T.G., K.R.B., L.S., M.F., and B.W.V.V.; validation, T.G., K.R.B., L.S., M.F., and B.W.V.V.; formal analysis, L.S.; investigation, T.G. and B.W.V.V.; data curation, L.S.; writing—original draft preparation, T.G. and K.R.B.; writing—review and editing, T.G., K.R.B., M.F., M.L., L.S., and B.W.V.V.; supervision, T.G. and B.W.V.V.; project administration, M.L.; funding acquisition, T.G. and B.W.V.V. All authors have read and agreed to the published version of the manuscript.

Acknowledgments: Content is solely the responsibility of the authors and does not necessarily represent the official views of the National Institutes of Health. Ethical bodies that approved this study include: Wellesley College Institutional Review Board (IRB), University of Illinois at Chicago IRB, Advocate Health Care IRB, Franciscan St. Mary IRB, Northwestern IRB and NorthShore University Health Systems IRB. Methods developed under Robert Wood Johnson (Project Curb "Chicago Urban Resiliency Building": Reducing Life Course Disparities in Depression Outcomes in Urban Youth Through Early Preventive Intervention) supported and informed the implementation process. Thank you to Brady Goodwin, Joselyn Williams, Hendricks Brown, David A. Aaby, Mark Reinecke, Joshua Fogel, Emily Sykes, William R. Beardslee, Amy Kane, and Sophia Rintell for their contributions. B.W.V.V. would like to acknowledge the interest of Asok K. Ray, MD FRCS (Edin), Purnima Ray and Malika Ray in this research is appreciated.

References

1. Rushton Jerry, L.; Michelle, F.; Schectman Robin, M. Epidemiology of depressive symptoms in the National Longitudinal Study of Adolescent Health. *J. Am. Acad. Child Adolesc. Psychiatry* **2002**, *41*, 199–205. [CrossRef] [PubMed]
2. Lewinsohn, P.M.; Rohde, P.; Klein, D.N.; Seeley, J.R. Natural course of adolescent major depressive disorder: I. Continuity into young adulthood. *J. Am. Acad. Child Adolesc. Psychiatry* **1999**, *38*, 56. [CrossRef] [PubMed]
3. Weissman, M.M.; Wolk, S.; Goldstein, R.B.; Moreau, D.; Adams, P.; Greenwald, S.; Klier, C.M.; Ryan, N.D.; Dahl, R.E.; Wickramaratne, P. Depressed adolescents grown up. *JAMA* **1999**, *281*, 1707. [CrossRef] [PubMed]
4. Birmaher, B.; Ryan, N.D.; Williamson, D.E.; Brent, D.A.; Kaufman, J.; Dahl, R.E.; Perel, J.; Nelson, B. Childhood and adolescent depression: A review of the past 10 years. Part I. *J. Am. Acad. Child Adolesc. Psychiatry* **1996**, *35*, 1427. [CrossRef]

5. Pine, D.S.; Goldstein, R.B.; Wolk, S.; Weissman, M.M. The Association Between Childhood Depression and Adulthood Body Mass Index. *Pediatrics* **2001**, *107*, 1049–1056. [CrossRef]
6. Balázs, J.; Miklósi, M.; Keresztény, Á.; Hoven, C.W.; Carli, V.; Wasserman, C.; Apter, A.; Bobes, J.; Brunner, R.; Cosman, D.; et al. Adolescent subthreshold-depression and anxiety: Psychopathology, functional impairment and increased suicide risk. *J. Child Psychol. Psychiatry* **2013**, *54*, 670–677. [CrossRef]
7. Georgiades, K.; Lewinsohn, P.M.; Monroe, S.M.; Seeley, J.R. Major depressive disorder in adolescence: The role of subthreshold symptoms. *J. Am. Acad. Child Adolesc. Psychiatry* **2006**, *45*, 936–944. [CrossRef]
8. Birmaher, B.; Ryan, N.D.; Williamson, D.E.; Brent, D.A.; Kaufman, J. Childhood and adolescent depression: A review of the past 10 years. Part II. *J. Am. Acad. Child Adolesc. Psychiatry* **1996**, *35*, 1575. [CrossRef]
9. Buntrock, C.; Berking, M.; Smit, F.; Lehr, D.; Nobis, S.; Riper, H.; Cuijpers, P.; Ebert, D. Preventing depression in adults with subthreshold depression: Health-economic evaluation alongside a pragmatic randomized controlled trial of a web-based intervention. *J. Med. Internet Res.* **2017**, *19*, e5. [CrossRef]
10. Hetrick, S.E.; Cox, G.R.; Witt, K.G.; Bir, J.J.; Merry, S.N. Cognitive behavioural therapy (CBT), third-wave CBT and interpersonal therapy (IPT) based interventions for preventing depression in children and adolescents. *Cochrane Database Syst. Rev.* **2016**. [CrossRef]
11. Brown, C.H.; Brincks, A.; Huang, S.; Perrino, T.; Cruden, G.; Pantin, H.; Howe, G.; Young, J.F.; Beardslee, W.; Montag, S. Two-year impact of prevention programs on adolescent depression: An integrative data analysis approach. *Prev. Sci.* **2018**, *19*, 74–94. [CrossRef]
12. Gladstone, T.; Terrizzi, D.; Stinson, A.; Nidetz, J.; Canel, J.; Ching, E.; Berry, A.; Cantorna, J.; Fogel, J.; Eder, M.; et al. Effect of Internet-based Cognitive Behavioral Humanistic and Interpersonal Training vs. Internet-based General Health Education on Adolescent Depression in Primary Care: A Randomized Clinical Trial. *JAMA Netw. Open* **2018**, *1*, e184278. [CrossRef]
13. Saulsberry, A.; Marko-Holguin, M.; Blomeke, K.; Hinkle, C.; Fogel, J.; Gladstone, T.; Bell, C.; Reinecke, M.; Corden, M.; Van Voorhees, B.W. Randomized Clinical Trial of a Primary Care Internet-based Intervention to Prevent Adolescent Depression: One-year Outcomes. *J. Can. Acad. Child Adolesc. Psychiatry* **2013**, *22*, 106–117. [PubMed]
14. Conejo-Cerón, S.; Moreno-Peral, P.; Rodríguez-Morejón, A.; Motrico, E.; Navas-Campaña, D.; Rigabert, A.; Martín-Pérez, C.; Rodríguez-Bayón, A.; Ballesta-Rodríguez, M.I.; Luna, J.d.D.; et al. Effectiveness of Psychological and Educational Interventions to Prevent Depression in Primary Care: A Systematic Review and Meta-Analysis. *Ann. Fam. Med.* **2017**, *15*, 262–271. [CrossRef] [PubMed]
15. Garber, J.; Clarke, G.N.; Weersing, V.R.; Beardslee, W.R.; Brent, D.A.; Gladstone, T.R.G.; DeBar, L.L.; Lynch, F.L.; D'Angelo, E.; Hollon, S.D.; et al. Prevention of depression in at-risk adolescents: A randomized controlled trial. *JAMA* **2009**, *301*, 2215. [CrossRef]
16. Beardslee, W.R.; Brent, D.A.; Weersing, V.R.; Clarke, G.N.; Porta, G.; Hollon, S.D.; Gladstone, T.R.G.; Gallop, R.; Lynch, F.L.; Iyengar, S.; et al. Prevention of depression in at-risk adolescents: Longer-term effects. *JAMA Psychiatry* **2013**, *70*, 1161. [CrossRef]
17. Gillham, J.E.; Hamilton, J.; Freres, D.R.; Patton, K.; Gallop, R. Preventing Depression Among Early Adolescents in the Primary Care Setting: A Randomized Controlled Study of the Penn Resiliency Program. *J. Abnorm. Child Psychol.* **2006**, *34*, 195–211. [CrossRef]
18. Merikangas, K.R.; He, J.-P.; Burstein, M.; Swanson, S.A.; Avenevoli, S.; Cui, L.; Benjet, C.; Georgiades, K.; Swendsen, J. Lifetime prevalence of mental disorders in U.S. adolescents: Results from the National Comorbidity Survey Replication—Adolescent Supplement (NCS-A). *J. Am. Acad. Child Adolesc. Psychiatry* **2010**, *49*, 980. [CrossRef] [PubMed]
19. Merikangas, K.R.; Nakamura, E.F.; Kessler, R.C. Epidemiology of mental disorders in children and adolescents. *Dialogues Clin. Neurosci.* **2009**, *11*, 7–20. [PubMed]
20. Kessler, R.C.; Berglund, P.; Demler, O.; Jin, R.; Merikangas, K.R.; Walters, E.E. Lifetime prevalence and age-of-onset distributions of DSM-IV disorders in the National Comorbidity Survey Replication. *Arch. Gen. Psychiatry* **2005**, *62*, 593–602. [CrossRef]
21. Kessler, R.; Avenevoli, S.; McLaughlin, K.; Green, J.; Lakoma, M.; Petukhova, M.; Pine, D.; Sampson, N.; Zaslavsky, A.; Merikangas, K. Lifetime co-morbidity of DSM-IV disorders in the US national comorbidity survey replication adolescent supplement (NCS-A). *Psychol. Med.* **2012**, *42*, 1997–2010. [CrossRef] [PubMed]

22. Keenan, K.; Feng, X.; Hipwell, A.; Klostermann, S. Depression begets depression: Comparing the predictive utility of depression and anxiety symptoms to later depression. *J. Child Psychol. Psychiatry* **2009**, *50*, 1167–1175. [CrossRef]
23. Snyder, J.; Bullard, L.; Wagener, A.; Leong, P.K. Childhood Anxiety and Depressive Symptoms: Trajectories, Relationship, and Association with Subsequent Depression. *J. Clin. Child Adolesc. Psychol.* **2009**, *38*, 837. [CrossRef]
24. Hale III, W.W.; Raaijmakers, Q.A.; Muris, P.; Van Hoof, A.; Meeus, W.H. One factor or two parallel processes? Comorbidity and development of adolescent anxiety and depressive disorder symptoms. *J. Child Psychol. Psychiatry* **2009**, *50*, 1218–1226. [CrossRef] [PubMed]
25. Lavigne, J.V.; Lavigne, J.V.; Hopkins, J.; Hopkins, J.; Gouze, K.R.; Gouze, K.R.; Bryant, F.B.; Bryant, F.B. Bidirectional Influences of Anxiety and Depression in Young Children. *J. Abnorm. Child Psychol.* **2015**, *43*, 163–176. [CrossRef] [PubMed]
26. Merikangas, K.R.; Avenevoli, S. Epidemiology of mood and anxiety disorders in children and adolescents. In *Textbook in Psychiatric Epidemiology*; Wiley-Liss: Hoboken, NJ, USA, 2002.
27. Copeland, W.E.; Wolke, D.; Shanahan, L.; Costello, E.J. Adult functional outcomes of common childhood psychiatric problems: A prospective, longitudinal study. *JAMA Psychiatry* **2015**, *72*, 892–899. [CrossRef] [PubMed]
28. Copeland, W.E.; Alaie, I.; Jonsson, U.; Shanahan, L. Associations of Childhood and Adolescent Depression With Adult Psychiatric and Functional Outcomes. *J. Am. Acad. Child Adolesc. Psychiatry* **2020**. [CrossRef]
29. Weller, B.E.; Blanford, K.L.; Butler, A.M. Estimated Prevalence of Psychiatric Comorbidities in U.S. Adolescents With Depression by Race/Ethnicity, 2011–2012. *J. Adolesc. Health* **2018**, *62*, 716–721. [CrossRef]
30. Costello, E.J.; Mustillo, S.; Erkanli, A.; Keeler, G. Prevalence and development of psychiatric disorders in childhood and adolescence. *Arch. Gen. Psychiatry* **2003**, *60*, 837–844. [CrossRef]
31. Melton, T.; Croarkin, P.; Strawn, J.; Mcclintock, S. Comorbid Anxiety and Depressive Symptoms in Children and Adolescents: A Systematic Review and Analysis. *J. Psychiatr. Pract.* **2016**, *22*, 84–98. [CrossRef]
32. Avenevoli, S.; Swendsen, J.; He, J.-P.; Burstein, M.; Merikangas, K.R. Major depression in the national comorbidity survey-adolescent supplement: Prevalence, correlates, and treatment. *J. Am. Acad. Child Adolesc. Psychiatry* **2015**, *54*, 37. [CrossRef]
33. Angold, A.; Costello, E.J. Depressive comorbidity in children and adolescents. *Am. J. Psychiatry* **1993**, *150*, 1779–1791. [PubMed]
34. Garber, J.; Weersing, V.R. Comorbidity of Anxiety and Depression in Youth: Implications for Treatment and Prevention. *Clin. Psychol.* **2010**, *17*, 293–306. [CrossRef] [PubMed]
35. Clark, L.A.; Watson, D. Tripartite model of anxiety and depression: Psychometric evidence and taxonomic implications. *J. Abnorm. Psychol.* **1991**, *100*, 316. [CrossRef] [PubMed]
36. Dozois, D.J.; Beck, A.T. Cognitive schemas, beliefs and assumptions. In *Risk Factors in Depression*; Elsevier: Amsterdam, The Netherlands, 2008; pp. 119–143.
37. Kranzler, A.; Young, J.F.; Hankin, B.L.; Abela, J.R.; Elias, M.J.; Selby, E.A. Emotional awareness: A transdiagnostic predictor of depression and anxiety for children and adolescents. *J. Clin. Child Adolesc. Psychol.* **2016**, *45*, 262–269. [CrossRef]
38. Schäfer, J.Ö.; Naumann, E.; Holmes, E.A.; Tuschen-Caffier, B.; Samson, A.C. Emotion regulation strategies in depressive and anxiety symptoms in youth: A meta-analytic review. *J. Youth Adolesc.* **2017**, *46*, 261–276. [CrossRef]
39. Ehrenreich, J.T.; Goldstein, C.R.; Wright, L.R.; Barlow, D.H. Development of a Unified Protocol for the Treatment of Emotional Disorders in Youth. *Child Fam. Behav. Ther.* **2009**, *31*, 20–37. [CrossRef]
40. Barlow, D.H.; Allen, L.B.; Choate, M.L. Toward a unified treatment for emotional disorders. *Behav. Ther.* **2004**, *35*, 205–230. [CrossRef]
41. Garber, J.; Brunwasser, S.M.; Zerr, A.A.; Schwartz, K.T.; Sova, K.; Weersing, V.R. Treatment and prevention of depression and anxiety in youth: Test of cross-over effects. *Depress. Anxiety* **2016**, *33*, 939–959. [CrossRef]
42. Van Voorhees, B.W.; Watson, N.; Bridges, J.F.P.; Fogel, J.; Galas, J.; Kramer, C.; Connery, M.; McGill, A.; Marko, M.; Cardenas, A.; et al. Development and pilot study of a marketing strategy for primary care/internet-based depression prevention intervention for adolescents (the CATCH-IT intervention). *Prim. Care Companion J. Clin. Psychiatry* **2010**, *12*, PCC.09m00791. [CrossRef]

43. Gladstone, T.G.; Marko-Holguin, M.; Rothberg, P.; Nidetz, J.; Diehl, A.; DeFrino, D.T.; Harris, M.; Ching, E.; Eder, M.; Canel, J.; et al. An internet-based adolescent depression preventive intervention: Study protocol for a randomized control trial. *Trials* **2015**, *16*, 203. [CrossRef] [PubMed]
44. Van Voorhees, B.W.; Fogel, J.; Reinecke, M.A.; Gladstone, T.; Stuart, S.; Gollan, J.; Bradford, N.; Domanico, R.; Fagan, B.; Ross, R.; et al. Randomized clinical trial of an Internet-based depression prevention program for adolescents (Project CATCH-IT) in primary care: 12-week outcomes. *J. Dev. Behav. Pediatrics* **2009**, *30*, 23–37. [CrossRef] [PubMed]
45. Richards, K.; Marko-Holguin, M.; Fogel, J.; Anker, L.; Ronayne, J.; Van Voorhees, B.W. Randomized clinical trial of an internet-based intervention to prevent adolescent depression in a primary care setting (Catch-It): 2.5-year outcomes. *J. Evid. Based Psychother.* **2016**, *16*, 113. [PubMed]
46. Christensen, H.; Griffiths, K.M. The prevention of depression using the Internet. *Med. J. Aust.* **2002**, *177*, S122–S125. [CrossRef] [PubMed]
47. Ip, P.; Chim, D.; Chan, K.L.; Li, T.M.; Ho, F.K.W.; Van Voorhees, B.W.; Tiwari, A.; Tsang, A.; Chan, C.W.L.; Ho, M. Effectiveness of a culturally attuned Internet-based depression prevention program for Chinese adolescents: A randomized controlled trial. *Depress. Anxiety* **2016**, *33*, 1123–1131. [CrossRef] [PubMed]
48. Van Voorhees, B.G.T.; Sobowale, K.; Brown, C.H.; Aaby, D.; Terrizzi, D.; Canel, J.; Ching, E.; Berry, A.; Cantorna, J. 24-Month Outcomes of Primary Care Web-Based Depression Prevention Intervention in Adolescents: Randomized Clinical Trial. *J. Med. Internet Res.* **2020**, *22*. [CrossRef]
49. Curran, G.M.; Bauer, M.; Mittman, B.; Pyne, J.M.; Stetler, C. Effectiveness-implementation hybrid designs: Combining elements of clinical effectiveness and implementation research to enhance public health impact. *Med. Care* **2012**, *50*, 217. [CrossRef]
50. Mahoney, N.; Gladstone, T.; DeFrino, D.; Stinson, A.; Nidetz, J.; Canel, J.; Ching, E.; Berry, A.; Cantorna, J.; Fogel, J.; et al. Prevention of Adolescent Depression in Primary Care: Barriers and Relational Work Solutions. *Calif. J. Health Promot.* **2017**, *15*, 1–12. [CrossRef]
51. Stuart, S.; Robertson, M. *Interpersonal Psychotherapy: A Clinician's Guide*; Oxford University Press: New York, NY, USA, 2003.
52. Jacobson, N.S.; Martell, C.R.; Dimidjian, S. Behavioral activation treatment for depression: Returning to contextual roots. *Clin. Psychol.* **2001**, *8*, 255–270. [CrossRef]
53. Gagne, R.M.; Briggs, L.J.; Wagner, W. *Principles of Instructional Design*; HBJ College: Fort Worth, TX, USA, 1992.
54. Van Voorhees, B.W.; Gladstone, T.; Cordel, S.; Marko-Holguin, M.; Beardslee, W.; Kuwabara, S.; Kaplan, M.A.; Fogel, J.; Diehl, A.; Hansen, C.; et al. Development of a technology-based behavioral vaccine to prevent adolescent depression: A health system integration model. *Internet Interv.* **2015**, *2*, 303–313. [CrossRef]
55. Kaufman, J.; Birmaher, B.; Brent, D.; Rao, U.; Flynn, C.; Moreci, P.; Williamson, D.; Ryan, N. Schedule for affective disorders and schizophrenia for school-age children-present and lifetime version (K-SADS-PL): Initial reliability and validity data. *J. Am. Acad. Child Adolesc. Psychiatry* **1997**, *36*, 980–988. [CrossRef] [PubMed]
56. Radloff, L.S. The use of the Center for Epidemiologic Studies Depression Scale in adolescents and young adults. *J. Youth Adolesc.* **1991**, *20*, 149–166. [CrossRef] [PubMed]
57. Birmaher, B.; Khetarpal, S.; Brent, D.; Cully, M.; Balach, L.; Kaufman, J.; Neer, S.M. The screen for child anxiety related emotional disorders (SCARED): Scale construction and psychometric characteristics. *J. Am. Acad. Child Adolesc. Psychiatry* **1997**, *36*, 545–553. [CrossRef] [PubMed]
58. Silva, R.R.; Alpert, M.; Pouget, E.; Silva, V.; Trosper, S.; Reyes, K.; Dummit, S. A rating scale for disruptive behavior disorders, based on the DSM-IV item pool. *Psychiatr. Q.* **2005**, *76*, 327–339. [CrossRef] [PubMed]
59. Weissman, M.M.; Orvaschel, H.; Padian, N. Children's symptom and social functioning: Self-report scales. *J. Nerv. Ment. Disord.* **1980**, *168*, 736–740. [CrossRef]
60. Beck, A.T.; Weissman, A.; Lester, D.; Trexler, L. The measurement of pessimism: The hopelessness scale. *J. Consult. Clin. Psychol.* **1974**, *42*, 861. [CrossRef]
61. Schaefer, E.S. A configurational analysis of children's reports of parent behavior. *J. Consult. Psychol.* **1965**, *29*, 552. [CrossRef]
62. Armitage, C.J.; Conner, M. Efficacy of the theory of planned behaviour: A meta-analytic review. *Br. J. Soc. Psychol.* **2001**, *40*, 471–499. [CrossRef]
63. Prochaska, J.O.; Velicer, W.F.; DiClemente, C.C.; Fava, J. Measuring processes of change: Applications to the cessation of smoking. *J. Consult. Clin. Psychol.* **1988**, *56*, 520. [CrossRef]

64. Hankin, B.L.; Abramson, L.Y. Measuring cognitive vulnerability to depression in adolescence: Reliability, validity, and gender differences. *J. Clin. Child Adolesc. Psychol.* **2002**, *31*, 491–504. [CrossRef]
65. Van Voorhees, B.W.; Vanderplough-Booth, K.; Fogel, J.; Gladstone, T.; Bell, C.; Stuart, S.; Gollan, J.; Bradford, N.; Domanico, R.; Fagan, B. Integrative internet-based depression prevention for adolescents: A randomized clinical trial in primary care for vulnerability and protective factors. *J. Can. Acad. Child Adolesc. Psychiatry* **2008**, *17*, 184. [PubMed]
66. Compton, S.N.; March, J.S.; Brent, D.; Albano, A.M.; Weersing, V.R.; Curry, J. Cognitive-behavioral psychotherapy for anxiety and depressive disorders in children and adolescents: An evidence-based medicine review. *J. Am. Acad. Child Adolesc. Psychiatry* **2004**, *43*, 930–959. [CrossRef] [PubMed]
67. Hudson, J.L.; Rapee, R.M.; Deveney, C.; Schniering, C.A.; Lyneham, H.J.; Bovopoulos, N. Cognitive-behavioral treatment versus an active control for children and adolescents with anxiety disorders: A randomized trial. *J. Am. Acad. Child Adolesc. Psychiatry* **2009**, *48*, 533–544. [CrossRef] [PubMed]
68. Martin, F.; Oliver, T. Behavioural activation for children and young people: A systematic review of progress and promise. *Eur. Child Adolesc. Psychiatry* **2019**, *28*, 427–441. [CrossRef] [PubMed]
69. Gladstone, T.R.; Diehl, A.; Thomann, L.O.; Beardslee, W.R. The Association Between Parental Depression and Child Psychosocial Intervention Outcomes: Directions for Future Research. *Harv. Rev. Psychiatry* **2019**, *27*, 241–253. [CrossRef] [PubMed]
70. Eckshtain, D.; Marchette, L.K.; Schleider, J.; Weisz, J.R. Parental depressive symptoms as a predictor of outcome in the treatment of child depression. *J. Abnorm. Child Psychol.* **2018**, *46*, 825–837. [CrossRef] [PubMed]
71. Legerstee, J.; Huizink, A.; Van Gastel, W.; Liber, J.M.; Treffers, P.; Verhulst, F.C.; Utens, E. Maternal anxiety predicts favourable treatment outcomes in anxiety-disordered adolescents. *Acta Psychiatr. Scand.* **2008**, *117*, 289–298. [CrossRef]
72. Toren, P.; Wolmer, L.; Rosental, B.; Eldar, S.; Koren, S.; Lask, M.; Weizman, R.; Laor, N. Case series: Brief parent-child group therapy for childhood anxiety disorders using a manual-based cognitive-behavioral technique. *J. Am. Acad. Child Adolesc. Psychiatry* **2000**, *39*, 1309–1312. [CrossRef]
73. Gordon, M.; Antshel, K.M.; Lewandowski, L. Predictors of treatment outcome in a child and adolescent psychiatry clinic: A naturalistic exploration. *Child. Youth Serv. Rev.* **2012**, *34*, 213–217. [CrossRef]
74. Solanto, M.V. Commentary: Development of a new, much-needed, cognitive-behavioral intervention for adolescents with ADHD–a reflection on Sprich et al.(2016). *J. Child Psychol. Psychiatry* **2016**, *57*, 1227–1228. [CrossRef]

5

Is this My Own Body? Changing the Perceptual and Affective Body Image Experience among College Students Using a New Virtual Reality Embodiment-Based Technique

Bruno Porras Garcia [1], Marta Ferrer Garcia [1], Agata Olszewska [1], Lena Yilmaz [1], Cristina González Ibañez [1], Mireia Gracia Blanes [1], Gamze Gültekin [1], Eduardo Serrano Troncoso [2,3] and José Gutiérrez Maldonado [1,*]

1 Department of Clinical Psychology and Psychobiology, University of Barcelona, Passeig de la Vall d'Hebron, 171, 08035 Barcelona, Spain
2 Child and Adolescent Psychiatry and Psychology Department, Hospital Sant Joan de Déu of Barcelona; Passeig de Sant Joan de Déu, 2, 08950 Esplugues de Llobregat, Barcelona, Spain
3 Children and Adolescent Mental Health Research Group, Institut de Recerca Sant Joan de Déu, Passeig de Sant Joan de Déu, 2, 08950 Esplugues de Llobregat, Barcelona, Spain
* Correspondence: jgutierrezm@ub.edu

Abstract: Body image disturbances (BIDs) have been widely studied using virtual reality (VR) devices that induce a full body illusion (FBI) and allow manipulation of the individual's perceptual and affective experiences of the body. This study aimed to assess whether the induction of the FBI over a virtual body would produce changes in body-related anxiety and BIDs using a new whole-body visuo-tactile stimulation procedure. Fifty non-clinical participants were randomly assigned to synchronous or asynchronous visuo-tactile groups. During the pre-assessment, all participants filled in BIDs and body-anxiety questionnaires. Then, they were embodied into two virtual bodies (VBs): firstly, with their real measurements, and secondly, with a larger-size body. Body image disturbances, body anxiety, fear of gaining weight, and FBI levels were assessed after exposure to each avatar. All participants in both conditions showed higher levels of BIDs and body anxiety after owning the larger-size VB than after owning the real-size VB ($p < 0.05$). The synchronous visuo-tactile group had higher scores, although the differences did not reach statistical significance. This study provides evidence of the usefulness of this new embodiment-based technique to induce changes in BIDs or body anxiety in a non-clinical sample, being suitable for use in future body image interventions.

Keywords: virtual reality; body image disturbances; body anxiety; fear of gaining weight; full body illusion

---

1. Introduction

Body image has been described as a multi-dimensional construct reflecting the mental representation a person has of their physical appearance [1], including perceptual, cognitive, attitudinal, and affective components [2,3]. Likewise, body image disturbances (BIDs) involve dysfunctional cognitions, attitudes, and emotions related to the way in which an individual experiences their own body shape or weight. Body image distortion (the perceptual component) and body image dissatisfaction (the affective component) are the most commonly studied and assessed BIDs [4,5]. Body image distortion refers to the difficulty of precisely estimating one's own body size, whereas body image dissatisfaction refers to the degree a person likes or dislikes their own body [6]. Body image disturbances have also been related to avoidance behaviors and negative checking strategies [7].

Other studies have suggested that body image may be a state rather than a trait and may, therefore, be modifiable, depending on the situation or emotional variables [6,8]. One emotional variable directly related to BID is fear of gaining weight and the resulting state body anxiety. Similarly, an excessive concern with having a thinner body is related to high anxiety levels, and that, consequently, affects BID [9].

Body image disturbances have a high prevalence among eating disorder patients, as well as in non-clinical populations. Regarding body dissatisfaction, previous studies found that 44% of women and 17% of men in European adult samples would like to lose weight [10]. In Spanish college students, 84.2% of young women were not satisfied with their physical appearance and that 70% of women and 52.8% of men desired to reduce their weight [11]. In relation to perceptual body image distortion, previous studies found that both eating disorder (ED) patients and healthy individuals overestimated their BMI by more than two points [12].

Virtual reality (VR) has been successfully used in the assessment and treatment of BID [13]. This technology allows researchers to create real-size 3D simulations of participants' bodies with their specific physical characteristics and place them in VR immersive environments that reproduce real-life situations related to their body image concerns [13,14]. Recent studies have progressed to assessing the effect of inducing the ownership illusion of a virtual body on the experience of one's own body (e.g., [15–18]). To do so, the avatar must elicit feelings of ownership and the participants must recognize themselves in the virtual avatar [17].

To induce these illusory feelings of ownership, it is necessary to synchronize the stimulation of the real body and the false body using different sensory modalities (e.g., visual, tactile, motor, and vestibular) [18]. Visuo-tactile synchronization is one of the most widely studied and best-known methods of eliciting this full body illusion (FBI) and is based on the paradigm of the rubber hand illusion (RHI) [19]. In this paradigm, the participant was first seated in front of a rubber hand which was positioned in the place of their real hidden hand. Next, the participant's non-visible hand was touched as they saw the fake rubber hand being touched synchronously, thus eliciting an illusion of ownership over the fake rubber hand. According to Botvinick and Cohen [19], asynchronous tactile and visual stimulation would significantly reduce this illusion.

Immersive VR devices have been widely used to investigate several important aspects related to FBI, such as the type of multisensory stimulation applied to produce it (e.g., visuo-tactile versus visuomotor stimulation) [20], or the sort of visual perspective from which the virtual body is observed (first versus third person perspective) [16]. Regarding the type of multisensory stimulation, there is no definite agreement in the literature at present about the best method to elicit the illusion. Several authors suggested that this illusion can be elicited using a synchronous visuo-tactile stimulation, in which the participant observes the virtual body or some specific virtual body parts being touched while also feeling touches on their own real body [15,18,21–23]. Other studies have also elicited the FBI by performing synchronous visuomotor stimulation [20,24,25]. Therefore, the results suggest that both visuomotor and visuo-tactile synchronous stimulation can induce the FBI [20], and that the illusion can be strengthened by combining vision, touch, motor control, and proprioception inputs in the same interventions [26].

Regarding the role of visual perspective, participants can either look at themselves in a first-person perspective (1PP) or in a mirror perspective, by observing their virtual bodies in a mirror. While some studies suggest that 1PP is necessary for eliciting FBI [21,25,27], others have also induced it by using a mirror view [16] or third person perspective [28]. Therefore, not only first-person visual perspectives can play an important role in creating the FBI [16].

A considerable number of studies have investigated the role of the FBI in attempts to modify body image disturbances (for extensive recent reviews, see Gutiérrez–Maldonado et al., 13,14), by changing the perceptual experiences of the size and shape of certain body parts [16]. For instance, the FBI was elicited in participants within a virtual avatar with enlarged arms [29]. Similarly, in another study participants felt an enlarged virtual abdomen as their own [22]. In a non-clinical sample, the FBI was elicited in a virtual avatar whose body mass index had been previously modified to have an enlarged or a thinner body [17].

Preston and Ehrsson [15] elicited the FBI in individuals who were exposed to a virtual mannequin body that was manipulated to be slimmer or wider than the individual's real body. In addition, they achieved significant reductions in individuals' perceived body size and increases in body satisfaction levels when participants owned a slim mannequin body. Similarly, Serino et al. [18,30] showed how non-clinical participants [18] and a single case patient with anorexia nervosa (AN) [30], reported significant reductions in the ratio between estimated and actual measurements of body parts after they were embodied into a VR avatar with a skinny abdomen. In a study with a clinical sample, Keizer et al. [23] found that owning a skinny virtual body significantly reduced the perceived body size in AN patients as well as in healthy participants. Additionally, this change in perceived body size was preserved two hours later, especially among the healthy participants. Finally, two previous studies with healthy samples found that owning a larger-size virtual body can produce changes in body representations [22] and can also elicit higher body anxiety levels [31]. Therefore, the use of FBI in VR environments may be a suitable method for manipulating the perceptual and emotional experiences of the body image.

In order to extend our knowledge of the usefulness of VR techniques to modify body image disturbances and body-related anxiety, this study presents a novel VR embodiment-based technique. Among the novelties of the current study are: the use of a visuo-tactile stimulation procedure over the whole body, in both 1PP and mirror view; the reproduction of a real-size virtual body, based on each participant's frontal silhouette, resulting in accurate representations of their actual body; and a realistic simulation of their weight gain through different body parts (e.g., stomach, hips, waist, etc.) based on their real silhouette.

The main aim of the study was to assess whether the induction of the FBI of a virtual body produced changes in body-related anxiety and body image disturbances of non-clinical participants. Participants owned two different virtual bodies (VBs): one with the same body size as their own and another with a larger body size. In addition, participants were randomly assigned to the synchronous or asynchronous visuo-tactile condition.

Based on previous studies (e.g., [22,31]), we expected: first, that owning a larger-size VB would elicit higher body anxiety and body image disturbances than owning the real-size VB in both synch/asynch groups (and that the synchronous group would have higher scores); second, that the visuo-tactile synchronous group would show higher FBI levels in the real-size and larger-size VBs than the asynchronous group.

2. Materials and Methods

2.1. Participants

This study was approved by the ethical committee of the University of Barcelona. The sample was composed of 50 undergraduate students at the University of Barcelona, recruited through campus flyers and advertisements in social network groups. Forty women and 10 men (M_{age} = 21.8, SD = 2.55, M_{BMI} = 22.5, SD = 2.51) participated in the study. Exclusion criteria were self-reported diagnosis of a current ED, a BMI under 17 (moderate thinness) or over 30 (obesity) according to the World Health Organization [32] or a current self-reported severe mental disorder diagnosis (e.g., schizophrenia or bipolar disorder). Each participant was given an identification code in order to guarantee the confidentiality of the data.

2.2. Measures

2.2.1. Assessment of Body Image Disturbances and Body Anxiety

Figural Drawing Scale for Body Image Assessment (BIAS-BD) [12]: This questionnaire allows the use of physical anthropometric dimensions of adult women and men by providing a series of human silhouettes. This questionnaire has two versions (A and B) in which silhouettes are randomized differently to avoid order effect bias. Participants selected, among a set of human silhouettes, the one that was perceived as their body size (perceived silhouette) and the one that was desired to have (desired body size). Then, according to their BMI, the real silhouette was also selected. Body dissatisfaction (BIAS-O) was assessed by calculating the discrepancy between the perceived and desired body sizes. Body distortion (BIAS-X) was assessed by calculating the discrepancy between the perceived and real body sizes. This questionnaire presents good psychometric properties, with a good reliability test-retest ($r = 0.86$) and a good concurrent validity ($r = 0.76$) [12].

Physical Appearance State and Trait Anxiety Scale (PASTAS) [33]: This body anxiety questionnaire comprises two separate self-report scales which measure weight-related and non-weight-related anxiety. In this study, we used the weight scale (W). This questionnaire presents good internal reliability, with a Cronbach's alpha that ranges from 0.82 to 0.92, good test–retest ($r = 0.87$) and good convergent validity indices for the W scale ($r = 0.74$ EDI-BD, $r = 0.62$ EDI-DT) [34].

Visual Analog Scale (VAS)-FGW: This scale ranging from 0 (zero) to 100 (complete) assesses the fear of weight gain that the individual is feeling at a specific moment. The following question was posed to the participants: "On a scale from 0 to 100, rate how afraid you are of gaining weight right now".

2.2.2. Assessment of the Full-Body Illusion (FBI)

VAS-FBI: This visual analog scale ranging from 0 (zero) to 100 (complete) assesses the level of FBI of the virtual body that the individual is feeling at a specific moment. The following question was posed to the participants: "On a scale from 0 to 100, indicate to what extent you felt that the virtual body was your own body". In case a participant asked about the meaning of the previous question, it was clarified that the expression "feeling the virtual body as your own body" referred to whether they had the sense of being the owner of the virtual body.

2.3. Hardware and Software Features

Participants were exposed to an immersive virtual scenario using a head-mounted display (HMD) HTC-VIVE connected to a computer with enough graphic and processor power to move VR environments. Two programs were used to develop the virtual simulations: Blender 2.78 to create the virtual avatars (a man and a woman), and Unity 3D 5.5 to integrate all the elements within a virtual environment, which consisted of an unfurnished room with a large mirror placed in front of the participant's avatar, 1.5 meters away. It was not visible at the beginning of the experiment (first-person perspective) and was activated only during the mirror view condition. In the back part of the room there was a small door, slightly open, which was placed there to avoid any feeling of being trapped inside.

Both male and female avatars wore a standard black t-shirt with black jeans and black trainers, as well as a swimming cap to reduce the idiosyncratic influence of hairstyle.

2.4. Procedure

Pre-assessment: Once they signed the informed consent form, all participants completed a test battery which included the BIAS-BD and PASTAS trait and state questionnaires. All participants were weighed and measured after completing the two questionnaires in order to avoid the possibility that anxiety might affect the questionnaire responses. The BMI was calculated using the classical formula (BMI = weight (kg)/height (m)^2).

Creating the real-size virtual avatar (whole body photograph): The first step in creating the virtual avatar with the real measurements of the participants was to take a frontal view photograph of the whole body of the participant. A high-definition (HD) Logitech camera was used. All participants had to remain still in a marked position, two meters away from the camera, with their arms slightly raised and their legs slightly separated. Once the participant's photo was taken and processed in our program, the experimenters manually overlapped the photo and the virtual body by adapting the height and different body measures of the virtual avatar (e.g., arms, legs, hip, waist, chest, shoulder, etc.)

to the silhouette of the participant. The resulting virtual avatar, which represented the participant's frontal body measurements, will be referred to from now on as the "real-size virtual body". Finally, all participants were located within the avatar's body during the exposure to an immersive VR environment.

Visuo-tactile stimulation procedure: To enhance the illusion of owning the virtual body, an adaptation of the visuo-tactile stimulation procedure used by Keizer et al. [23] was conducted. While the Keizer et al. [23] procedure consisted of applying a tactile stimulation only to the abdomen for 90 seconds, in our study we also induced tactile stimulation over other specific body parts (the upper and lower limbs). Therefore, a series of continuous touches were applied to specific body parts, with a total duration of a minute and a half (15″ each for left and right arm, 30″ to the abdomen, and 15″ each for left and right leg). The experimenter used one of the HTC-VIVE controllers to deliver the touches, while the participants looked at themselves (first-person perspective) while in their virtual bodies. Additionally, after the first-person perspective procedure (1PP), a mirror appeared on the wall in front of the avatar; the participants were asked to look at their avatars reflected in the mirror, while the same visuo-tactile procedure was repeated (mirror view). The complete duration of the visuo-tactile stimulation procedure was three minutes.

The control group asynchronous condition followed the procedure just described (1PP and mirror view) but the experimenter delivered the continuous touches, with a two-second delay, so that the visual feedback was inconsistent between what participants saw and what they really felt. For example, when they were feeling the touch to their forearm, they saw their avatar being touched on the shoulders.

In sum, both groups (synch/asynch) initially answered the test battery in the pre-assessment, then all participants were exposed to two virtual bodies: the first with the same body size as the participant and the second one larger than the participant (see Figure 1). In each body size condition, a visuo-tactile stimulation procedure was applied, using first a 1PP and second using a mirror view. Then, once they had finished the visuo-tactile stimulation procedure, participants answered the VAS-FBI and VAS-FGQ questions orally. Finally, after the last of each body size exposures, they left the VR environment and answered the BIAS-BD and PASTAS questionnaires.

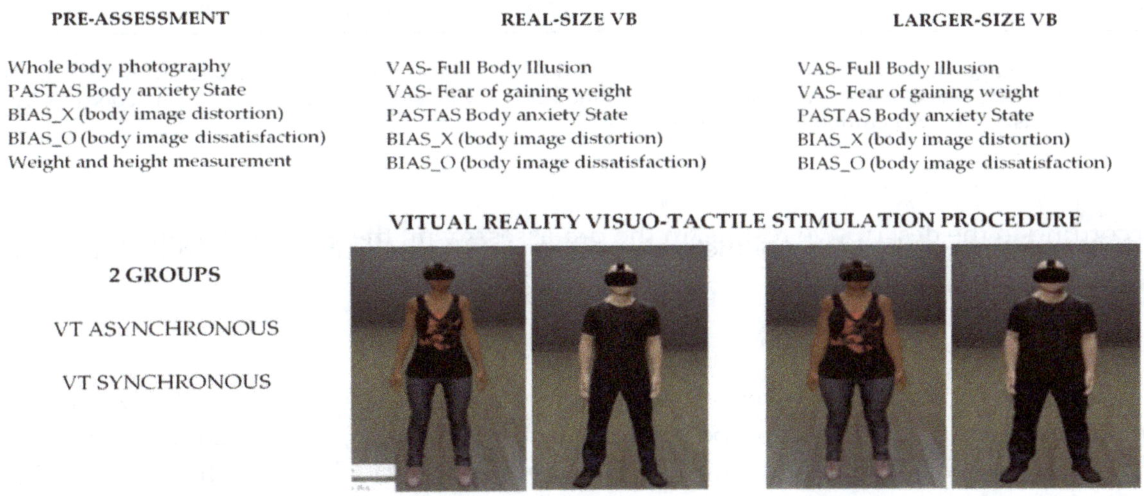

Figure 1. Experimental design scheme. Between-subjects group condition (synchronous versus asynchronous), within-subjects assessment condition (pre-assessment, real-size and larger-size virtual bodies), and dependent variables reported. VT = visuo-tactile, VB = virtual body, VAS = visual analog scales.

2.5. Statistical Analysis

The outcome of the intervention was analyzed with the statistical software IBM SPSS Statistics v.23. Mixed between (group)–within (assessment condition) analyses of variance (ANOVA) were conducted. The assumptions were partially met, since there was homogeneity of variances ($p > 0.05$) as assessed by the Levene's test. The assumption of sphericity was not completely met ($p < 0.05$) for some variables

(VAS_Fear of weight gain), therefore, it was decided to use the Green–House–Geisser corrected test for sphericity instead of this variable. Data were not normally distributed in all the variables assessed by the Kolmogorov–Smirnov test. However, it was decided to run the test regardless, as ANOVA is considered a robust test even in the case of a deviation from normality [35]. Finally, few outliers were detected in both BIDs measures, as assessed by inspection of a boxplot. Statistical analyses were conducted with and without the outliers, and since the results did not significantly differ, it was decided to include them in the analyses.

3. Results

3.1. Descriptive Results

A two-way mixed ANOVA was conducted. Means and standard deviations of all dependent variables were specified for each experimental condition at the different assessment times (Table 1).

Table 1. Descriptive outcomes, means, and standard deviations stated in the visuo-tactile group condition (asynchronous group versus synchronous group) at the different assessment conditions.

	Pre-Assessment		**Real-Size VB**		**Larger-Size VB**	
	Asyn-Group $n = 24$ **M (SD)**	**Syn-Group** $n = 26$ **M (SD)**	**Asyn-Group** $n = 24$ **M (SD)**	**Syn-Group** $n = 26$ **M (SD)**	**Asyn- Group** $n = 24$ **M (SD)**	**Syn-Group** $n = 26$ **M (SD)**
PASTAS	5.00 (5.87)	5.92 (5.31)	4.96 (5.46)	6.23 (5.77)	5.71 (6.07)	9.15 (6.89)
BIAS_X	9.58 (16,68)	13.65 (16.40)	9.17 (12.22)	12.50 (15.25)	18.54 (18.56)	19.62 (18.92)
BIAS_O	8.75 (18.72)	14.40 (21.81)	7.29 (14.06)	10.60 (19.22)	16.67 (18.57)	18.40 (22.39)
VAS-FBI	-		48.33 (20.44)	65.46 (19.15)	42.71 (28.97)	55.58 (23.07)
VAS-FGW	-		23.33 (26.77)	33.00 (29.34)	29.79 (29.39)	48.77 (29.48)

Note: Body Image Disturbances (Body Image Distortion-BIAS_X, Body Image Dissatisfaction- BIAS_O), Body Anxiety (PASTAS), fear of gaining weight (VAS-FWG), and full-body illusion (VAS-FBI). VB = Virtual body, Async = Asynchronous, Sync = Synchronous group conditions.

According to the descriptive results, in the pre-assessment, there were no statistically significant group differences ($p > 0.05$) in any of the body anxiety or BID measures. Therefore, it was decided to continue the statistical analyses.

3.2. Statistical Analyses

As shown in Table 2, there were no statistically significant interactions between group and assessment conditions ($p > 0.05$) on body dissatisfaction (BIAS_O), body distortion (BIAS_X), fear of gaining weight (VAS-FGW), and full body illusion (VAS-FBI). However, there was a significant interaction between group and assessment conditions in body anxiety (PASTAS) F (2, 96) = 3.297, $p = 0.041$, partial $\eta^2 = 0.064$.

Regarding body anxiety (PASTAS), three additional between-subjects ANOVAs were conducted separately in each assessment condition to follow up the simple effects of group on assessment time. Mean differences (*MD*) ± standard error (*SE*) are specified. Body anxiety scores did not differ significantly between the two groups ($p > 0.05$) in the pre-assessment and the real-size virtual body conditions (see Figure 2a). With the larger size virtual body, even though differences between the groups did not reach statistically significance F (1, 48) = 3.492, $p = 0.07$, partial $\eta^2 = 0.068$, with a medium effect size according to Cohen [36]; body anxiety scores were higher in the synchronous than in the asynchronous group condition ($MD = 3.446 \pm SE = 1.84$).

Table 2. Mixed between–within subject analysis of variance comparing groups (Group 1-Asynchronous group versus Group 2-Synchronous group) with the different assessment conditions.

	Time x Group			Time of Assessment		
	F	*p*	η^2	*F*	*p*	η^2
PASTAS	3.297	0.041 *	0.064	8.554	0.001 *	0.151
BIAS_X	0.347	0.707	0.007	11.798	0.001 *	0.197
BIAS_O	0.410	0.665	0.009	8.177	0.001 *	0.148
VAS-FBI	0.312	0.579	0.006	4.130	0.048 *	0.079
VAS-FGW	3.855	0.055	0.074	21.968	0.001 *	0.314

Note: Green–House–Geisser corrected test for sphericity used. * Significant p-values < 0.05.

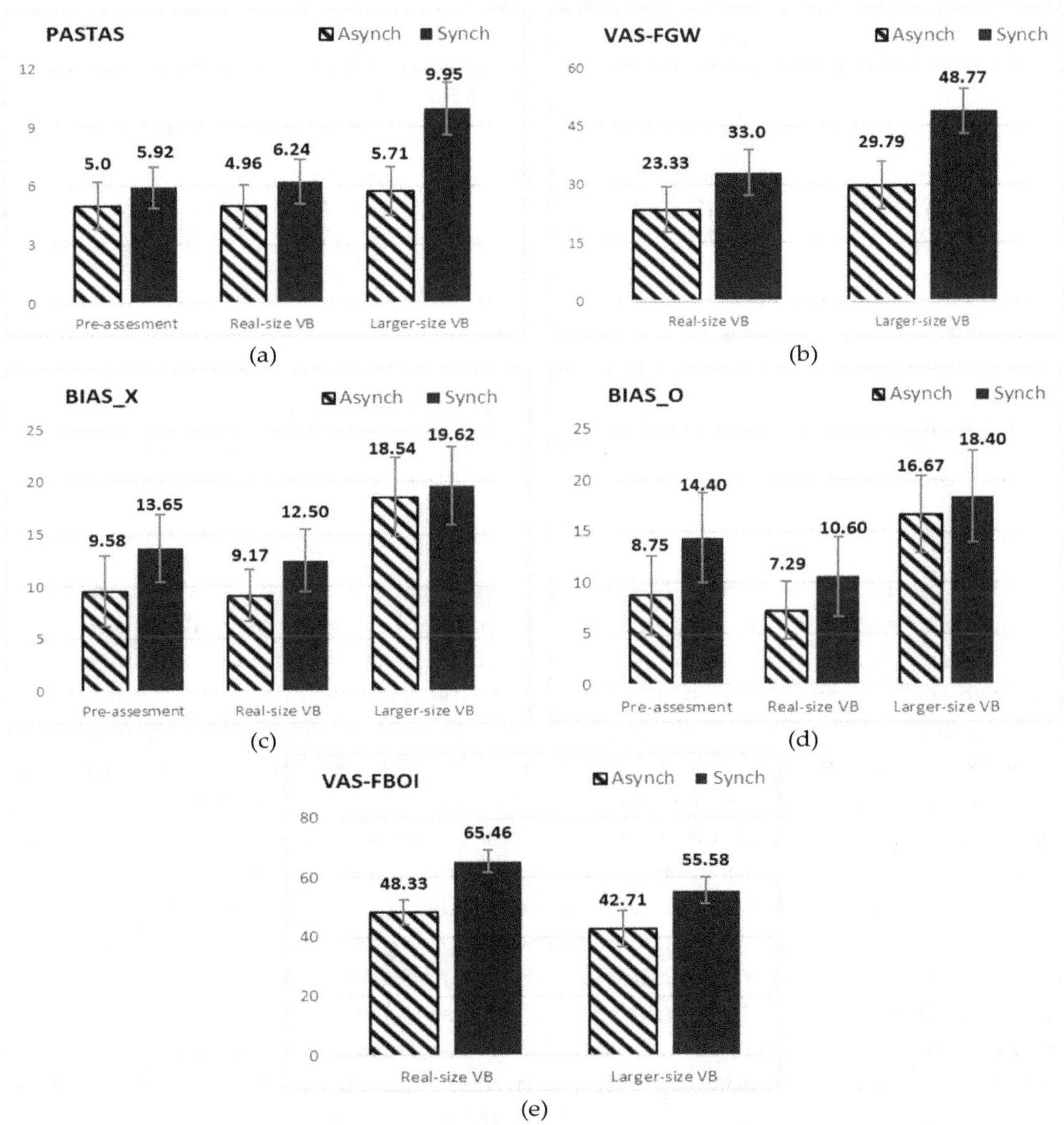

Figure 2. (**a**)Body anxiety mean scores, (**b**) fear of weight gain mean scores, (**c**) body image distortion mean scores, (**d**) body image dissatisfaction mean scores, (**e**) full-body ownership illusion mean scores. Means of the asynchronous and synchronous groups in the three assessment conditions (pre-assessment, real-size virtual body, larger-size virtual body). Error bars represent standard errors. Body image disturbances (Body Image Distortion-BIAS_X, Body Image Dissatisfaction-BIAS_O), Body anxiety (PASTAS), fear of gaining weight (VAS-FWG), and full-body ownership illusion (VAS-FBI). VB = Virtual body.

The main effect of assessment condition (see Table 2) showed that there were statistically significant differences ($p < 0.05$) in body anxiety (PASTAS), body image disturbances (BIAS_X or BIAS_O), fear of weight gain (VAS-FWG), and full body ownership illusion (VAS-FBI) measures.

To analyze the outcomes in more detail, multiple post-hoc tests (pairwise comparisons) were conducted. Mean differences (*MD*) ± standard error (*SE*) were specified. As can be seen in Table 3, all the measures were significantly higher in the larger-size VB condition than in both the real-size VB and the pre-assessment (for illustrations see Figure 2a–d). However, the VAS-FBI scores decreased compared with the real-size VB.

Table 3. Post-hoc analyses (pairwise comparison) at the different assessment times (pre-assessment, real-size virtual body and larger-size virtual body).

	Assessment Time Conditions					
	Pre-Assessment versus Real-Size VB		**Larger-Size VB versus Real-Size VB**		**Larger-Size VB versus Pre-Assessment**	
	MD	**SE**	**MD**	**SE**	**MD**	**SE**
PASTAS	0.133	0.491	1.837 *	0.517	1.970 *	0.584
BIAS_X	0.785	1.717	8.245 *	1.957	7.460 *	1.938
BIAS_O	2.629	1.915	8.588 *	2.133	5.958	2.448
VAS-FBI			−7.755 *	3.816		
VAS-FGW			11.114 *	2.371		

Note: MD = Mean differences, SE = Standard Error. * Significant *p*-values < 0.05. VB = Virtual body.

Finally, there was a statistically significant main effect of group on the VAS-FBI $F(1, 48) = 7940$, $p = 0.007$, partial $\eta^2 = 0.142$. Regardless of the assessment condition, the synchronous group showed higher levels of FBI than the asynchronous group (see Figure 2e).

4. Discussion

This study aimed to assess whether a visuo-tactile embodiment-based procedure could elicit changes in the body anxiety and body image disturbance responses of healthy participants when owning two different-size virtual bodies. In addition, two different visuo-tactile group conditions were compared (synchronous versus asynchronous visuo-tactile stimulation).

As expected, all participants, regardless of group, showed higher levels of body image disturbances (BIDs) and body anxiety after owning the larger-size virtual body (VB) than after owning with the real-size VB, and the scores were higher in the synchronous visuo-tactile group. Our results support previous findings suggesting that body image is a state rather than a trait, and can, thus, be modified by internal and external stimuli [6], such as owning a larger-size VB. Jakatdar, Cash, and Engle [37] suggested that malleability of the body image is more frequent in ED patients but also occurs in healthy participants, as our data show. Our results contrast with those of previous studies which did not report significant differences on body size estimating tasks before and after owning a larger mannequin/virtual body [15,17]. The differences in the results may be explained by differences in the methodological procedures used. For instance, even though in all the studies there was a larger-size/overweight virtual body condition, in our study, participants previously owned a real-size virtual body that represented their own silhouette, while in two previous studies [15,17], thin/underweight virtual bodies or mannequins were used instead.

In addition, the appearance of the virtual body, i.e., the body shape, may also explain the differences between the present study and previous studies. The appearance of the virtual body may play an important role not only in the eliciting of the illusory feelings of ownership [38,39], but also in eliciting emotional responses in healthy participants [15]. In our study a weight gain proportionally spread over the whole body (e.g., the belly, thighs, waist, arms) was reproduced, resulting in a more realistic increase of weight across the body, and consequently evoking higher anxiety and body image disturbance levels in participants when owning the larger virtual body than when owning the real-size virtual body. In contrast, other studies may have not found similar results because the weight gain was represented less proportionally, for example, by increasing only the stomach size of the mannequin [15]. Additionally, the increase in the weight of our avatar was previously based on the real-size virtual body with the participant's silhouette, allowing a more accurate and natural weight increase in the larger-size virtual body.

Regarding body anxiety levels, our results are in line with those of a previous study by our group [31], in which healthy college students undergoing a synchronous visuomotor procedure reported higher levels of body anxiety and fear of weight gain after owning a larger-size VB than after owning their real-size VB. However, the current study has attempted to overcome some of the limitations reported there, such as the small sample size, the lack of an asynchronous visuomotor procedure, and the lack of a baseline pre-assessment time condition. Furthermore, BID and body anxiety levels did not differ significantly after owning a virtual avatar with participants' real measurements (real-size VB) compared with the pre-assessment. This suggests that, regardless of the type of visuo-tactile stimulation, all participants delivered, perceived, and felt the real-size VB as their own body, even without being aware of it.

According to the differences between the synchronous and asynchronous visuo-tactile groups, there were not statistically significant group differences in BID and body anxiety measures. Interesting non-significant tendencies were found in body anxiety measures. Participants who underwent a synchronous visuo-tactile procedure reported higher body anxiety and fear of gaining weight levels than those in the asynchronous condition, at the larger size VB. One possible explanation for these tendencies, is that some of the body parts that were (in)congruently stimulated (e.g., the stomach or the thighs) are usually reported as body areas of higher concern [40] or weight-related body areas [33]. Previous studies have reported that individuals with ED [40,41] show an attentional preference towards these self-reported unattractive body areas. Therefore, it might be expected that a synchronous visuo-tactile stimulation over those salient body areas with a significant weight gain might elicit a higher more unpleasant anxious response that was not observed at equal levels in the asynchronous group. Consequently, our results suggest that the specific influence of the FBI induced by a synchronous visuo-tactile stimulation over specific body parts may differentially affect body anxiety and BID measures after owning a larger-size VB. Regarding BID measures, our results are in line with previous studies in which inducing a synchronous or asynchronous visuo-tactile stimulation did not affect body distortion levels after owning a skinny virtual body [18], or an underweight or overweight virtual body [17].

Regarding the FBI levels, the synchronous visuo-tactile group showed significantly greater FBI levels in both the real-size VB and larger-size VB than the asynchronous group. Our results are in line with previous studies that compared synchronous versus asynchronous visuo-tactile stimulation procedures for eliciting FBI by owning either a slim virtual body or mannequin body (e.g., [15,16,21,23]) or an overweight virtual body [15,17,22]. However, some important differences between our study and previous research should be noted, such as, for example, the type of visual perspective displayed. In the present study, a combination of both 1PP and a mirror view perspective were used successively in order to strengthen the FBI, in comparison to previous studies that have used only a first-person perspective to elicit the FBI (e.g., [15,21,23]).

Another important difference is the sort of tactile stimulation delivered. A visuo-tactile stimulation procedure over the whole body (abdomen, upper and lower extremities) was delivered in this study, in contrast to previous studies in which the only stimulated body parts were the abdomen or the belly [18,23], or the upper and lower limbs [17]. Additionally, the body posture was also different from the study conducted by Piryankova et al. [17], in which the participants were seated while the upper and lower virtual limbs were touched. In our study, all participants were in a standing position, in which the realism of the virtual avatar is less likely to be affected.

The current study presents some limitations that should be addressed in future research. Body mass index (BMI) was not controlled. Although we excluded participants with obesity (BMI > 30) or who were moderate-to-severely underweight (BMI < 17), previous literature suggested that overweight, compared to healthy weight, individuals present higher body dissatisfaction levels [42]. Another important limitation is that no screening questionnaire or clinical structured interview was used to properly assess the presence of an ED diagnosis or other mental disorders. It should be noted that even though our participants were allocated randomly, the synchronous visuo-tactile group reported slightly higher BID levels than the asynchronous group at the pre-assessment time condition. However, as the group differences did not reach significance, it was decided to continue the statistical analyses. As regards the length of the experiment, participants generally spent one hour in the laboratory. We realize that it may cause fatigue, especially because participants were asked to stand still while the experimenter was running the tactile-stimulation procedure for each body size condition. Following the previous argument, and so as not to lengthen the experiment further, it was decided not to include other body-size conditions such as a slimmer virtual body, as the studies by Preston et al. [15] or Piryankova et al. [17] had done.

These results may have different implications in clinical practice. In the near future, it would be interesting to apply FBI and VR embodiment-based techniques to treat the fear of gaining weight and body anxiety in ED patients, and specifically in anorexia nervosa (AN) patients. One possibility would be to develop an exposure therapy to one's own body, in which an AN patient could own an avatar with their own body silhouette and their BMI would increase gradually, according to a pre-established hierarchy. Additionally, our results support those of previous studies suggesting that VR embodiment-based techniques may be a useful tool for interventions that aim to modify or improve BID levels among healthy participants, or in clinical ED patients (e.g., [23]).

Another interesting approach would be to use VR embodiment-based procedures not only to treat BID, but also to assess it. Following a similar procedure to paper-based figural drawing scale questionnaires (e.g., BIAS-BD, [12]) or human-based 3D computer scales [43,44], participants or ED patients could own a virtual avatar and modify different body parts (or the whole body of the avatar) according to their perceived or desired body size. Additionally, using a VR assessment procedure would also allow the generation of more ecologically valid experimental settings that represent daily life situations: for instance, looking at one's own body in a mirror.

5. Conclusions

This study provides new evidence of the usefulness of VR embodiment-based techniques to induce changes in body image disturbances or body anxiety in a non-clinical sample of college students. Specifically, our findings provide new information about how the influence of the FBI, induced by a synchronous visuo-tactile stimulation, may not only strengthen the FBI when participants own their real-size VB, but may also elicit higher BID and body anxiety levels after owning a larger-size VB, with body anxiety measures being particularly affected by a congruent visuo-tactile stimulation. In addition, a new VR visuo-tactile stimulation procedure over the whole body, which combines first-person perspective and mirror view, is presented and discussed. Finally, this study presents a novel procedure for adapting our virtual avatar bodies based on the real-size frontal silhouettes of our participants, allowing the recreation of a realistic real-size virtual avatar, but even more importantly, the simulation of a more realistic weight gain in our virtual bodies.

The use of VR embodiment-based techniques opens up new possibilities in body image research, some of which are presented and briefly discussed in this article. However, considering the high prevalence of BID among ED patients [12] and among non-clinical populations [10,11], future interventions should continue to focus on understanding and improving the disturbed representations that so many individuals have of their body appearance.

Author Contributions: Conceptualization, B.P.G., M.F.G., A.O., L.Y., C.G.I., M.G.B., G.G., and J.G.M.; methodology, B.P.G.; validation, B.P.G., C.G.I., and M.G.B.; formal analysis, B.P.G..; investigation, B.P.G., M.F.G., C.G.I., M.G.B.; resources, M.F.G., J.G.M.; data curation, B.P.G.; writing—original draft preparation, B.P.G. A.O., L.Y., and G.G. writing—review and editing, B.P.G., M.F.G., E.S.T., J.G.M.; visualization, B.P.G., M.F.G., A.O., L.Y., G.G.; supervision, M.F.G., E.S.T., and J.G.M.; project administration, J.G.M.; funding acquisition, J.G.M.

References

1. Cash, T.F. Cognitive-behavioural perspectives on body image. In *Body Image: A Handbook of Theory, Research, and Clinical Practice*; Cash, T.F., Pruzinsky, T., Eds.; Guilford Press: New York, NY, USA, 2002; pp. 38–46.
2. Cash, T.F. Cognitive-Behavioral Perspectives on Body Image. In *Body Image: A Handbook of Science, Practice, and Prevention*; Cash, T.F., Smolak, L., Eds.; Guilford Press: New York, NY, USA, 2012; pp. 39–47.
3. Gaudio, S.; Quattrocchi, C.C. Neural basis of a multidimensional model of body image distortion in anorexia nervosa. *Neurosci. Biobehav. Rev.* **2012**, *36*, 1839–1847. [CrossRef] [PubMed]
4. Cash, T.F.; Deagle, E.A. The nature and extent of body-image disturbances in anorexia nervosa and bulimia nervosa: A meta-analysis. *Int. J. Eat. Disord.* **1997**, *22*, 107–126. [CrossRef]
5. Hagman, J.; Gardner, R.M.; Brown, D.L.; Gralla, J.; Fier, J.M.; Frank, G.K.W. Body size overestimation and its association with body mass index, body dissatisfaction, and drive for thinness in anorexia nervosa. *Eat. Weight Disord.* **2015**, *20*, 449–455. [CrossRef] [PubMed]
6. Ferrer-García, M.; Gutiérrez-Maldonado, J. The use of virtual reality in the study, assessment, and treatment of body image in eating disorders and nonclinical samples: A review of the literature. *Body Image* **2012**, *9*, 1–11. [CrossRef] [PubMed]
7. Legenbauer, T.; Thiemann, P.; Vocks, S. Body image disturbance in children and adolescents with eating disorders: Current evidence and future directions. *Z. Kinder. Jugendpsychiatr. Psychother.* **2014**, *42*, 51–59. [CrossRef] [PubMed]
8. Espeset, E.M.S.; Gulliksen, K.S.; Nordbø, R.H.S.; Skårderud, F.; Holte, A. The link between negative emotions and eating disorder behaviour in patients with anorexia nervosa. *Eur. Eat. Disord. Rev.* **2012**, *20*, 451–460. [CrossRef]
9. Maganto Mateo, C.; Cruz Saez, S. La insatisfacción corporal como variable explicativa de los trastornos alimenticios. *Rev. Psicol.* **2002**, *10*, 197–223.
10. Bellisle, F.; Monneuse, M.O.; Steptoe, A.; Wardle, J. Weight concerns and eating patterns: A survey of university students in Europe. *Int. J. Obes. Relat. Metab. Disord.* **1995**, *19*, 723–730.
11. Lameiras Fernández, M.; Calado Otero, M.; Rodríguez Castro, Y.; Fernández Prieto, M. Hábitos alimentarios e imagen corporal en estudiantes universitarios sin trastornos alimentarios. *Rev. Int. Psicol. Clín. Salud* **2003**, *3*, 23–33.
12. Gardner, R.M.; Jappe, L.M.; Gardner, L. Development and validation of a new figural drawing scale for body-image assessment: The BIAS-BD. *J. Clin. Psychol.* **2009**, *65*, 113–122. [CrossRef]
13. Gutiérrez-Maldonado, J.; Wiederhold, B.K.; Riva, G. Future Directions: How Virtual Reality Can Further Improve the Assessment and Treatment of Eating Disorders and Obesity. *Cyberpsychol. Behav. Soc. Netw.* **2016**, *19*, 148–153. [CrossRef] [PubMed]
14. Gutiérrez-Maldonado, J.; Ferrer-García, M.; Dakanalis, A.; Riva, G. Virtual Reality: Applications to Eating Disorders. In *The Oxford Handbook of Eating Disorders*, 2nd ed.; Agras, W.S., Robinson, A.H., Eds.; Oxford University Press: Oxford, UK, 2018; Volume 19, pp. 148–153.
15. Preston, C.; Ehrsson, H.H. Illusory changes in body size modulate body satisfaction in a way that is related to non-clinical eating disorder psychopathology. *PLoS ONE* **2014**, *9*, e85773. [CrossRef] [PubMed]
16. Preston, C.; Kuper-Smith, B.J.; Henrik Ehrsson, H. Owning the body in the mirror: The effect of visual perspective and mirror view on the full-body illusion. *Sci. Rep.* **2015**, *5*, 18345. [CrossRef]

17. Piryankova, I.V.; Wong, H.Y.; Linkenauger, S.A.; Stinson, C.; Longo, M.R.; Bülthoff, H.H.; Mohler, B.J. Owning an overweight or underweight body: Distinguishing the physical, experienced and virtual body. *PLoS ONE* **2014**, *9*, e103428. [CrossRef] [PubMed]
18. Serino, S.; Pedroli, E.; Keizer, A.; Triberti, S.; Dakanalis, A.; Pallavicini, F.; Chirico, A.; Riva, G. Virtual Reality Body Swapping: A Tool for Modifying the Allocentric Memory of the Body. *Cyberpsychol. Behav. Soc. Netw.* **2016**, *19*, 127–133. [CrossRef] [PubMed]
19. Botvinick, M.; Cohen, J. Rubber hands "feel" touch that eyes see. *Nature* **1998**, *301*, 756. [CrossRef] [PubMed]
20. Kokkinara, E.; Slater, M. Measuring the effects through time of the influence of visuomotor and visuotactile synchronous stimulation on a virtual body ownership illusion. *Perception* **2014**, *43*, 43–58. [CrossRef]
21. Petkova, V.I.; Ehrsson, H.H. If I were you: Perceptual illusion of body swapping. *PLoS ONE* **2008**, *3*, e3832. [CrossRef]
22. Normand, J.M.; Giannopoulos, E.; Spanlang, B.; Slater, M. Multisensory stimulation can induce an illusion of larger belly size in immersive virtual reality. *PLoS ONE* **2011**, *6*, e16128. [CrossRef]
23. Keizer, A.; van Elburg, A.; Helms, R.; Dijkerman, H.C. A virtual reality full body illusion improves body image disturbance in anorexia nervosa. *PLoS ONE* **2016**, *11*, e0163921. [CrossRef]
24. Gonzalez-Franco, M.; Perez-Marcos, D.; Spanlang, B.; Slater, M. The contribution of real-time mirror reflections of motor actions on virtual body ownership in an immersive virtual environment. In Proceedings of the IEEE Virtual Reality Conference (VR), Waltham, MA, USA, 20–24 March 2010. [CrossRef]
25. Slater, M.; Spanlang, B.; Sanchez-Vives, M.V.; Blanke, O. First person experience of body transfer in virtual reality. *PLoS ONE* **2010**, *5*, e10564. [CrossRef] [PubMed]
26. Ehrsson, H.H. The Concept of Body Ownership and Its Relation to Multisensory Integration. In *The New Handbook of Multisensory Processes*; Stein, B.E., Ed.; MIT Press: Cambridge, MA, USA, 2012; pp. 775–792.
27. Petkova, V.I.; Khoshnevis, M.; Ehrsson, H.H. The perspective matters! Multisensory integration in ego-centric reference frames determines full-body ownership. *Front. Psychol.* **2011**, *2*, 35. [CrossRef] [PubMed]
28. Preston, C.; Newport, R. How long is your arm? Using multisensory illusions to modify body image from the third person perspective. *Perception* **2012**, *41*, 247–249. [CrossRef] [PubMed]
29. Kilteni, K.; Normand, J.M.; Sanchez-Vives, M.V.; Slater, M. Extending body space in immersive virtual reality: A very long arm illusion. *PLoS ONE* **2012**, *7*, e40867. [CrossRef]
30. Serino, S.; Polli, N.; Riva, G. From avatars to body swapping: The use of virtual reality for assessing and treating body-size distortion in individuals with anorexia. *J. Clin. Psychol.* **2018**, *75*, 313–322. [CrossRef]
31. Ferrer-Garcia, M.; Porras-Garcia, B.; Gonzalez-Ibanez, C.; Gracia-Blanes, M.; Vilalta-Abella, F.; Pla-Sanjuanelo, J.; Gutierrez-Maldonado, J.; Achotegui-Loizate, J.; Riva, G.; Dakanalis, K.; et al. Does owning a "fatter" virtual body increase body anxiety in college students? *Annu. Rev. Cyber Ther. Telemed.* **2017**, *15*, 147–153.
32. World Health Organization. *ICD-10 International Statistical Classification of Diseases and Related Health Problems: Tenth Revision*, 2nd ed.; World Health Organization: Geneva, Switzerland, 2004; Volume 3, ISBN 9241546492.
33. Reed, D.L.; Thompson, J.K.; Brannick, M.T.; Sacco, W.P. Development and validation of the physical appearance state and trait anxiety scale (PASTAS). *J. Anxiety Disord.* **1991**, *5*, 323–332. [CrossRef]
34. Garner, D. *Eating Disorder Inventory-3: Professional Manual*; Psychological Assessment Resources: Lutz, FL, USA, 2004.
35. Schmider, E.; Ziegler, M.; Danay, E.; Beyer, L.; Bühner, M. Is it really robust? Reinvestigating the robustness of ANOVA against violations of the normal distribution assumption. *Methodol. Eur. J. Res. Methods Behav. Soc. Sci.* **2010**, *6*, 147–151. [CrossRef]
36. Cohen, J. *Statistical Power Analysis for the Behavioral Sciences*, 2nd ed.; Lawrence Erlbaum Associates: Hillsdale, NJ, USA, 1988.
37. Jakatdar, T.; Cash, T.; Engle, E. Body-image thought processes: The development and initial validation of the Assessment of Body-Image Cognitive Distortions. *Body Image* **2006**, *3*, 325–333. [CrossRef]
38. Maselli, A.; Slater, M. The building blocks of the full body ownership illusion. *Front. Hum. Neurosci.* **2013**, *7*, 83. [CrossRef]
39. Tsakiris, M.; Carpenter, L.; James, D.; Fotopoulou, A. Hands only illusion: Multisensory integration elicits sense of ownership for body parts but not for non-corporeal objects. *Exp. Brain Res.* **2010**, *204*, 343–352. [CrossRef] [PubMed]
40. Jansen, A.; Nederkoorn, C.; Mulkens, S. Selective visual attention for ugly and beautiful body parts in eating disorders. *Behav. Res. Ther.* **2005**, *43*, 183–196. [CrossRef]

41. Tuschen-Caffier, B.; Bender, C.; Caffier, D.; Klenner, K.; Braks, K.; Svaldi, J. Selective visual attention during mirror exposure in anorexia and bulimia nervosa. *PLoS ONE* **2015**, *10*, e0145886. [CrossRef] [PubMed]
42. Weinberger, N.A.; Kersting, A.; Riedel-Heller, S.G.; Luck-Sikorski, C. Body Dissatisfaction in Individuals with Obesity Compared to Normal-Weight Individuals: A Systematic Review and Meta-Analysis. *Obes. Facts* **2017**, *9*, 424–441. [CrossRef] [PubMed]
43. Cornelissen, K.; Bester, A.; Cairns, P.; Tovée, M.; Cornelissen, P. The influence of personal BMI on body size estimations and sensitivity to body size change in anorexia spectrum disorders. *Body Image* **2015**, *13*, 75–85. [CrossRef] [PubMed]
44. Cornelissen, K.; McCarty, K.; Cornelissen, P.; Tovée, M. Body size estimation in women with anorexia nervosa and healthy controls using 3D avatars. *Sci. Rep.* **2017**, *7*, 15773. [CrossRef] [PubMed]

6

Characterizing Body Image Distortion and Bodily Self-Plasticity in Anorexia Nervosa via Visuo-Tactile Stimulation in Virtual Reality

Luca Provenzano [1,2,†], Giuseppina Porciello [1,2,†,*], Sofia Ciccarone [1,2], Bigna Lenggenhager [3], Gaetano Tieri [2,4], Matteo Marucci [1,2,5], Federico Dazzi [6], Camillo Loriedo [7] and Ilaria Bufalari [2,8,*]

1 Department of Psychology, "Sapienza" University of Rome, 00185 Rome, Italy; luca.provenzano@uniroma1.it (L.P.); sofia.ciccarone@uniroma1.it (S.C.); matteo.marucci@uniroma1.it (M.M.)
2 IRCCS, Santa Lucia Foundation, 00142 Rome, Italy; gaetano.tieri@gmail.com
3 Department of Psychology, University of Zurich, 8050 Zurich, Switzerland; bigna.lenggenhager@gmail.com
4 Virtual Reality Lab, University of Rome Unitelma-Sapienza, 00161 Rome, Italy
5 BrainTrends Ltd., Applied Neuroscience, Gallicano nel Lazio (RM), 00010 Rome, Italy
6 Department of Human Sciences, Lumsa University, 00193 Rome, Italy; federicodazzi@hotmail.com
7 Clinica Psichiatrica, "Sapienza" University of Rome, 00185 Rome, Italy; camillo.loriedo@uniroma1.it
8 Department of Developmental and Social Psychology, "Sapienza" University of Rome, 00185 Rome, Italy
* Correspondence: ilaria.bufalari@uniroma1.it (I.B.); giuseppina.porciello@uniroma1.it (G.P.)
† These authors contributed equally to this work.

Abstract: We combined virtual reality and multisensory bodily illusion with the aim to characterize and reduce the perceptual (body overestimation) and the cognitive-emotional (body dissatisfaction) components of body image distortion (BID) in anorexia nervosa (AN). For each participant (20 anorexics, 20 healthy controls) we built personalized avatars that reproduced their own body size, shape, and verisimilar increases and losses of their original weight. Body overestimation and dissatisfaction were measured by asking participants to choose the avatar that best resembled their real and ideal body. Results show higher body dissatisfaction in AN, caused by the desire of a thinner body, and no body-size overestimation. Interpersonal multisensory stimulation (IMS) was then applied on the avatar reproducing participant's perceived body, and on the two avatars which reproduced increases and losses of 15% of it, all presented with a first-person perspective (1PP). Embodiment was stronger after synchronous IMS in both groups, but did not reduce BID in participants with AN. Interestingly, anorexics reported more negative emotions after embodying the fattest avatar, which scaled with symptoms severity. Overall, our findings suggest that the cognitive-emotional, more than the perceptual component of BID is severely altered in AN and that perspective (1PP vs. 3PP) from which a body is evaluated may play a crucial role. Future research and clinical trials might take advantage of virtual reality to reduce the emotional distress related to body dissatisfaction.

Keywords: anorexia nervosa; body image distortion; body dissatisfaction; embodiment; virtual reality; interpersonal multisensory stimulation

1. Introduction

Anorexia nervosa (AN) affects mostly adolescent and young women [1], has the highest mortality rate among all psychiatric disorders [2] and is largely resistant to currently available treatments [3]. A core clinical symptom of AN is body image distortion (BID), which impacts onset, prognosis, and relapse [4]. Body image is a multifaceted construct that comprises body-related perception, expectations, thoughts, feelings, and actions [5,6] which are represented in dedicated neural circuitries [7–10]. In AN, BID affects both perceptual and cognitive-emotional components of the body representation [11], i.e., patients typically overestimate their body size [12] and report higher body dissatisfaction [13] than healthy controls (HC) [14].

The use of new sophisticated and biometrically plausible distortion methods, made possible by immersive virtual reality contexts, has paved the way for precisely measuring body overestimation e.g., [15], whereas the development of interpersonal multisensory stimulation (IMS) paradigms has increased insights into the plasticity of the bodily self [15,16]. In IMS paradigms, participants typically experience a tactile stimulation on their own body synchronously with an observed touch at the corresponding body part on another individual's body [17–19] which leads to the illusory sensation of ownership toward the latter (termed embodiment), as evidenced by subjective, behavioral, and physiological measures [20–24].

IMS paradigms have been extended to virtual avatars observed from a first-person perspective (1PP) [25], even of different sizes [26], which might lead to a change in one's own body perception according to the avatar size [27]. Specifically, in HC identification with a slim virtual body reduces not only the overestimation of the own body size but also increases body satisfaction [28], while identification with an obese avatar induces body dissatisfaction [28].

Embodiment illusions might thus represent a promising tool to reduce BID in AN. Preliminary results in this field suggest that, in AN patients, illusory ownership of a fake hand is enhanced [29] and leads to a reduction in hand-size overestimation [30]. Also, embodying a normal body mass index (BMI) avatar reduces overestimation of shoulders, abdomen, and hips [31]. However, this effect occurs after both synchronous (experimental condition) and asynchronous (control condition) IMS, suggesting that it might not be due to the embodiment per se, but rather to purely visual effects.

Thus, the few existing studies using embodiment illusions in AN patients tentatively suggest that a normalization of BID is possible. Yet, it is still unclear how robust the effect is, to what degree it is linked to embodiment per se and how such illusions affect and interact with the affective-emotional components of body representation, which are central to BID [11,32].

Here, we addressed these issues by: (i) individualizing the avatars for each of our participant' body (unlike previous studies); (ii) assessing the embodiment strength both at the explicit (questionnaires, e.g., [19,33]) and implicit level (body temperature, e.g., [34], but see [35] for a critical account), and (iii) measuring both perceptual and emotional aspects of BID before and after the embodiment of three different sized avatars was induced. We tested young females with AN and low-BMI age-matched HC with no diagnosis of eating disorders.

We expected AN patients to overestimate their body size [12] and to show higher body dissatisfaction than HC [13], as indexed by clinical measures (clinical questionnaires' scores) and by the higher discrepancy between one's own perceived and ideal body [36]. Furthermore, according to Eshkevari and colleagues [29], we expected higher bodily self-plasticity (namely higher embodiment measured both at the implicit and explicit level) in AN patients compared to HC. Importantly, we hypothesized that body dissatisfaction would decrease in AN patients as an effect of embodying a body which corresponds or is thinner than the perceived one [28]. Lastly, we expected that embodying an avatar larger than the perceived one would enhance negative emotions in AN patients more than HC.

2. Materials and Methods

2.1. Participants

A total of 21 female patients diagnosed with AN and 22 age-matched HC were recruited. All AN patients were diagnosed with anorexia nervosa (restricting type) by the Department of Psychiatry and Eating Disorder of the Hospital Policlinico Umberto I, which followed the criteria of Diagnostic and Statistical Manual of Mental Disorder—5 [37]. One AN patient was later excluded because of diagnostic migration, i.e., the diagnosis changed from AN to major depression as primary disorder with a secondary eating disorder component. Two HC were excluded for technical problems. A total of 20 AN patients ((mean ± standard error (SE)) (age = 23.30 ± 7.61, BMI = 15.87 ± 1.12)) and 20 HC (age = 23.85 ± 3.23, BMI = 18.98 ± 1.01) finally participated in the study. For the HC, the presence and/or history of any eating disorder and/or other psychiatric disorders constituted an exclusion criterion, whereas a BMI score in the lower normal range (i.e., between 17 and 21) was an inclusion criterion. The study was approved by the Ethical Committees of Policlinico Umberto I and IRCCS Santa Lucia Foundation and in accordance with the ethical standards of the 2013 Declaration of Helsinki. All the participants read and signed the informed consent.

2.2. *Procedure*

The experiment consisted of two sessions: a pre-experimental (Section 2.3) and an experimental session (Section 2.4), with about one week break in between, in which the individualized avatars were created.

2.3. *Pre-Experimental Session*

This session lasted about one hour. Participants filled out a series of questionnaires presented in randomized order on a computer using E-Prime® 2.0 software. The Eating Disorder Inventory—2 (EDI-2) [38], the Body Shape Questionnaire (BSQ) [39], the Body Uneasiness Test (BUT) [40], and the Bulimic Investigatory Test, Edinburgh (BITE) [41] were used to assess the symptoms severity of the eating disorder pathology, whereas the Symptom Checklist-90-R (SCL-90-R) [42] was used to check for the presence of others psychiatric symptoms (see Supplementary Materials for detailed information).

Subsequently, a female experimenter measured circumferences and lengths of selected body parts of each participants and took pictures of participants' body standing up (front, back, and profile view) with a Nikon D40 mounted on a tripod. Participants' pictures and body measures served to create the avatars personalized for each participant.

Avatars Modelling

A 3D modelling software (MakeHumans, open source tool for making 3d characters) was used to recreate the personalized avatar that matched participants' real body in terms of height, shape, and body size and two more avatars that reproduced verisimilar loss of 30% and gain of 50% of the original weight (Figure 1, panel A). Specifically, Adobe Photoshop 7.0 (Adobe Systems Incorporated, San Jose, CA, USA) was used to create highly detailed skin, clothes, and material textures. Subsequently, these three avatars were imported into 3dsMax (Autodesk Inc., Mill Valley, CA), a 3D modelling and animation software, which we used to create a continuum of 28 avatars incrementing in size in steps of 3%, starting from the thinnest (−30%) to the fattest avatar (+50%). One set of 28 standing avatars facing the participants was created for subsequent task, i.e., the Avatar selection task (please see Section 2.4.1) in which participants could choose the avatar that best resembled their own body by observing it from a 3PP). We decided to present a set of avatars going from −30% to +50% of the original body size in order to not end up with unrealistically thin bodies (especially in the case of the AN) and to be able to measure the presence of body overestimation in the range suggested by a recent meta-analysis [12]. Another set of avatars was created lying on a deck chair (Figure 1, panel B) and used for inducing the embodiment (please see Section 2.4.3).

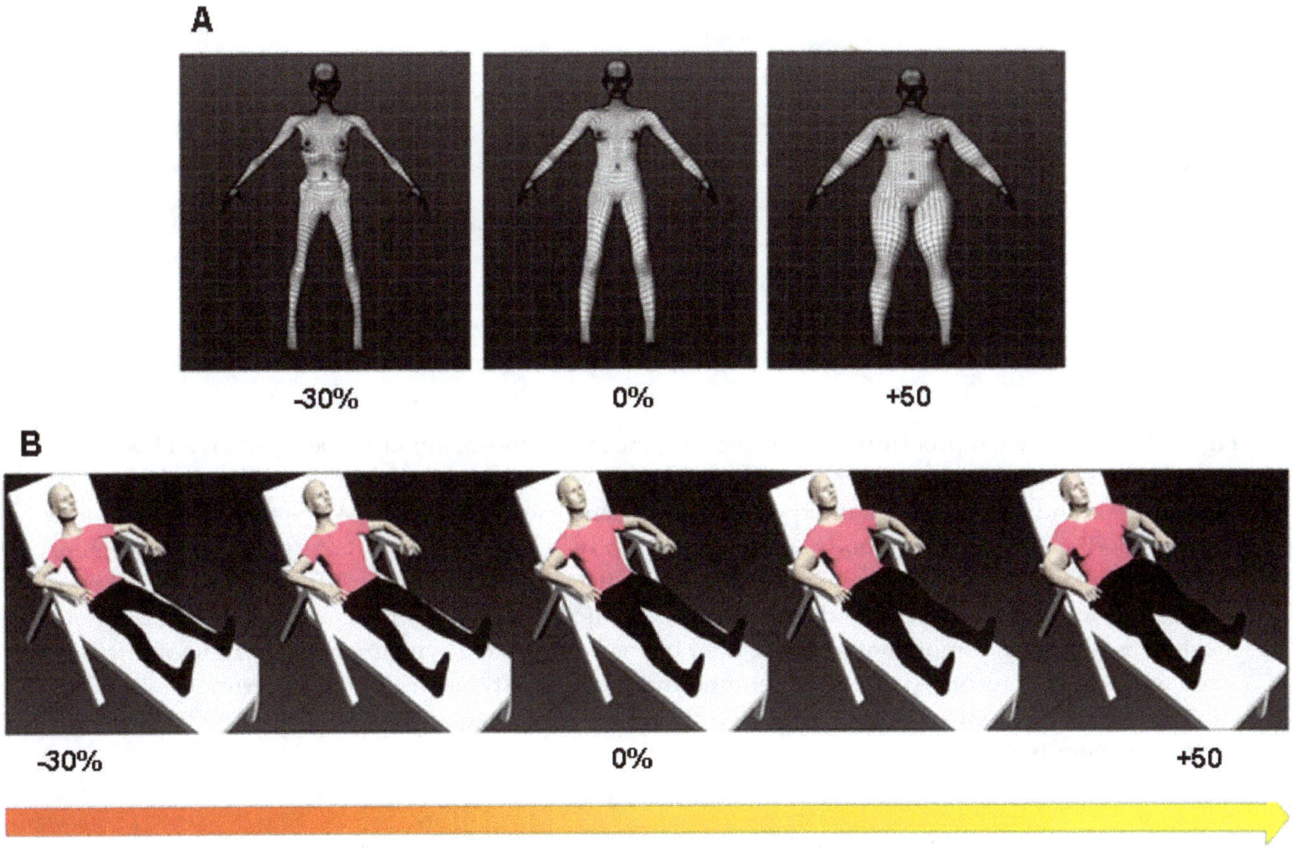

Figure 1. Creation of 3D Stimuli. (**A**) Example of three customized avatars built according to the participant's body measures and pictures: an avatar that reproduced participant's real body (avatar 0%), a thinner avatar (avatar −30%), and fatter avatar (+50%). (**B**) Example of avatars selection extracted from the continuum of avatars lying on a deck chair and increasing in size in steps of 3%, starting from the thinnest (−30%) to the fattest avatar (+50%).

2.4. Experimental Session

This session lasted about two hours (see Figure 2 for an illustration of the procedure). Participants first performed the Avatar selection task (Section 2.4.1). Then they put on clothes that matched the avatar's outfit and lay down on the deck chair to perform the perceived and ideal body tasks (Section 2.4.2). Afterward, participants experienced synchronous and asynchronous IMS (Section 2.4.3) with three different body size avatars (Avatar 0%., i.e., the avatar they chose in the Avatar selection task; Avatar −15% and Avatar +15%, i.e., an avatar 15% thinner and one 15% fatter than the one reproducing their own perceived body) in separate runs, counterbalanced across participants. Within each run participants received synchronous and asynchronous IMS in separate blocks (counterbalanced across participants) with the same avatar size. Immediately after each IMS block, participants performed the perceived body task (first 6 blocks) or the ideal body task (second 6 blocks, or vice versa). Then, we collected explicit and implicit measurements of embodiment (Section 2.4.4) and the emotional response (Section 2.4.5) to the IMS. At the end participants were also asked to rate the avatars in terms of similarity and attractiveness (Section 2.4.6).

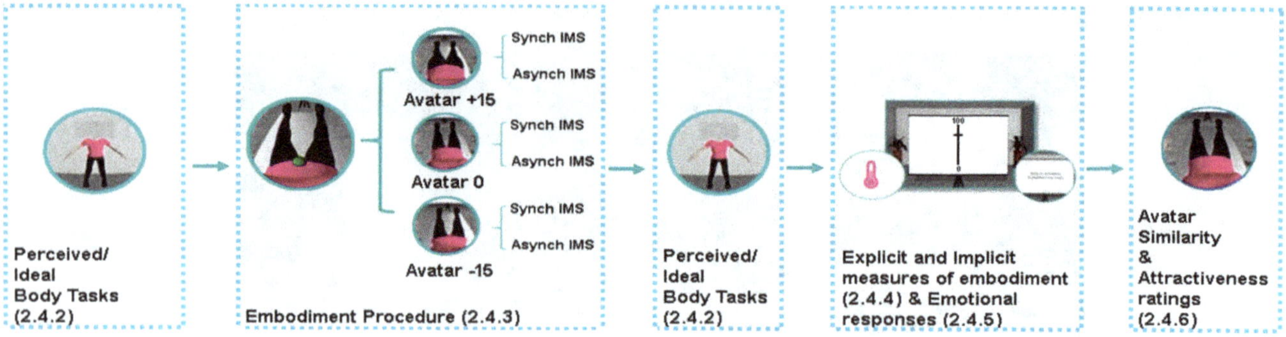

Figure 2. Experimental procedure. After selecting the avatar most similar to their perceived body and the one most resembling their ideal body, participants were enrolled in embodiment blocks in which synchronous and asynchronous interpersonal multisensory stimulation (IMS) were applied to three different bodies (the perceived body, −15% thinner body, +15% fatter body). After each embodiment block participants repeated the perceived and ideal body tasks to measure the effects of the embodiment of different sized avatars on body dissatisfaction. Explicit and implicit measures of the embodiment illusion, as well as the emotional response after being exposed to a/synchronous touching of different sized avatars were recorded after each embodiment block. At the end of the experiment we asked participants to rate from a first-person perspective the three avatars in terms of similarity to their own body and overall attractiveness.

All the experimental tasks were done in a virtual scenario that reproduced the actual experimental room, i.e., a 5 × 8 meters furnished room with a deck chair, identical to the one participant sat on during the experiment, and a 1.5 × 1.5 meters screen where questionnaires were projected.

2.4.1. Avatar Selection Task

Participants were asked to choose the avatar that best fits their own body from a continuum ranging from a body that was 30% thinner to another one that was +50% fatter than the actual body, i.e., the body that was reproduced on the bases of each participant's body size and shape. Participants initially saw the avatar in the middle of this continuum and were specifically instructed to explore all the continuum before choosing the avatar's body that best resembled their own in terms of shape and size. In this task, participants were standing up and the avatars were presented in a specular congruence with respect to their actual body, i.e., from a 3PP, as if they were looking at themselves in a mirror. The selected avatar (0% Avatar), the one 15% fatter (+15% Avatar) and the one 15% thinner (−15% Avatar) than the 0%, were used as virtual body stimuli for the embodiment blocks (Section 2.4.3).

2.4.2. Perceived and Ideal Body Tasks: Body Dissatisfaction

To assess participants' body dissatisfaction immediately before and after the IMS we asked them to choose the avatar which best resembled their real (perceived body task) and ideal (ideal body task) body in terms of size/shape/weight along the −30%–+50% continuum (Figure 3A). Differently from the avatar selection task, however, judgments were performed while participants were laying down on the deck chair and avatars were projected standing up in front of them, i.e., from a 3PP. As these tasks were performed before and immediately after IMS, participants were left lying on the desk chair to avoid disrupting any induced feelings of ownership over the avatar's body.

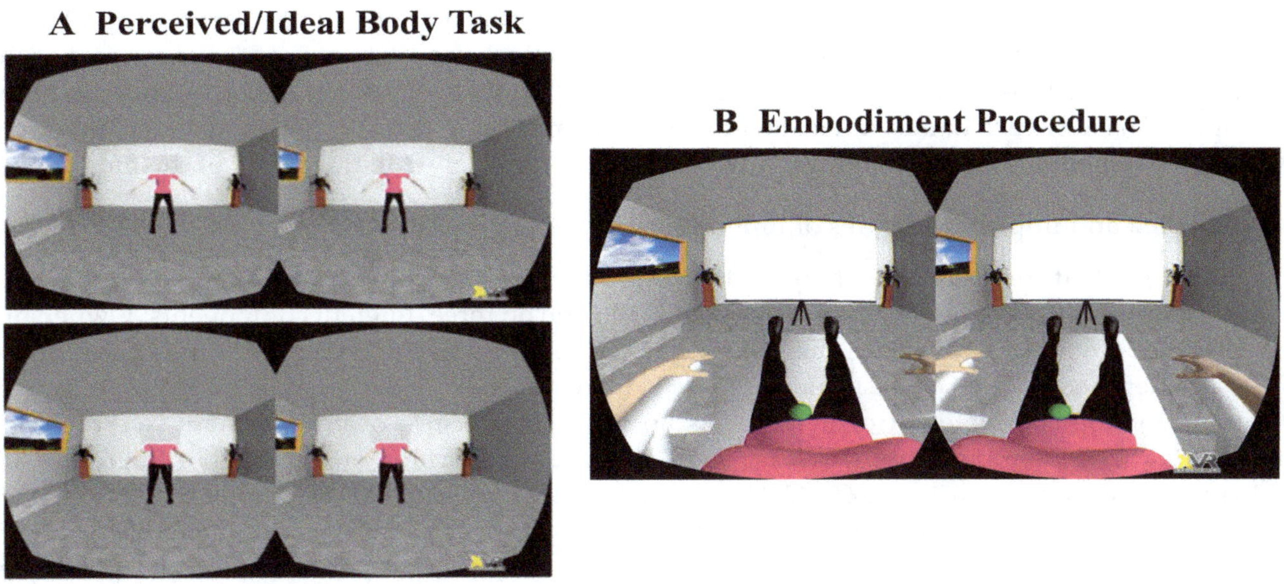

Figure 3. (**A**) Perceived/ideal body task. In separate blocks, participants choose the avatar which was the most similar to their own body (perceived body task) and the avatar which best resembled their ideal body (ideal body task) along a continuous of avatars presented from a third-person perspective (3PP). Each task comprised two trials presented in counterbalanced order: in one trial participants started the selection from the thinnest avatar (upper part of panel A), in the other from the fattest one (lower part of panel A). (**B**) Embodiment procedure. During the embodiment procedure a three minute of a/synchronous visuo-tactile stimulation was delivered. During the embodiment participants observed one of three different avatars from a first-person perspective (1PP). A virtual ball was programmed to touch the avatar on three different spots around the belly button in eight different ways (single touches and stroking movements).

Each task (perceived and ideal body task) comprised two trials, presented in counterbalanced order: in one trial participants started the selection from the thinnest avatar, in the other from the fattest one. Trials' scores were then averaged for the final score. The discrepancy between the size of the ideal and the perceived body, calculated as the absolute difference between the two, was considered an index of participants' body dissatisfaction.

2.4.3. Embodiment Procedure

During the IMS procedure participants saw the body from a 1PP (Figure 3B) through a head-mounted display (Oculus Rift Developers Kit Dk1, Oculus VR, Menlo Park, CA, USA). Thus, the virtual body replaced the participant's body in space. A calibration was performed to assure a proper positioning of the virtual camera and a precise overlap between the touch felt on the abdomen and the one observed on the avatar. Then, three minutes of visuo-tactile IMS were applied to the participant's and the avatar's body. The IMS was performed by a female experimenter, who received through headphones audio cues indicating the time and the location of each touch.

For the experimental condition (Synchronous-IMS), we aimed to reach the maximal multisensory congruence between the real and the virtual body. Thus, in the synchronous condition the observed and felt touch matched in time and location, and we tracked participants' head movements online to adjust visual perspective. However, as the visuo-proprioceptive congruence given by observing an avatar from a 1PP can be enough to induce feelings of ownership over a virtual body [43], we also aimed to reduce the possible occurrence of such illusory effects in the asynchronous control condition. Thus, we tried to boost the discrepancy in the control condition by delivering touches that were asynchronous in both time and location, as previous studies found that this stimulation was effective in maximizing the difference between synchronous and asynchronous conditions (see for example [44,45]) and we locked participant's head tracking during the asynchronous IMS.

During visual-tactile stimulation, the participants were asked not to move their head and look at the belly that was stimulated. Before starting the stimulation, the experimenter made sure that the participant always looked at the virtual abdomen by continuously checking: (i) the orientation of the participants' head (which had to be directed toward their real belly), and (ii) the virtual scenario on the PC monitor (where the virtual abdomen always had to be positioned in the center of the monitor).

2.4.4. Explicit and Implicit Measures of Embodiment

As an explicit measure of embodiment, we used a self-reported questionnaire adapted from previous studies [19,33] assessing the strength of the illusion on three different components: Ownership, i.e., the sense of virtual body being one's own; Agency i.e., the sense of being in control of the virtual body; and Referred Touch, i.e., the feeling of directly being touched by the seen ball (see Supplementary Materials for the complete list of items). As an implicit measure of embodiment, we recorded participants' body temperature, taken through an infrared thermometer (IFR 100, Microlife AG, Widnau, CH, precision: ± 0.2 °C, 32.0–42.2 °C) under participants' right armpit immediately after each block of IMS to compare ratings taken after synchronous vs. asynchronous embodiment blocks. Since we wanted to exclude participants with altered body temperature (due for example to febrile illness) we also took the body temperature before the experimental session started.

2.4.5. Measure of Emotional Response Induced by Embodiment

Valence and intensity of the emotional response induced by being exposed to a/synchronous touching of the three differently sized avatars were assessed by a visual analogue scale (VAS) ranging from "very negative" (0) to "very positive" (100) presented after both synchronous and asynchronous IMS.

2.4.6. Similarity and Attractiveness Ratings of the Avatars

As part of the final debriefing procedure, we checked how the −15%, 0%, and +15% avatars used during the embodiment blocks were actually perceived by the participants. Therefore, we asked participants to verbally rate on 0–100 VAS how much the three avatars resembled their own body (similarity ratings) and how attractive they thought these were (attractiveness ratings). The avatars were presented from a 1PP while participants were still laying down on the deck chair. Thus, ratings were collected while there was a spatial congruence between the actual participant's body and the avatar's body, i.e., while participants observed the three avatars replacing their own body in space.

3. Results

Data were analyzed using STATISTICA version 8.0 (StatSoft, Tulsa, OK, USA). Significance was set at $p < 0.05$. The Duncan test was used for post-hoc comparisons. Bayes Factors were calculated by means the open-source software JASP [46] which allows quantification of evidence in favor of the alternative or null hypothesis.

3.1. Baseline Measures

Descriptive statistics and independent sample t-tests were used for group comparisons of the demographical variables, eating disorder pathology and all the other baseline measures (Table 1).

Patients with anorexia nervosa (AN) reported higher symptoms severity scores in all scales (the Eating Disorder Inventory (EDI)—drive for thinness, EDI—body dissatisfaction scales, Body Shape Questionnaire (BSQ), Body Uneasiness Test—Global Severity Score (BUT GSI), but not at the EDI—bulimia, and at the Bulimic Investigatory Test, Edinburgh (BITE)). Patients with AN also had a lower body mass index (BMI) compared to healthy controls (HC). Body dissatisfaction (calculated as perceived minus ideal body) was higher in AN patients than in HC. While both groups were accurate and did not differ on the estimation of their perceived body, AN patients considered a thinner body as ideal compared to HC (see Table 2 for detailed statistics).

Table 1. Means (M) and standard deviations (SD) of demographic and eating disorders variables for the two groups (healthy controls-HC, and anorexics-AN), and results of the *t*-tests.

Demographic and Eating Disorder Variables							
	HC (N = 20)		AN (N = 20)				
	M	SD	M	SD	t	df	*p*
Age	23.85	3.23	23.30	7.60	0.29	38	0.767
BMI	18.94	0.98	15.86	1.12	9.22	38	0.001
EDI—drive for thinness	2.00	3.54	13.05	7.42	−6.01	38	0.001
EDI—bulimia	0.40	0.99	0.95	2.19	−1.02	38	0.313
EDI—body dissatisfaction	4.00	3.66	13.10	7.15	−5.07	38	0.001
BSQ	64.55	17.13	118.75	32.89	−6.54	38	0.001
BUT GSI	0.93	0.28	2.58	1.01	−7.07	37	0.001
BITE Symptoms	6.10	3.97	11.80	6.41	−3.38	38	0.002
BITE Severity	1.15	1.18	2.80	3.96	−1.79	38	0.082

BMI = Body Mass Index; EDI = Eating Disorder Inventory; BSQ = Body Shape Questionnaire; BUT GSI = Body Uneasiness Test, General Symptom Index subscale, BITE = Bulimic Investigatory Test, Edinburgh.

Table 2. Means (M) and standard deviations (SD) of perceived body, ideal body, and body dissatisfaction (perceived body minus ideal body) tasks measured at the baseline of the two groups (healthy controls-HC, and anorexic patients-AN), and results of the *t*-tests, i.e., *p*-values (p) and Bayesian factors (BF). Values are expressed as a % of the real bodies of the participants (100 is the real body size).

Perceived, Ideal and Body Dissatisfaction Measures								
	HC		AN					
Task	M	SD	M	SD	t	df	*p*	BF
Perceived Body	101.65	8.02	102.85	14.06	−0.33	38	0.742	0.32
Ideal Body	94.65	1.38	87.10	1.59	2.28	38	0.028	2.26
Body Dissatisfaction	8.45	7.85	19.95	12.97	−3.39	38	0.002	20.90

3.2. *Explicit and Implicit Measures of Embodiment*

Three separate 2 × 2 × 3 ANOVAs were run for each component (i.e., Ownership, Agency, and Referral of Touch) of the illusion, each with the factors Group, IMS, and Avatar. They revealed a main effect of IMS for the Ownership, Agency, and Referral of Touch (all Fs > 13.34; all ps < 0.001; all ηs2 > 0.259), suggesting a stronger illusion for synchronous as compared to the asynchronous IMS. We also found a main effect of Avatar on Ownership (F (1,38) = 7.85, *p* < 0.001, η2= 0.171)), with participants reporting higher scores for the +15% Avatar ((mean ± SE) (39.38 ±1.89)) compared to the 0% (33.78 ± 2.26) and to the −15% (32.08 ± 2.27) (all ps < 0.001). All the other main and interaction effects were not significant (all Fs< 3.35 all ps > 0.084).

The same 2 × 2 × 3 ANOVA run on the body temperature revealed a main effect of IMS (F (1,38) = 1.80, *p* = 0.002, η2 = 0.221)) showing a lower body temperature after the synchronous stimulation (34.91 ± 0.14) compared to the asynchronous one (35.02 ± 0.13). None of the other main and interaction effects were significant (all Fs < 1.27, all ps > 0.287). Please see Supplementary Materials for additional analyses.

These results suggest that there was no group dependent difference in how avatars were embodied and therefore a comparable level of bodily self-plasticity between AN and HC.

3.3. Body Dissatisfaction after Embodiment

A 2 × 2 × 3 ANOVA with Group (AN, HC) as between-and IMS (synchronous, asynchronous) and Avatar (−15%, 0%, +15%) as within-subjects factors showed no significant main or interaction effects (all Fs < 3.39, all ps > 0.073, all $\eta 2 < 0.065$). Given that classical null hypothesis testing is not the ideal statistical tool for drawing conclusions about non-significant results [47,48], we also performed a Bayesian ANOVA which allows quantification of evidence in favor of the alternative or null hypothesis. The full model including main effects and the interaction between them provides evidence in favor of the null hypothesis ($BF_{10} = 8.131 \times 10^{-5}$), suggesting that embodiment of avatars of different body sizes did not change body dissatisfaction in AN and HC.

3.4. Emotional Response after Embodiment

The 2 × 2 × 3 ANOVA on the emotional ratings with the factors Group, IMS, and Avatar revealed a main effect of IMS ($F(1,38) = 18.01, p < 0.001, \eta 2 = 0.321$), explained by more positive emotions following synchronous (59.44 ± 3.34) compared to the asynchronous (44.34 ± 2.93) IMS. The Avatar × Group interaction was also significant ($F(2,76) = 7.21, p < 0.001, \eta 2 = 0.159$) (Figure 4) and shows that independently of the IMS, AN patients felt more negative emotions after being exposed to the +15% Avatar (44.71 ± 3.95) compared to the −15% Avatar (53.59 ± 4.50) ($p = 0.017$). The opposite trend was true for the HC who showed significantly more negative emotional response after being exposed to the −15% (50.02 ± 4.49) compared to the +15% (58.60 ± 3.95; $p = 0.020$) and marginally to the 0% Avatar (56.88 ± 3.99; $p = 0.057$). Finally, AN patients experienced more negative emotions to the +15% Avatar (44.71 ± 3.95) than HC (58.60 ± 3.95; $p = 0.040$). No other main or interaction effects were significant (all Fs < 3.73, all ps > 0.061). These results suggest that differently from the HC group, AN patients experienced negative emotions when they observed an avatar replacing their own body in space which reproduced a verisimilar increase in weight of 15%, with respect to the one that reproduced verisimilar decrease of weight of the same magnitude. This happened independently from the type of IMS used to induce the embodiment.

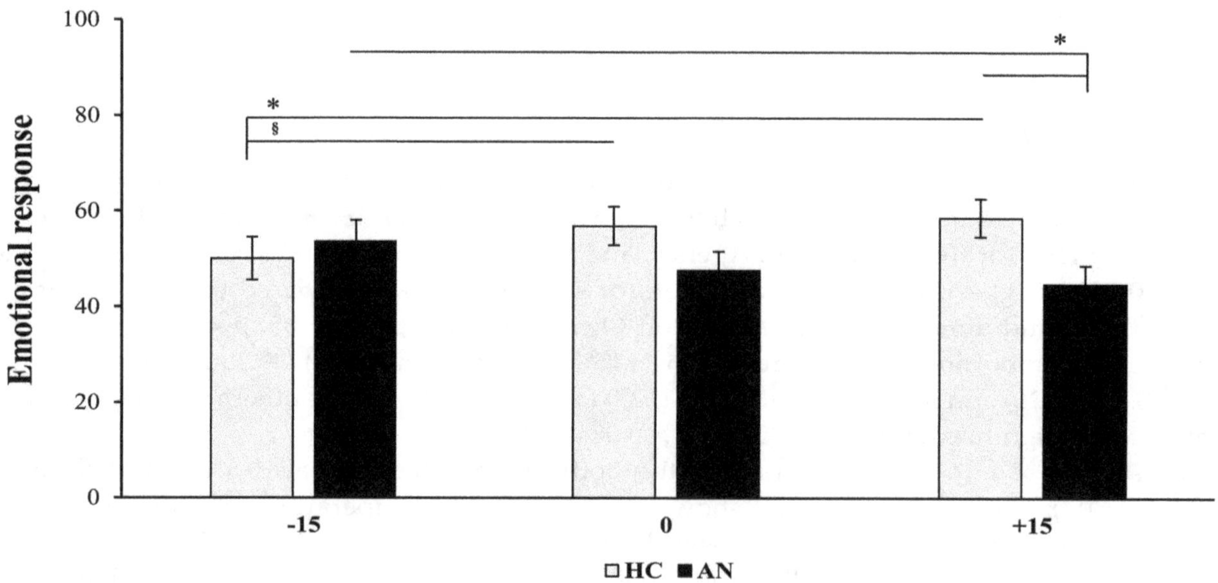

Figure 4. Emotional response after embodiment. Graph showing the effect of the interaction between avatar size (−15%; 0%; +15%) and group (healthy controls—HC; patients with anorexia nervosa—AN) on the emotional scale ranging from 0 (very negative emotions) to 100 (very positive emotions). Error bars represent standard error of mean. * = $p < 0.05$, § = marginally significant ($p = 0.057$).

3.5. Avatars' Similarity and Attractiveness Ratings

The 2 × 3 ANOVA with the factors Group and Avatar performed on the similarity ratings revealed a main effect of the Avatar ($F(2,76) = 39.14$, $p < 0.001$, $\eta 2 = 0.50$): participants perceived the 0% (66.82 ± 3.26) and the +15% Avatar (69.37 ± 3.91) as more similar to their real body than the −15% Avatar (33.72 ± 4.52) (all ps < 0.001) (Figure 5, panel A). All the other main and interaction effects were not significant (all Fs < 0.59; all ps > 0.446). These results show that an increase in weight of 15% with respect to one's own perceived body size might pass unobserved in both patients and controls, while a loss of weight of similar magnitude is detected.

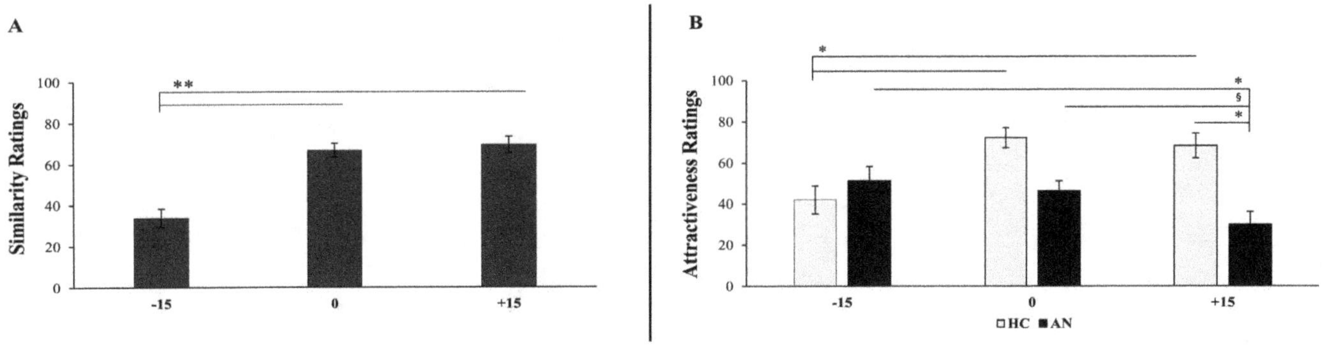

Figure 5. (**A**) Avatars' similarity ratings. Graph showing the main effect of Avatar size (−15%; 0%; +15%) on similarity ratings given during the observation of the avatars from a 1PP. (**B**) Avatars' attractiveness ratings. Graph showing the effect of the interaction between Avatar size (−15%; 0%; +15%) and Group (healthy controls, HC; patients with anorexia nervosa, AN) on attractiveness ratings given during the observation of the avatars from a 1PP. Error bars represent standard error of mean. ** = $p < 0.001$, * = $p < 0.05$, § = marginally significant, i.e., $p = 0.058$.

The same ANOVA performed on the attractiveness ratings revealed a main effect of Group ($F(1,38) = 12.07$, $p = 0.001$, $\eta 2 = 0.241$). HC rated the avatars as more attractive than AN (60.87 ± 3.71 vs. 42.63, ± 3.71). The Avatar × Group interaction was also significant ($F(2,76) = 9.47$, $p < 0.001$, $\eta 2 = 0.119$) (Figure 5, panel B). AN considered the +15% Avatar as the least attractive ((30.10 ± 5.99) vs. the −15% Avatar (51.45 ± 6.83; $p = 0.016$) and the 0% Avatar (46.35 ± 4.82; $p = 0.058$. HC instead considered the −15% Avatar as the least attractive ((42.00 ± 6.83) vs. the 0% Avatar (72.25 ± 4.82; $p < 0.001$) and +15% Avatar (68.35 ± 5.99; $p = 0.002$)). The main effect of Avatar was not significant ($F(2,76) = 2.74$, $p = 0.070$). These results show that a loss of 15% of body weight is associated in AN patients to an increase in body attractiveness with respect to the perceived body weight (even though marginally) and to a verisimilar gain of the same magnitude in body weight, while it results in a decrease in body attractiveness with respect to the same categories of virtual bodies in HC participants.

3.6. Correlations between +15% Avatar Emotional Response and Symptoms Severity

Finally, we tested, separately for each group, whether the emotions experienced with the exposure to the +15% Avatar (which was considered highly similar to the self and minimally attractive (Section 3.5)), was associated to self-reported body shape preoccupations, as indexed by the Body Shape Questionnaire (BSQ), and to the presence of abnormal body image concerns and eating behaviors, as indexed by the global severity index of the Body Uneasiness Test (BUT-GSI). We found that in AN patients, there was a significant correlation between the emotions experienced with the +15% Avatar and the strength of the concerns about the body shape ($r = 0.62$; $p = 0.004$; $BF_{10} = 14.05$). Also, the correlation between the emotions experienced with the +15% Avatar and the BUT-GIS was significant ($r = 0.69$; $p = 0.001$; $BF_{10} = 37.07$). These correlations therefore suggested that the higher the symptoms' severity was, the higher the negative emotional experience with the +15% Avatar (Figure 6, right panels). No significant correlation was found in the HC group (all rs < 0.05; all ps > 0.826; $BFs_{10} < 0.283$), Figure 6, left panels).

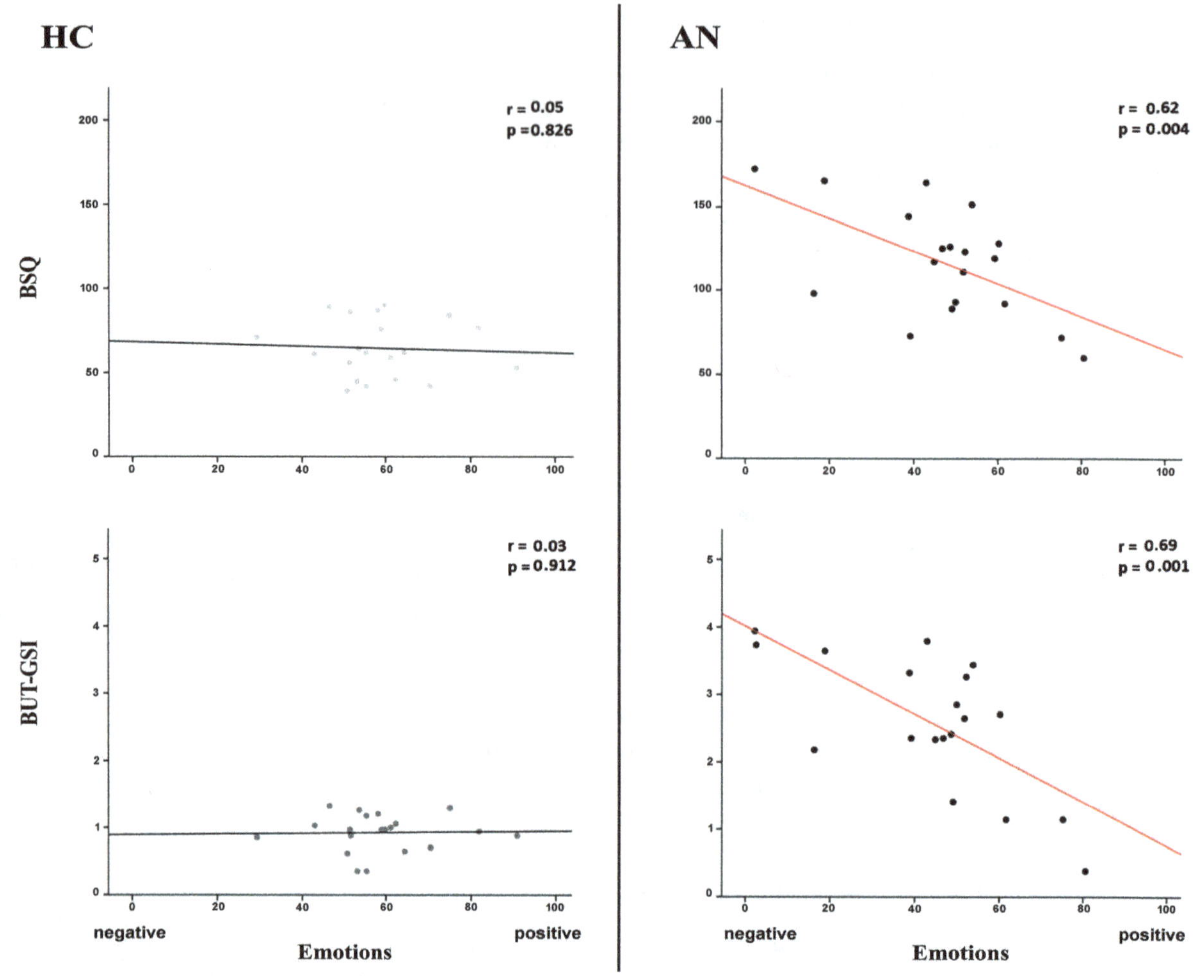

Figure 6. Correlations between +15% Avatar emotional response and symptoms severity. Scatterplots showing correlations between emotional changes after the exposure to the +15% Avatar and severity symptoms scores in the two groups. In the group of patient with anorexia nervosa (AN), the +15% Avatar emotional index correlated significantly with scores at the Body Shape Questionnaire (BSQ) and with the global severity index of the Body Uneasiness Test (BUT-GSI), while correlations were not significant in the healthy control (HC) group.

4. Discussion

We aimed to characterize, and eventually reduce, perceptual and cognitive-emotional components of body image distortion (BID) in AN using virtual bodies and embodiment illusion. To the best of our knowledge, only one study [49] investigated the body image in AN by: (i) using biometric self-avatars and (ii) reproducing the daily life experience of looking at oneself in the mirror. No studies instead coupled the creation of biometric self-avatars with multisensory bodily illusion paradigms.

Our results confirm that AN patients show higher body weight/shape concerns, drive for thinness (self-report questionnaires) and body dissatisfaction (perceptual minus ideal body size) compared to HC. However, body dissatisfaction in AN was not caused by a body overestimation, as suggested by previous literature [12]. Indeed, both AN patients and HC were accurate and did not differ in estimating the size of their real bodies, but AN patients desired a thinner body than HC. Although unexpected, these results are in line with a recent study [49] that adopted a virtual reality (VR) approach similar to the present one. Molbert and colleagues [49] measured body overestimation in AN by using a body scanner to create 3D avatars that faithfully reproduced participants' real body and then manipulated these avatars to reproduce weight gains and losses. Analogously to our findings, results from this study show that AN patients perceived their body similar to the HC but, differently from them, they desired a thinner body. Thus, all together these results support the idea that BID in AN is characterized by distorted attitudes concerning the desired body rather than by perceptual overestimation of the body size. Moreover, in agreement with the results of a recent meta-analysis [14], our findings also support the idea that estimation of one's own body size based on depictive methods (i.e., when participants estimate their body size by selecting a visual representation of their own body, like in this study) is less adapt to capture body size overestimation with respect to metric methods (i.e., when participants estimate their body size using quantifiable spatial estimations). This might be due to different features characterizing body representation that are targeted by these two types of methods. According to the body model proposed by Longo [50], the metric measures use both explicit and implicit knowledge of the body while the depictive measures, rely on explicit knowledge only, therefore they might be less automatic and more controllable.

The main aim of the present study was to investigate whether embodiment of differently sized avatars could reduce BID in AN. Therefore, we coupled virtual reality with a visuo-tactile IMS setup to induce embodiment of differently sized avatars, and measured embodiment strength and changes in perceptual and cognitive-emotional components of BID after embodiment induction. We adopted a controlled IMS procedure that differed from previous studies in several ways [15,28] and had the final aim of maximizing the congruence of virtual and real bodily signals. Thus we adopted both the 1PP and the head tracking during the synchronous IMS condition. This was particularly relevant in case of embodiment of bodies that patients might consider unattractive, as the ones reproducing their own weight and maximally in those reproducing a gain of 15% of this weight.

However, differently from [28], we used both synchronous and asynchronous IMS in order to disentangle the effects of embodiment and of observing the avatars from a 1PP. To this aim, we adopted a particular asynchronous control condition, in which we tried to maximize the incongruence between the virtual and real bodily signals. Indeed, the simple visuo-proprioceptive congruence between the real body and avatar's body given by presenting the avatars from a 1PP might result per-se in illusory feelings of ownership of the observed body. Thus, to reduce the possible occurrence of such illusory effects also in the asynchronous control condition, we applied spatio-temporal asynchronous touches as in [44,45]. Also, we locked the head tracking of the virtual camera (differently from [15]), to reduce the visuo-motor congruency between the self and the virtual body and further disrupt possible illusory embodiment in the control condition (see Section 2.4.3 of the methods for details). Instead of using the same avatar size for all participants [28], we created customized avatars, matching actual weight, height, and body parts' dimensions/shape and induced embodiment with the avatar reproducing participant's perceived body size/shape and avatars reproducing realistic loss and gain in weight of 15% with respect to the perceived weight.

Both explicit (scores at the embodiment questionnaire) and implicit (body temperature data) measures of the embodiment suggest that our synchronous visuo-tactile stimulation was effective in inducing higher embodiment compared to the asynchronous one. Specifically, the answers at the self-report questionnaire show higher ratings after the synchronous compared to the asynchronous visuo-tactile stimulation for all the three components of corporal awareness. Participants were more likely to: (i) feel that the avatar's body was their own one (Ownership), (ii) feel in control of its movements (Agency), and (iii) feel that the perceived touch was caused by the virtual one (Referral of Touch). These illusory sensations were independent of group and no interaction with the avatar size was found. Only for the Ownership component there was a main effect of the avatar size, with higher ratings attributed to the fatter avatars compared to both the 0% and the −15% avatar independently of group and type of IMS. Implicit measures of the embodiment mirror the explicit ones, as we found a change in body temperature between synchronous and asynchronous conditions independently of group and avatar size. However, the interpretation that this change in body temperature might be considered an implicit index of embodiment is currently highly debated in the literature [35] and we believe future studies are needed to clearly attribute the occurrence of such change to any evident factor (please see Supplementary Materials for a more detailed discussion on body temperature changes).

All in all, our measures on embodiment strength converge in showing that plasticity of body representation was similar in AN and HC. This result apparently contradicts previous literature which showed stronger bodily illusion for body parts (i.e., hands) in AN compared to HC participants [30]. It has been shown that bodily illusion negatively correlated with interoceptive abilities [29] and that higher bodily plasticity in AN plausibly results from altered multisensory integration of extero-and interocepetive signals [51]. In line with our results, HC and AN showed similar levels of embodiment of full bodies [31]. A conceivable reason for these contrasting results (rubber hand vs. full body illusion) might reside in the body part where touch is delivered. During the full body illusion touch is delivered to a highly salient and problematic body part for AN, i.e., the area around the abdomen. This may cause unpleasant sensations and negative emotions that in turn may dampen the embodiment in AN patients, making it similar to the level experienced by HC. Even though unpleasantness of the touch was not directly assessed in this study, AN patients anecdotally reported it.

An interesting finding of the present study is the fact that, independently of IMS type, AN patients showed more negative feelings after being exposed to the fatter avatar and that the strength of this effect correlated with clinical symptoms' severity. HC, instead, showed more negative emotional reactions toward the thinner avatar, which were unrelated to body concerns and eating disorder measures. This is even more interesting when considering how much the three differently sized avatars were retrospectively considered physically attractive and similar to the self. Both AN and HC participants rated the perceived and the fatter avatars as most similar to themselves (compared to the −15%). However, AN patients found them to be the least attractive (and the −15% as the maximally attractive), while HC rated them as the most attractive (and the −15% as the minimally attractive). Thus, anorexics reacted negatively to fatter avatars which were considered highly self-resembling and less attractive. These results mirror results from a previous study in HC who embodied obese avatars (BMI of 32.3) observed from 1PP [52]. This experience increased body dissatisfaction and negative emotional reactions, and at a neural level changed activity of anterior cingulate cortex and anterior insula. Such regions are known to mediate negative body-related emotional and affective experiences, such as pain and disgust [53,54]. While these results may shed light on negative emotions experienced by anorexics, it is worth noticing that we did not include obese avatars. The personalized avatars increased by 15% were still below the over-weight range, considering the average BMI (18.98) in HC. We would like to notice that both in the synchronous and in the asynchronous IMS blocks the avatars were presented in the 1PP. As we reported above, simple visuo-proprioceptive congruence (1PP) may induce some illusory feelings of embodiment even during asynchronous visuo-tactile stimulation. Even though we introduced spatio-temporal incongruent touches and motor discrepancy to get illusory sensations in the asynchronous condition as low as possible, it is possible that such sensations were able to trigger an emotional response as in the synchronous condition.

Importantly, contrary to our predictions embodiment of differently sized avatars did not significantly change participants' body dissatisfaction. This result stands in contrast with the results of a previous study by Preston and Ehrsson [28] conducted in HC only, which found that embodiment of a standardized slim body decreased body size perception and increased body satisfaction. Several differences may acknowledge for the discrepant results. Here, we measured body size perception with a task based on a visual representation of the body, i.e., participants had to estimate their body size on a customized avatar presented from a 3PP (body image). Instead, in the study by Preston and Ehrsson [28], perception of hip size was estimated by asking participants to indicate the distance on a ruler which reproduced their hip size in the absence of visual feedback (body schema). Participants were quite accurate in our body size estimation task, while participants in Preston and Ehrsson's study [28] overestimated the size of their hips. In line with the above-mentioned discussion about the effectiveness of metric vs. depictive measures in detecting body size overestimation, these contrasting results suggest that IMS might be able to change body schema more than body image.

Absence of changes in body dissatisfaction might also be explained from a theoretical point of view by considering differences between the egocentric frame of reference [55,56], i.e., body perceived from the 1PP based on its present state constituted by interoceptive and exteroceptive inputs, vs. the allocentric frame of reference, i.e., a somatic representation of the body as a 3PP based on beliefs and attitudes related to the body. According to the Allocentric Lock Theory [57], people with AN are locked in their allocentric representation of the body and are unable to update it through egocentric sensory inputs. Indeed, in our study participants experienced embodiment of avatars of different sizes from an egocentric frame of reference, whereas the estimation of real/ideal body size was performed from an allocentric frame of reference. We can speculate that, even if the embodiment of differently sized avatars could have been successful in affecting the body image as experienced from an egocentric frame of reference, the inability for the AN patients to update their allocentric representation of the body through egocentric sensory inputs might have led to no changes in body dissatisfaction induced by the embodiment.

Related to the point above, our results also let us speculate that observing one's own body from a 1PP (as it usually happens when we look down to our own body) or observing its reproduction from a 3PP (as it usually happens in front of a mirror, in pictures or videos) might bias our perception of its dimension. Indeed, when participants judge 3D reproduction of themselves without spatial or specular congruence with the self-body (as in the perceived body task), they are quite good at estimating their own body size. However, when they observe their own body by looking directly at it (as in similarity ratings task) they are more sensible to detect a loss than an increase in weight. Indeed, results from the similarity ratings show that an increase in weight of 15% with respect to one's own perceived body size might pass unobserved in both patients and controls, while a loss of weight of similar magnitude is detected. This shows an asymmetry in how weight loss and gain might be considered by our perceptual system that seems to be detectable only when the to-be-judged body replaces our own in space. Also, our results suggest that the above-mentioned perceptual asymmetry is probably due to how we affectively experience our own body. Indeed, loss of weight is associated in controls to a decrease in body attractiveness, while in anorexic patients it is associated to an increase in body attractiveness. An increase of 15% in body weight is instead considered as attractive as the perceived body weight, both in patients and controls. If we focus on patients only, our results also suggest that when dealing with the affective component of the body, it does not matter whether one's own body size is observed from a detached third-person perspective (ideal body task) or through directly looking at it (attractiveness ratings). One's own perceived body size seem to be considered less desirable and attractive than a simulated loss of weight of 15%. On the same line, the simulated illusory experience of a gain in one's own body weight is negatively experienced by anorexic patients, but not by controls (results from the emotional response task).

Overall, the present study suggests that the cognitive-emotional component of body image and not the perceptual one is severely altered in AN. Despite the inability to reduce body dissatisfaction in AN patients, our procedure was successful in inducing a strong embodiment of differently sized avatars, as measured at both the explicit and implicit level, and in enhancing negative emotional responses of anorexics to the fattest avatar which scaled with symptoms' severity.

Future research and clinical trials should aim at changing the distorted cognitive-emotional components of body image through the internalization of a normal weight body and the reduction of the emotional distress caused by weight gain, more than at changing the perceptual ones. Additionally, even if one should be cautious in using stimuli of enlarged bodies, virtual reality could be used to gradually expose and habituate AN patients to healthier versions of their bodies and to act as an intermediary step prior to the in vivo body image exposure, as some therapeutic protocols are already showing (see [58] for a review).

Author Contributions: G.P. and I.B. designed research; G.T. and M.M. implemented the virtual reality setup; L.P., S.C., I.B. and G.P. created the experimental stimuli; L.P. and S.C. collected and processed the experimental data; L.P., G.P., S.C., and I.B. analyzed data; F.D. and C.L. verified the diagnosis and provided clinical support to the anorexic patients; I.B. supervised the work. All authors discussed the results and commented on the manuscript. L.P., G.P. and I.B. wrote the manuscript, B.L. critically revised it. All authors have read and agreed to the published version of the manuscript.

Acknowledgments: We thank all participants who took part in this study. Particular thanks go to those with AN who, make research on AN possible. I.B. was funded by the Italian Ministry of Health (GR-2011-02351798). B.L. was supported by the Swiss National Science Foundation (nr. 170511), GP was supported "Progetti per Avvio alla Ricerca 2019", "Sapienza" University of Rome (Prot. Num. AR21916B890A9214) and SC was supported by "Progetti per Avvio alla Ricerca 2019", "Sapienza" University of Rome (Prot. Num. AR11916B88D6817C).

References

1. Gaudio, S.; Brooks, S.J.; Riva, G. Nonvisual multisensory impairment of body perception in anorexia nervosa: A systematic review of neuropsychological studies. *PLoS ONE* **2014**, *9*, e110087. [CrossRef] [PubMed]
2. Arcelus, J. Mortality Rates in Patients with Anorexia Nervosa and Other Eating Disorders. *Arch. Gen. Psychiatry* **2011**, *68*, 724. [CrossRef] [PubMed]
3. Cornelissen, K.K.; Bester, A.; Cairns, P.; Tovée, M.J.; Cornelissen, P.L. The influence of personal BMI on body size estimations and sensitivity to body size change in anorexia spectrum disorders. *Body Image* **2015**, *13*, 75–85. [CrossRef] [PubMed]
4. Farrell, C.; Lee, M.; Shafran, R. Assessment of body size estimation: A review. *Eur. Eat. Disord. Rev.* **2005**, *13*, 75–88. [CrossRef]
5. Urgesi, C.; Fornasari, L.; Canalaz, F.; Perini, L.; Cremaschi, S.; Faleschini, L.; Thyrion, E.Z.; Zuliani, M.; Balestrieri, M.; Fabbro, F.; et al. Impaired configural body processing in anorexia nervosa: Evidence from the body inversion effect. *Br. J. Psychol.* **2014**, *105*, 486–508. [CrossRef]
6. Cash, T.F. Body image: Past, present, and future. *Body Image* **2004**, *1*, 1–5. [CrossRef]
7. Peelen, M.V.; Downing, P.E. The neural basis of visual body perception. *Nat. Rev. Neurosci.* **2007**, *8*, 636–648. [CrossRef]
8. Gandolfo, M.; Downing, P.E. Causal Evidence for Expression of Perceptual Expectations in Category-Selective Extrastriate Regions. *Curr. Biol.* **2019**, *29*, 1–5. [CrossRef]
9. Moreau, Q.; Pavone, E.F.; Aglioti, S.M.; Candidi, M. Theta synchronization over occipito-temporal cortices during visual perception of body parts. *Eur. J. Neurosci.* **2018**, *48*, 2826–2835. [CrossRef]
10. Moreau, Q.; Parrotta, E.; Era, V.; Martelli, M.; Candidi, M. Role of the occipito-temporal Theta rhythm in hand visual identification. *J. Neurophysiol.* **2019**. [Epub ahead of print]. [CrossRef]
11. Cash, T.F.; Deagle, E.A. The nature and extent of body-image disturbances in anorexia nervosa and bulimia nervosa: A meta-analysis. *Int. J. Eat. Disord.* **1997**, *22*, 107–125. [CrossRef]
12. Gardner, R.M.; Brown, D.L. Body size estimation in anorexia nervosa: A brief review of findings from 2003 through 2013. *Psychiatry Res.* **2014**, *219*, 407–410. [CrossRef] [PubMed]
13. Keel, P.K.; Dorer, D.J.; Franko, D.L.; Jackson, S.C.; Herzog, D.B. Postremission predictors of relapse in women with eating disorders. *Am. J. Psychiatry* **2005**, *162*, 1–6. [CrossRef] [PubMed]
14. Mölbert, S.C.; Klein, L.; Thaler, A.; Mohler, B.J.; Brozzo, C.; Martus, P.; Karnath, H.O.; Zipfel, S.; Giel, K.E. Depictive and metric body size estimation in anorexia nervosa and bulimia nervosa: A systematic review and meta-analysis. *Clin. Psychol. Rev.* **2017**, *57*, 21–31. [CrossRef] [PubMed]
15. Piryankova, I.V.; Wong, H.Y.; Linkenauger, S.A.; Stinson, C.; Longo, M.R.; Bülthoff, H.H.; Mohler, B.J. Owning an overweight or underweight body: Distinguishing the physical, experienced and virtual body. *PLoS ONE* **2014**, *9*, e103428. [CrossRef] [PubMed]
16. Berlucchi, G.; Aglioti, S.M. The body in the brain revisited. *Exp. Brain Res.* **2010**, *200*, 25–35. [CrossRef] [PubMed]
17. Porciello, G.; Bufalari, I.; Minio-Paluello, I.; Di Pace, E.; Aglioti, S.M. The 'Enfacement' illusion: A window on the plasticity of the self. *Cortex* **2018**, *104*, 261–275. [CrossRef]
18. Botvinick, M.; Cohen, J. Rubber hands "feel" touch that eyes see. *Nature* **1998**, *391*, 756. [CrossRef]

19. Lenggenhager, B.; Tadi, T.; Metzinger, T.; Blanke, O. Video ergo sum: Manipulating bodily self-consciousness. *Science* **2007**, *317*, 1096–1099. [CrossRef]
20. Sforza, A.; Bufalari, I.; Haggard, P.; Aglioti, S.M. My face in yours: Visuo-tactile facial stimulation influences sense of identity. *Soc. Neurosci.* **2010**, *5*, 148–162. [CrossRef]
21. Bufalari, I.; Sforza, A.L.; Di Russo, F.; Mannetti, L.; Aglioti, S.M. Malleability of the self: Electrophysiological correlates of the enfacement illusion. *Sci. Rep.* **2019**, *9*, 1–14. [CrossRef] [PubMed]
22. Fusaro, M.; Tieri, G.; Aglioti, S. Influence of cognitive stance and physical perspective on subjective and autonomic reactivity to observed pain and pleasure: An immersive virtual reality study. *Conscious. Cogn.* **2019**, *67*, 86–97. [CrossRef] [PubMed]
23. Porciello, G.; Holmes, B.S.; Liuzza, M.T.; Crostella, F.; Aglioti, S.M.; Bufalari, I. Interpersonal Multisensory Stimulation reduces the overwhelming distracting power of self-gaze. *Sci. Rep.* **2014**, *4*, 6669. [CrossRef] [PubMed]
24. Mino-Paluello, I.; Porciello, G.; Gandolfo, M.; Boukarras, S.; Aglioti, S.M. The Enfacement illusion boosts facial mimicry. *Cortex* **2019**, *123*, 113–123. [CrossRef] [PubMed]
25. Maselli, A.; Slater, M. The building blocks of the full body ownership illusion. *Front. Hum. Neurosci.* **2013**, *7*, 1–15. [CrossRef] [PubMed]
26. Van der Hoort, B.; Guterstam, A.; Ehrsson, H.H. Being barbie: The size of one's own body determines the perceived size of the world. *PLoS ONE* **2011**, *6*, e20195. [CrossRef]
27. Normand, J.M.; Giannopoulos, E.; Spanlang, B.; Slater, M. Multisensory stimulation can induce an illusion of larger belly size in immersive virtual reality. *PLoS ONE* **2011**, *6*, e16128. [CrossRef]
28. Preston, C.; Ehrsson, H.H. Illusory changes in body size modulate body satisfaction in a way that is related to non-clinical eating disorder psychopathology. *PLoS ONE* **2014**, *9*, e85773. [CrossRef]
29. Eshkevari, E.; Rieger, E.; Longo, M.R.; Haggard, P.; Treasure, J. Increased plasticity of the bodily self in eating disorders. *Psychol. Med.* **2012**, *42*, 819–828. [CrossRef]
30. Keizer, A.; Smeets, M.A.M.; Postma, A.; van Elburg, A.; Dijkerman, H.C. Does the experience of ownership over a rubber hand change body size perception in anorexia nervosa patients? *Neuropsychologia* **2014**, *62*, 26–37. [CrossRef]
31. Keizer, A.; Van Elburg, A.; Helms, R.; Dijkerman, H.C. A virtual reality full body illusion improves body image disturbance in anorexia nervosa. *PLoS ONE* **2016**, *11*, e0163921. [CrossRef] [PubMed]
32. Sepúlveda, A.R.; Botella, J.; León, J.A. Body-image disturbance in eating disorders: A meta-analysis. *Psychol. Spain* **2002**, *6*, 83–95.
33. Tieri, G.; Tidoni, E.; Pavone, E.F.; Aglioti, S.M. Body visual discontinuity affects feeling of ownership and skin conductance responses. *Sci. Rep.* **2015**, *5*, 17139. [CrossRef] [PubMed]
34. Tieri, G.; Gioia, A.; Scandola, M.; Pavone, E.F.; Aglioti, S.M. Visual appearance of a virtual upper limb modulates the temperature of the real hand: A thermal imaging study in Immersive Virtual Reality. *Eur. J. Neurosci.* **2017**, *45*, 1141–1151. [CrossRef] [PubMed]
35. De Haan, A.M.; Van Stralen, H.E.; Smit, M.; Keizer, A.; Van der Stigchel, S.; Dijkerman, H.C. No consistent cooling of the real hand in the rubber hand illusion. *Acta Psychol. (Amst.)* **2017**, *179*, 68–77. [CrossRef] [PubMed]
36. Mohr, H.M.; Röder, C.; Zimmermann, J.; Hummel, D.; Negele, A.; Grabhorn, R. Body image distortions in bulimia nervosa: Investigating body size overestimation and body size satisfaction by fMRI. *Neuroimage* **2011**, *56*, 1822–1831. [CrossRef]
37. American Psychiatric Association. *Diagnostic and Statistical Manual of Mental Disorder*, 5th ed.; American Psychiatric Association: Arlington, VA, USA, 2013.
38. Garner, D. *Eating Disorder Inventory-2: Professional Manual*; Psychological Assessment Resources Inc: Odessa, Finland, 1991.
39. Cooper, P.; Taylor, M.; Sc, B.; Cooper, Z.; Fairburn, C.G. The Development and Validation of the Body Shape Questionnaire. *Int. J. Eat. Disord.* **1987**, *6*, 485–494. [CrossRef]
40. Cuzzolaro, M.; Vetrone, G.; Marano, G.; Garfinkel, P.E. The Body Uneasiness Test (BUT): Development and validation of a new body image assessment scale. *Eat. Weight Disord.* **2006**, *11*, 1–13. [CrossRef]
41. Henderson, M.; Freeman, C.P.L. A Self-rating Scale for Bulimia the "BITE". *Br. J. Psychiatry* **1987**, *150*, 18–24. [CrossRef]

42. Derogatis, L.R. *Symptom Checklist-90-R: Administration, Scoring & Procedure Manual for the Revised Version of the SCL-90*; National Computer Systems: Minneapolis, MN, USA, 1994.
43. Slater, M.; Spanlang, B.; Sanchez-Vives, M.V.; Blanke, O. First person experience of body transfer in virtual reality. *PLoS ONE* **2010**, *5*, e10564. [CrossRef]
44. Apps, M.A.J.; Tsakiris, M. The free-energy self: A predictive coding account of self-recognition. *Neurosci. Biobehav. Rev.* **2014**, *44*, 85–97. [CrossRef] [PubMed]
45. Bufalari, I.; Lenggenhager, B.; Porciello, G.; Holmes, B.S.; Aglioti, S.M. Enfacing others but only if they are nice to you. *Front. Behav. Neurosci.* **2014**, *8*, 1–12. [CrossRef] [PubMed]
46. Love, J.; Selker, R.; Marsman, M.; Jamil, T.; Dropmann, D.; Verhagen, J.; Ly, A.; Gronau, Q.F.; Šmíra, M.; Epskamp, S.; et al. JASP: Graphical statistical software for common statistical designs. *J. Stat. Softw.* **2019**, *88*, 1–17. [CrossRef]
47. Dienes, Z. Using Bayes to get the most out of non-significant results. *Front. Psychol.* **2014**, *5*, 1–17. [CrossRef] [PubMed]
48. Dienes, Z. How Bayes factors change scientific practice. *J. Math. Psychol.* **2016**, *72*, 78–89. [CrossRef]
49. Mölbert, S.C.; Thaler, A.; Mohler, B.J.; Streuber, S.; Romero, J.; Black, M.J.; Zipfel, S.; Karnath, H.O.; Giel, K.E. Assessing body image in anorexia nervosa using biometric self-avatars in virtual reality: Attitudinal components rather than visual body size estimation are distorted. *Psychol. Med.* **2017**, *48*, 1–12. [CrossRef]
50. Longo, M.R. *Perceptual and Emotional Embodiment: Foundations of Embodied Cognition Volume 1*; Routledge: London, UK, 2015.
51. Pollatos, O.; Kurz, A.L.; Albrecht, J.; Schreder, T.; Kleemann, A.M.; Schöpf, V.; Kopietz, R.; Wiesmann, M.; Schandry, R. Reduced perception of bodily signals in anorexia nervosa. *Eat. Behav.* **2008**, *9*, 381–388. [CrossRef]
52. Preston, C.; Ehrsson, H.H. Illusory obesity triggers body dissatisfaction responses in the insula and anterior cingulate cortex. *Cereb. Cortex* **2016**, *26*, 4450–4460. [CrossRef]
53. Jabbi, M.; Bastiaansen, J.; Keysers, C. A Common Anterior Insula Representation of Disgust Observation, Experience and Imagination Shows Divergent Functional Connectivity Pathways. *PLoS ONE* **2008**, *3*, e2939. [CrossRef]
54. Wiech, K.; Lin, C.; Brodersen, K.H.; Bingel, U.; Ploner, M.; Tracey, I. Anterior Insula Integrates Information about Salience into Perceptual Decisions about Pain. *J. Neurosci.* **2010**, *30*, 16324–16331. [CrossRef]
55. Galati, G.; Lobel, E.; Vallar, G.; Berthoz, A.; Pizzamiglio, L.; Le Bihan, D. The neural basis of egocentric and allocentric coding of space in humans: A functional magnetic resonance study. *Exp. Brain Res.* **2000**, *133*, 156–164. [CrossRef] [PubMed]
56. Haggard, P.; Longo, M.R.; Aza, E. More than skin deep: Body representation beyond primary somatosensory cortex. *Neuropsychologia* **2010**, *48*, 655–668.
57. Riva, G. Neuroscience and eating disorders: The allocentric lock hypothesis. *Med. Hypotheses* **2012**, *78*, 254–257. [CrossRef] [PubMed]
58. Koskina, A.; Campbell, I.C.; Schmidt, U. Reviews Exposure therapy in eating disorders revisited. *Neurosci. Biobehav. Rev.* **2013**, *37*, 193–208. [CrossRef] [PubMed]

7

The Use of New Digital Information and Communication Technologies in Psychological Counseling during the COVID-19 Pandemic

Artemisa R. Dores [1,2,*], Andreia Geraldo [2], Irene P. Carvalho [3] and Fernando Barbosa [2]

1 Center for Rehabilitation Research, School of Health, Polytechnic Institute of Porto, 4200-072 Porto, Portugal
2 Laboratory of Neuropsychophysiology, Faculty of Psychology and Education Sciences of University of Porto, 4200-135 Porto, Portugal; g.andreia9@gmail.com (A.G.); fbarbosa@fpce.up.pt (F.B.)
3 CINTESIS and Department of Clinical Neurosciences and Mental Health, School of Medicine, University of Porto (FMUP), 4200-319 Porto, Portugal; irenec@med.up.pt
* Correspondence: artemisa@ess.ipp.pt

Abstract: The use of digital information and communication technologies (ICTs) has enabled many professionals to continue to provide their services during the COVID-19 pandemic. However, little is known about the adoption of ICTs by psychologists and the impact of such technologies on their practice. This study aimed to explore psychologists' practices related with the use of ICTs before and during the COVID-19 lockdown, to identify the main changes that the pandemic has brought and the impact that such changes have had on their practice with clients, and also identify the factors that potentially have affected such changes. The Portuguese Psychologists Association announced the study, and 108 psychologists responded to an online survey during the mandatory lockdown. The results showed that these professionals continued to provide their services due to having adopted ICTs. Comparing with face-to-face interventions, psychologists recognized that additional precautions/knowledge were needed to use such technologies. Despite the challenges identified, they described the experience with the use of ICTs as positive, meeting clients' adherence, and yielding positive results. Psychologists with the most years of professional experience maintained their services the most, but those with average experience showed the most favorable attitudes toward the use of technologies and web-based interventions.

Keywords: digital information and communication technologies; psychological counseling; therapy; COVID-19; coronavirus SARS-CoV-2; digital literacy

---

1. Introduction

The coronavirus disease (COVID-19) pandemic represents an unprecedented global challenge in our era, strongly affecting people's lives, namely, the exercise of various professional activities [1,2]. This unique circumstance, associated with the current availability of several digital tools, has contributed exponentially to the digital revolution that we have witnessed in recent years, with impact on the social, economic, and professional domains of life [3].

In this scenario, e-Health has emerged as one viable solution to allow the continuity of the provision of health services, particularly considering the public health measures that have been taken as a result of the National Emergency State, which has limited people's access to in-person services [4]. E-Health is broadly defined as the provision of services related to health supported by a safe and cost-effective use of information and communications technologies (ICTs) [5].

The path toward the progressive adoption of ICTs in the field of psychology had already begun before the COVID-19 pandemic, albeit in varied degrees across different countries. If documentation guiding and/or regulating professional practice is already available in some countries, a legal or normative void still exists in others. This has implications regarding the availability of the psychological services offered, which are still quite scarce in some countries, as is the case in Portugal. For example, before the COVID-19 pandemic, few Portuguese psychologists adopted guided and unguided psychological internet interventions (1.3% and 1.5%, respectively) [6], despite the already recognized advantages of this type of intervention [7–11].

Many of the guidelines for the online practice of psychology are the result of the work of several national and international associations and bodies (e.g., the American Psychological Association and European Federation of Psychologists' Associations), in an effort to set forth a consensus about the practices that they aim to guide. In Portugal, after a first approval of at-distance interventions by the Ordem dos Psicólogos Portugueses (OPP; transl.: Portuguese Psychologists Association) in 2015, the OPP issued a document with the guidelines for these types of services very recently, precisely at the peak of the COVID-19 pandemic [12,13].

In its first issue, this association claimed that psychological intervention should always be conducted within the same obligations and responsibilities (i.e., ethical principles and deontological and legal norms), regardless of the format of the intervention, as defined in the Code of Ethics. Although the OPP recognized the potential benefits of web-based interventions and use of ITCs, it also launched warnings about the need for a better understanding of the effects of the different modalities of remote intervention (e.g., written, audio or audiovisual support) compared to face-to-face intervention. The OPP additionally warned of the fact that the specificities of cyber space could elude the means of control available to psychologists, which could put privacy and confidentiality at risk [12]. In its second document, entitled "OPP guidelines for professional practice: Provision of psychology services mediated by ICTs" [13], a set of recommendations for the adoption of these technological and digital resources were presented.

In addition to the OPP, other projects have been carried out in Portugal (and elsewhere) with the aim to issue good practices to be adopted for the use of these digital and technological means in the area of health in general, and of psychology in particular. As an example, the European project THERAPY 2.0—Counseling and Therapeutic Interactions with Digital Natives, financed by the ERASMUS + program, sought to issue the appropriate integration of ICTs in counseling and therapy, especially for younger populations and refugees [14,15].

In several countries, an increasing number of studies have also sought to characterize the attitudes of psychologists toward the inclusion of ICTs in their professional practice and to gather evidence about the efficacy and effectiveness of psychological interventions mediated by ICTs (e.g., [7,16–21]). Regarding the psychologists' attitudes, the results of the studies are not consistent (e.g., [6,22]). In Portugal, a recent study assessing psychologists' attitudes revealed a slightly negative/neutral position regarding internet interventions and greater acceptability of blended treatment interventions when compared to standalone internet interventions. However, these attitudes seem to depend on different factors, such as knowledge and training [6]. A study in other countries revealed that, among those who have employed any online means of practicing counseling and therapy, 52.97% had a positive or very positive opinion about the use of these tools. In this study, e-mail was the most widely used online tool, and the computer and smart phone were the most frequently used equipment [14]. Different circumstances and factors seem to contribute to explain the different attitudes and the adoption (or not) of this type of resources [23]. Such factors include the therapist's theoretical model/orientation, geographic area, previous experience with the use of these resources, presence or absence of previous training, perception about the usefulness of these tools, ease with their use, and years of clinical practice [24–31].

Regarding the effectiveness of these online means, in general, studies allow us to conclude that internet interventions may be efficacious and cost-effective [6,16,17,19,20,32–35]. They seemed to be at least as effective as face-to-face interventions in a large group of clients receiving treatment for psychological disorders, namely, for generalized anxiety and other types of anxiety disorders [36–42], depression [43–52], and stress [53,54].

The recognized advantages of using ICTs do not refer merely to their power to compensate for the limitations of traditional interventions (e.g., travelling requirements for customers or therapists), nor to their use as complementary means. There are several advantages associated with implementing internet interventions [8–11,13,14,55]. These include easy accessibility, high adaptability, flexibility and convenience, evolution at the client's pace, easy adherence and treatment monitoring, privacy and possibility of anonymity, cultural adaptability, low cost, and high potential for dissemination [55]. Conversely, the main challenges identified in the use of ICTs include ethical concerns (e.g., security, privacy, confidentiality, and an absence or lack of deontological orientation), clients' ICT illiteracy, and negative attitudes toward internet interventions [6]. Others can be added, such as a lack of access to technological and digital tools by some users, technological problems in their use, and changes to the setting and regarding the therapeutic relationship [8,10,14,26,55–58].

Because different circumstances and factors seem to contribute to explain psychologists' attitudes and the adoption (or not) of this type of resources, it is important to identify potential changes in the use of ICTs during the COVID-19 pandemic. Given the measures of physical distance and isolation that most governments imposed with the state of emergency (e.g., [4]), how have psychologists dealt with the provision of counseling and therapy to their clients? The aims of this work were to (a) analyze how the attitudes of professionals in the field of psychology have changed in relation to the use of ICTs in the context of psychological monitoring during the lockdown; (b) assess whether the practice of psychological counseling and therapy includes greater use of ICTs during the lockdown period; (c) identify the factors that potentially have affected such changes; and (d) study the possible adoption of guidelines for at-distance psychological monitoring by psychologists who are using ICTs during the period of physical distance

2. Materials and Methods

2.1. Participants

The sample in this study comprised 108 psychologists who were registered in the OPP. Most were women (89, or 82.4%). The mean age was 37.20 years old (SD = 10.05; Min = 23, Max = 65), with 55 (50.9%) in the age group between 23 and 35 years, and 53 (49.1%) in the group between 36 and 65 years. The number of years of professional experience ranged between one or less and 33 (M = 11.52; SD = 8.60). The sample reflects national representation (including continental Portugal and islands), with 19 of the 20 Portuguese districts participating in the study. The most represented districts were Porto (n = 39; 36.8%), Lisbon (n = 21; 18.9%), Braga (n = 13; 12.3%), and Coimbra (n = 9; 8.5%). These cities comprehend the national OPP delegations with the most psychologists [59]. Most participants held master's degrees (n = 69; 63.9%). Most were specialists in clinical psychology (n = 60; 55.6%), and 23 (21.3%) had one or more advanced specialties, including in psychotherapy (n = 13; 12.0%), among others.

Participants worked mainly with adults (n = 81; 75.0%), followed by adolescents (n = 52; 48.1%), children (n = 46; 42.6%), and the elderly (n = 24; 22.2%), in the areas of anxiety disorders (n = 91; 84.3%), mood disorders (n = 72; 66.7%), personality disorders (n = 37; 34.3%), neurocognitive disorders (n = 30; 27.8%), among others. For more information, see Table 1.

Table 1. Socio-demographic characteristics of the participants.

	n/% *M*/*SD*
Gender	M: $n = 19$, 17.6% F: $n = 89$, 82.4%
Age	$M = 37.2$; $SD = 10.0$
Education	Graduation: $n = 26$, 24.1% Master: $n = 69$, 63.9% PhD: $n = 13$, 12.0%
Professional Experience	$M = 11.5$; $SD = 8.6$
Clinical and Health Specialty	Y: $n = 60$, 55.6% N: $n = 48$, 44.4%
Advanced Specialties	Neuropsychology: $n = 6$, 5.6% Psychogerontology: $n = 0$ Justice Psychology: $n = 2$, 1.9% Sports Psychology: $n = 0$ Psychotherapy: $n = 13$, 12.0% Sexology: $n = 1$, 0.9% Others: $n = 9$, 8.3%
Population	Children: $n = 46$, 42.6% Adolescents: $n = 52$, 48.1% Adults: $n = 81$, 75.0% Elderly: $n = 24$, 22.2%
Psychological Disorders	Neurodevelopment disorders: $n = 24$, 22.2% Mood disorders: $n = 72$, 66.7% Anxiety disorders: $n = 91$, 84.3% Personality disorders: $n = 37$, 34.3% Substance-related disorders and addictive behaviors: $n = 21$, 19.4% Sleep disorders: $n = 23$, 21.3% Neurocognitive disorders: $n = 30$, 27.8% Others: $n = 10$, 9.3%

2.2. Instruments

A questionnaire was developed for this study and a pilot test was conducted to check its comprehension level and adequacy for the current purposes. The questionnaire included 30 questions divided into three sections: (i) socio-demographic data, with 9 questions; (ii) experience before the COVID-19 pandemic, with 7 questions; and (iii) current experience using ICTs in psychology sessions (namely web-based interventions during the lockdown period), with 14 questions. The questions were designed based on a previous questionnaire developed for the purpose of studying the use of ICTs in the provision of therapy and counseling [14], as well as on the advantages and challenges identified in the literature about the use of these technologies on psychological counseling.

Socio-demographic data included gender, age, education level, number of years of professional experience, district where the respondent was practicing, area of specialization, and targeted population in the respondent's practice (including development stages and most frequent disorders). The remaining two sections of the questionnaire focused on information about the use of ICTs in the respondents' clinical practice. Questions included which tools and devices were used, clients' degree of satisfaction with the use of ICTs, advantages and difficulties identified by the professionals, impact on clients' adherence and on therapeutic results, among others (cf. Appendix A).

2.3. Procedure

This study was approved by the local ethics committee (Approval No.: CE0003A), and the questionnaire was made available at the web-based survey platform LimeSurvey [60]. OPP sent this anonymous online self-report questionnaire to its members via e-mail and published it on its webpage. The questionnaire was also sent to the authors' professional institutions via their mailing lists and was made available via professional social media, such as LinkedIn. This procedure ensured that all psychologists registered at OPP (a mandatory requirement for practicing psychology in Portugal) were invited to take part in this study. The e-mail containing the questionnaire included the study's description and aims, followed by an informed consent form. If the person agreed to participate, a link gave them access to the questionnaire. The data were collected during April and May 2020, precisely at the peak of the Covid-19 pandemic, and during the lockdown period. Data were exported from LimeSurvey [60] into IBM SPSS Statistics 25 Commuter License [61] for analysis.

2.4. *Statistical Analysis*

Descriptive statistics (e.g., frequency distributions) were conducted for the sample characteristics (e.g., age, gender, educational and professional background)) and for the data pertaining both to the period before and during the COVID-19 pandemic. Data before the COVID-19 pandemic included aspects such as the use of digital tools in professional practice, professional experience with this type of tool, and adherence of clients to therapeutic activities based on digital technologies. During the COVID-19 lockdown, analyses considered the following aspects: maintenance of psychological support services, percentage of clients who have maintained the use of psychological counseling or therapy, frequency and duration of the therapeutic sessions, therapeutic adherence, therapeutic relationship, feedback from the clients, and results of the at-distance sessions.

Additionally, a thematic analysis for the open-type questions was performed on the open-ended questions. Two independent raters (A.G. and I.P.C.) have proceeded to the classification of the categories in each answer. Conflicts were solved by a third rater (A.R.D.).

To explore the correlations between professional experience, age and the selected outcome variables, point-biserial and Spearman correlations were performed.

3. Results

3.1. *ICTs in Psychological Counseling and Therapy before the COVID-19 Pandemic*

3.1.1. Use of ICTs in Psychological Counseling and Therapy

Regarding the use of digital technologies for providing at-distance psychological counseling and therapy before the COVID-19 pandemic, most (n = 63; 58.3%) had rarely or never used digital tools in clinical practice before the COVID-19 pandemic (Table 2).

The reasons pointed out by Portuguese psychologists for never or rarely (n = 63) having used digital technologies in psychological counseling and therapy were they considered it very impersonal (n = 28; 44.4%), inefficient (n = 18; 28.6%), ineffective (n = 10; 15.9%), not safe enough (n = 9; 14.3%) or ethical (n = 8; 12.7%), and for their lack of knowledge on how to apply these technologies in psychological counseling and therapy (n = 1; 1.6%). Under "Other", participants additionally shared that they did not feel the need to use these means of providing counseling and therapy before, that these means were not part of their institutions' policies, and that they preferred in-presence interventions.

Table 2. Use of digital information and communication technologies in psychological counseling before and during the COVID-19 pandemic.

	Before the COVID-19	*n* (%)	During the COVID-19 Confinement Period	*n* (%)
ICTs use (*n* = 108)	never	37 (34.3%)	yes (sessions continued)	91 (84.3%)
	rarely	26 (24.1%)	no (sessions discontinued during this period)	15 (15.7%)
	sometimes	26 (24.1%)		
	frequently	14 (13.0%)		
	always	5 (4.6%)		
Tools (*n* = 71 before) (*n* = 91 after)	video conferences	50 (70.4%)	video conference	71 (78.0%)
	telephone calls	41 (57.7%)	telephone calls	48 (52.7%)
	e-mails	31 (43.7%)	social networks	35 (38.5%)
	social networks	23 (32.4%)	e-mails	33 (36.3%)
	audio conferences	14 (19.7%)	audio conference	16 (17.6%)
	online intervention platforms	6 (8.5%)	smartphones/tablet apps	7 (7.7%)
	smartphones/tablet apps	6 (8.5%)	online intervention platforms	3 (3.3%)
	online forums	4 (5.6%)	chats	3 (3.3%)
	chats	3 (4.2%)	online forums	1 (1.1%)
	short-message services	2 (1.8%)	virtual rooms	1 (1.1%)
	virtual rooms	1 (0.9%)		
Devices (*n* = 71 before) (*n* = 91 after)	computer	62 (87.3%)	computer	80 (87.9%)
	telephone/smartphone	58 (81.7%)	telephone/smartphone	66 (72.5%)
	tablets	9 (12.7%)	tablets	9 (9.9%)
Psychologists' experiences/results (*n* = 71 before) (*n* = 91 after)	positive	37 (52.1%)	more or less the same	65 (71.4%)
	neither negative nor positive	21 (29.6%)	better results	4 (4.4%)
	very positive	13 (18.3%)	worse results	22 (24.2%)
	very negative or negative	0 (0%)		
Clients' involvement/adherence (*n* = 71 before) (*n* = 91 after)	moderate	28 (39.4%)	more or less the same	52 (57.1%)
	high	18 (25.4%)	decreased	24 (26.4%)
	low involvement	12 (16.9%)	improved	10 (11.0%)
	very low	7 (9.9%)	significantly decreased	5 (5.5%)
	very high	6 (8.5%)	significantly improved	0 (0.0%)

Table 2. *Cont.*

	Before the COVID-19	n (%)	During the COVID-19 Confinement Period	n (%)
Advantages ($n = 108$)	geographic flexibility	74 (68.5%)	geographic flexibility	73 (80.2%)
	scheduling flexibility	55 (50.9%)	scheduling flexibility	57 (62.6%)
	reaching new groups	36 (33.3%)	reaching new groups	30 (33.0%)
	easier access to some target-groups	28 (25.9%)	cost-benefit relationship	24 (26.4%)
	cost-benefit relationship	27 (25.0%)	easier access to some target-groups	21 (23.1%)
	new business areas	10 (9.3%)	new business areas	11 (12.1%)
	no advantages	12 (11.1%)	no advantages	2 (2.2%)
	other		other	
Challenges ($n = 108$)	establishing/maintaining the therapeutic relationship	67 (62.0%)	non-verbal communication	58 (63.7%)
	non-verbal communication	66 (61.1%)	privacy	36 (39.6%)
	therapeutic adherence	52 (48.1%)	establishing/maintaining the therapeutic relationship	34 (37.4%)
	client engagement	50 (46.3%)	session interruptions	31 (34.1%)
	privacy	35 (32.4%)	therapeutic adherence	22 (24.2%)
	session interruption	29 (26.9%)	some problems/topics	19 (20.9%)
	ethical concerns	23 (21.3%)	ethical concerns	19 (20.9%)
	misunderstandings difficulties approach some problems/topics	22 (20.4%)	patient engagement in the sessions	18 (19.8%)
	sessions' frequency	20 (18.5%)	other	
	lack of security	20 (18.5%)		
	establishment of boundaries	19 (17.6%)		
	time management	19 (17.6%)		
	no challenges	12 (11.1%)		
	other	4 (3.7%)		

3.1.2. Tools and Technological Devices Used

Among the Portuguese psychologists who used ICTs to provide at-distance psychological counseling and therapy (n = 71), the most often used tools were video conferences (n = 50; 70.4%), telephone calls (n = 41; 57.7%), e-mails (n = 31; 43.7%), and social networks (n = 23; 32.4%). Other tools used were audio conferences (n = 14; 19.7%), online intervention platforms (n = 6; 8.5%), smartphones and tablet apps (n = 6; 8.5%), online forums (n = 4; 5.6%), chats (n = 3; 4.2%), short-message services (n = 2; 1.8%), and virtual rooms (n = 1; 0.9%). Concerning the technological devices used for providing at-distance psychological counseling and therapy, the most frequently used device was a computer (n = 62; 87.3%), followed by a telephone/smartphone (n = 58; 81.7%) and by tablets (n = 9; 12.7%) (Table 2).

3.1.3. Psychologists' Perceptions about Their Experiences and about Clients' Adherence

Among the psychologists that used digital technologies in psychological counseling and therapy previously to the COVID-19 pandemic (n = 71), none considered their experiences with these tools to be negative or very negative. Nevertheless, 21 (of these 71) psychologists (29.6%) considered their experiences to be neither negative nor positive. Most of the respondents considered their experience with digital technologies to be either positive (n = 37; 52.1%) or very positive (n = 13; 18.3%). Regarding the involvement of their patients in the therapeutic activities that were delivered through digital technologies, most of the psychologists rated it as moderate (n = 28; 39.4%), followed by high (n = 18; 25.4%) and low involvement (n = 12; 16.9%). Only six psychologists (8.5%) considered their patients' involvement in this type of activities very high, and seven psychologists (9.9%) rated their patients' involvement as very low (Table 2).

3.1.4. Advantages and Challenges of ICTs Use

With regard to the advantages that Portuguese psychologists considered might be experienced or already were experienced through the use of ICTs in psychological counseling and therapy, geographic flexibility was the most frequently selected advantage (n = 74; 68.5%), followed by scheduling flexibility (n = 55; 50.9%), the possibility of them reaching new groups of people in need of psychological counseling and therapy (n = 36; 33.3%), and by their easier access to some target-groups, such as persons with disability, refugees, among others (n = 28; 25.9%). They added the cost–benefit relationship (n = 27; 25.0%) and the possibility of obtaining new business areas (n = 10; 9.3%). Twelve (11.1%) of the respondents considered that they have never benefitted, or will never benefit, from any advantage through the use of ICTs in psychological counseling and therapy.

On the contrary, through the analysis of the challenges that psychologists had already faced or were afraid of facing when using new ICTs in psychological counseling and therapy, the most frequently referred challenge was the difficulty in establishing and/or maintaining the therapeutic relationship (n = 67; 62.0%), followed by the lack of non-verbal communication (n = 66; 61.1%), reduced therapeutic adherence (n = 52; 48.1%), reduced client engagement in the sessions (n = 50; 46.3%), and reduced privacy (n = 35; 32.4%). Other challenges referred by the psychologists were the interruption of the sessions (n = 29; 26.9%), ethical concerns (n = 23; 21.3%), possible misunderstandings (n = 22; 20.4%), difficulties in therapeutically approaching some problems/topics (n = 20; 18.5%), the substantial decrease or increase of the sessions' frequency (n = 20; 18.5%), lack of security (n = 19; 17.6%), establishment of boundaries (n = 19; 17.6%), and time management (n = 12; 11.1%). Under the category "Other", they also mentioned technical problems. Four (3.7%) respondents considered to never have faced or feared to face challenges in the future related to the use of digital technologies in their professional practice (Table 2).

3.2. ICTs in Psychological Counseling and Therapy during the COVID-19 Pandemic

3.2.1. Use of ICTs in Psychological Counseling and Therapy

During the COVID-19 pandemic, and specifically during the lockdown period, only 17 (15.7%) of the 108 psychologists discontinued the provision of psychological counseling and therapy to their clients (Table 2). These psychologists reported that the main reasons for interrupting their professional activities were the suspension of activities on the part of the institution where they worked, activity suspension on the part of their clients for various reasons (e.g., considering themselves to be info-excluded populations or presenting digital illiteracy, financial difficulties, or sensing that the clinical setting is lacking), psychologists' own personal unavailability during this period (e.g., due to new family responsibilities), and considering that digital means were inadequate for the target population (i.e., children) or clinical condition (e.g., attention deficits) that they were treating. All the other psychologists ($n = 91$, 84.3%) were able to continue the sessions with their cases due to the use of ICTs.

3.2.2. Readiness for the Use of ICTs

Among the 91 psychologists who continued to provide at-distance psychological services, 71 (84.3%) previously read guidelines and other documents that support their at-distance psychological practice. The documents that these psychologists consulted the most were materials made available by the OPP (e.g., written material, videos, and webinars), guidelines from APA and from the International Psychoanalytical Association (IPA), scientific papers, and manuals about online therapeutic interventions (including the Therapy2.0 project).

Regarding additional cautionary procedures implemented by the psychologists for at-distance interventions, respondents referred the careful definition of rules and ethical limits, namely in terms of privacy, confidentiality, security, schedules, forms of contact, session duration and frequency, as well as how to proceed when unforeseen situations occur (e.g., technical failures such as problems with the internet connection, technology problems such as problems with the tools/equipment used, or interruptions). Caution about the type of software and the type of technology used were mentioned, also related with non-exposure of personal life, as well as the conditions of the physical space and the psychologist's personal appearance/presentation, and personal well-being. Psychologists also referred several precautions and procedures associated with the actual therapeutic process, namely regarding verbal and non-verbal communication (e.g., minimizing the occurrence of overlaps, interruptions, and misunderstandings), greater session structuration and directivity (which involved greater previous preparation for some of them), avoidance of emotional themes that require in-person support, which distance prevents, parent follow-up in sessions with children, and assessment of clients' level of comfort with the new format.

3.2.3. Tools and Technological Devices

When focusing on the technological tools used to provide at-distance psychological counseling and therapy, video conference was the most frequently used ($n = 71$; 78.0%), followed by phone calls ($n = 48$; 52.7%), social networks ($n = 35$; 38.5%), e-mail ($n = 33$; 36.3%), audio conference ($n = 16$, 17.6%), smartphones and tablet apps ($n = 7$; 7.7%), online intervention platforms ($n = 3$; 3.3%), chats ($n = 3$; 3.3%), online forums ($n = 1$; 1.1%), and virtual rooms ($n = 1$; 1.1%). Computers were the most frequently used technological device to provide psychological services during the COVID-19 pandemic ($n = 80$; 87.9%), followed by telephones/smartphones ($n = 66$; 72.5%) and tablets ($n = 9$; 9.9%) (Table 2).

3.2.4. Impact of the COVID-19 on the Psychologists' Practice

Most of the respondents ($n = 53$; 58.2%) have continued to provide their services to most of their clients, i.e., twenty-seven (29.7%) of the psychologists continued to provide counseling and therapy to between 51% and 75% of their clients, and 26 psychologists (28.6%) to between 76% and 100% of their clients. However, for 23 psychologists (25.3%), the number of clients decreased to a range of between 0% and 25%, and for another 15 psychologists (16.5%) that number diminished to a range of between 26% and 50%. These psychologists referred, as main reasons for these reductions, low client adherence, lack of client's necessary privacy, confidentiality and non-interruption conditions at home, the fact that clients preferred in-presence contacts (considering such forms of intervention to be more effective than, or feeling uncomfortable with, the new format), had financial difficulties, had difficulties managing the new routines (including caring for the children at home), and lacked the technological means for at-distance sessions. In some cases, the client's condition was stable, and the therapeutic process had come to an end, or it was requiring no immediate sessions.

Considering the frequency of the counseling and therapy sessions among the clients who continued to use this service, a small majority of the psychologists (n = 48; 52.7%) referred that their clients have maintained the previous frequency, but 29 psychologists (31.9%) reported a decrease in the number of sessions, and six (6.6%) reported a significant decrease in that number. Despite that, seven psychologists (7.7%) reported an increase in the number of sessions during the COVID-19 pandemic, and one (1.1%) reported a significant increase. The same pattern was found for the duration of the counseling and therapy sessions, with 55 (60.4%) psychologists reporting a maintenance of the duration of each session, 20 (22.0%) reporting a decrease, and 4 (4.4%) reporting a significant decrease in the duration of the sessions. Nevertheless, 12 psychologists (13.2%) stated that the duration of the counseling and therapy sessions increased during the COVID-19 pandemic.

3.2.5. Psychologists' Perception about Their Experiences and about Clients' Adherence

Regarding the results of the current therapeutic sessions, when compared to former in-presence sessions, most psychologists (n = 65; 71.6%) considered the results to be more of less the same, four (4.4%) reported obtaining better results with at-distance sessions, and 22 (24.2%) considered that at-distance sessions have yielded worse results than in-presence sessions. Similarly, from the points of views that clients shared with their psychologists, at-distance and in-person sessions were more or less the same (n = 71; 78.0%). Six (6.6%) of the respondents reported receiving better feedback (i.e., the clients preferred the online sessions), and one (1.1%) received much better feedback. Even so, 13 (14.3%) psychologists received worse feedback from their clients about this type of intervention.

In what concerns therapeutic adherence to the ICT sessions, the majority of psychologists considered it to be more or less the same during the COVID-19 pandemic, comparing to the pre-COVID sessions (n = 52; 57.1%), and 10 psychologists (11.0%) reported an improvement. Nevertheless, other psychologists reported a decrease (n = 24; 26.4%) or a significant decrease (n = 5; 5.5%) in the therapeutic adherence of their clients (Table 2). The vast majority of respondents considered that the therapeutic relationship between the psychologists and their clients was maintained (n = 77; 84.6%), with only three (3.3%) psychologists reporting an improvement in those relationships. However, 11 (12.1%) psychologists considered that those relationships have worsened during this period.

3.2.6. Advantages and Challenges of the ICTs Use

Regarding the advantages that Portuguese psychologists viewed as associated with their current use of new ICTs in psychological counseling and therapy, geographic flexibility was the most frequently selected (n = 73; 80.2%), followed by scheduling flexibility (n = 57; 62.6%) and the possibility of reaching new groups of persons in need of psychological counseling and therapy (n = 30; 33.0%). Other advantages that they mentioned were the cost–benefit relationship (n = 24; 26.4%), the easier access of psychologists to some target groups, such as persons with disability and refugees, among others (n = 21; 23.1%), and the possibility of obtaining new business areas (n = 11; 12.1%). Under the category "Other", they further mentioned the possibility of providing secure interventions in the current COVID-19 pandemic context, which ensured the possibility of maintaining the interventions. Only two (2.2%) respondents considered that at-distance psychological counseling and therapy does not offer any advantages.

Through the analysis of the challenges that psychologists currently face when they provide at-distance psychological counseling and therapy sessions, the most frequently referred difficulty was lack of non-verbal communication ($n = 58$; 63.7%), followed by reduced privacy ($n = 36$; 39.6%), the difficulty in establishing and/or maintaining the therapeutic relationship ($n = 34$; 37.4%), session interruptions ($n = 31$; 34.1%), reduced therapeutic adherence ($n = 22$; 24.2%), difficulties in approaching some problems/topics therapeutically ($n = 19$; 20.9%), ethical concerns ($n = 19$; 20.9%), and a reduction in patient engagement in the sessions ($n = 18$; 19.8%) (Table 2). Other challenges that counsellors referred to (under the category "Other") were the establishment of boundaries ($n = 17$; 18.7%), the significant decrease or increase in session frequency ($n = 16$; 14.8%), the time management of the sessions ($n = 15$; 16.5%), possible misunderstandings ($n = 14$; 15.4%), and lack of security ($n = 10$; 11.0%). Under this category, they additionally mentioned technology problems (e.g., equipment adjustments) and technical failures (e.g., internet connection). Five respondents (5.5%) did not report any difficulty or challenge in providing at-distance psychological counseling and therapy.

In Table 2, the psychologists' practices are presented pre- and post-COVID-19 for easy comparison of the main results described previously.

3.3. *Variables Associated with Psychologist' Attitudes and Practices*

Significant point-biserial correlation coefficient were positive between the aspect "continue to provide psychological counseling to customers regularly" and years of professional experience, $r_{pb} = 0.296$, $p = 0.002$. Significant correlations were negative between "frequency of psychological counseling sessions" and both years of professional experience, $r_s = -0.341$, $p < 0.001$, and age, $r_s = -0.229$, $p = 0.017$. The aspect, "duration of psychological counseling sessions" also displayed a significant negative correlation with age, $r_s = -0.209$, $p = 0.030$. Thus, regarding respondents' professional experience, psychologists with more years of experience maintained their professional services during the COVID-19 pandemic more than professionals with less years of experience. Nevertheless, the frequency of the sessions decreased for the professionals who had more years of professional experience. Regarding age, older psychologists reported a decrease in session frequency and duration. No significant results were found in any of the other variables analyzed.

4. Discussion

This study aimed to explore psychologists' attitudes and practices related with the use of ICTs before and during the COVID-19 pandemic lockdown period, for identification of the main changes that have occurred in the provision of counseling and therapy. The impact of age and years of professional experience on the use of ICTs was also inspected.

In this study, psychologists' use of ICTs in their professional activity before the COVID-19 pandemic is in accordance with the literature, namely in terms of previous experience of their use, tools, devices, professionals' satisfaction with their use, advantages, and perceived challenges. These results reproduce those by Mendes-Santos (2020), in which only 29.6% of the inquired Portuguese psychologists admitted to having used digital technologies in their professional practice. The results of the present study also showed that most Portuguese psychologists had never or rarely used digital technologies as a means of delivering psychological counseling and therapy before the COVID-19 pandemic [6]. There is also a high degree of similarity between the tools most frequently used in our study and the tools used, the resources that psychologists most recommend to their clients (e.g., telephone calls, e-mails, video conferences, social networks, and apps) [6], and the most used devices (e.g., computers and smart phones) reported in other research (e.g., [14]). Additionally, according to previous studies, accessibility/geographic flexibility, convenience/(scheduling) flexibility, and cost-effectiveness/low cost are amongst the most recognized advantages of using ICTs (e.g., [6,55]). Regarding the disadvantages, the major challenges in this study, pertaining to ethical concerns and to the difficulty in establishing and/or maintaining the therapeutic relationship due to different reasons, were also identified in the literature [6,8,10,14,26,55–58].

The analysis of the reasons given for not using ICTs before the COVID-19 pandemic revealed that lack of knowledge and training about the correct use of ICTs was particularly relevant, which might explain professionals' concerns about efficiency, effectiveness, and ethical issues. These same factors were associated with more negative attitudes toward the use of technologies in a previous study [6]. Training thus seems to be a necessary step in order to increase the use of ICTs. However, before the COVID-19 pandemic, available training was scarce, perhaps also because the professionals themselves perceived the use of ICTs as unnecessary, as they indicated in this study.

The emergence of the COVID-19 pandemic brought about relevant changes in the use of ICTs. Barriers to their use by both professionals and clients have been reduced, as the availability of information about their use in various formats has increased. The percentage of psychologists who have adopted ICTs in their practice during the lockdown period was very high in this study, and the vast majority of respondents were able to maintain their professional activity due to the inclusion of these means in their practice. This shows an enormous capacity of adaptation and flexibility, both on the psychologists' and clients' parts. This phenomenon was observed not only in Portugal but in other countries too, such as the United States, where the provision of at-distance psychological services has been raised from 7.07% to 85.53% [62]. Additionally, other health services are also adopting the online modalities, namely in medicine [63,64], with the professionals reporting positive perceptions regarding the telehealth services. However, the implementation of ICTs in such a short period of time leads to questions about the conditions under which they were implemented.

Our results showed that more than half of the psychologists have read about the use of ICTs, and some had already used these tools, even if not exclusively, in their professional practice before, which is consistent with a previous study [6]. They additionally identified a number of materials that were informative of at-distance psychological practice. These materials also contained information on additional care that needs to be adopted in at-distance psychological monitoring sessions and that is different from the procedures that these professionals might have adopted in the use of digital technologies in the context of their social relationships.

Their concerns about web-based session pertained to a diversity of aspects considered to be critical in the e-Health literature (e.g., the clear definition of rules and ethical limits) that can be different from face-to-face services [13]. However, it is noteworthy that most professionals have not offered any input on any additional measures that they might have adopted (e.g., use end-to-end encrypted technology), nor has it been possible, within the scope of this work, to identify how psychologists were capable of responding effectively to the new requirements and specificities that they reported they have adopted. Despite the great availability of webinars and the training and specialty documents made available during this period (e.g., [13]) by accredited entities, often free of charge, little is known about how such information transfer to the professional contexts.

This study provides important information in that regard by confirming the pertinence and usefulness of such materials among the psychologists. In general, the tools and devices used before the lockdown period were the same that were used during the COVID-19 pandemic, although there was an increase in the use of several of them during the COVID-19 pandemic (e.g., video conferences, computers, and telephones/smartphones). The primary use of computers and smartphones in this study is in line with the findings from previous research, although psychologists in our study used mostly video conference and telephone calls, whereas e-mail was the most widely used tool in a previous study [14].

Psychologists who do use ICTs in their practice tended to report a positive or very positive experience regarding the use of these online technologies in counseling and therapy. Similarly, a study focused on the attitudes of psychotherapists towards online therapy during the COVID-19 pandemic have also found a positive attitude of the professionals with regard to this therapy modality [65]. Research has recognized several advantages associated with using ICTs in such contexts, and participants in our sample identified equivalent advantages [8–11,13,14,55]. Their reported advantages were the same before and during the lockdown period, although they added a new advantage during the lockdown period, i.e., the possibility to conduct secure interventions. The number of professionals who did not see any advantage in the use of ICTs after the pandemic decreased to a practically residual value. However, the implementation of these modalities was not without difficulties. Both before and during the pandemic, psychologists identified a set of challenges in the adoption of DICTS in professional practice. Some decreased during the pandemic, possibly due to the professionals' increased experience (e.g., establishing/maintaining the therapeutic adherence). However, others were particularly worsened during the period of mandatory lockdown (e.g., loss of privacy and risk of interruption).

Although generally positive, the results regarding psychologists' experiences/results and clients' adherence to therapeutic activities based on digital technologies were variable, as reported in previous studies (e.g., [36–54] and [6,55] respectively). It is important in the future to understand which ingredients explain this variability, both in relation to individual and to disorder aspects, and to work with the group of clients who have failed to adhere to the new format. From the limitations identified in this study, some clients might benefit from better advertisement of this type of services and of the scientific evidence of its effects, together with the possibility of receiving a reduction in the price of the services provided. Increasing clients' digital literacy will also contribute to their adherence to web-based interventions. This is already happening among the new generations, whose members are already known as digital natives [14,15], but it is still difficult when working with specific populations, such as the elderly and people that live in rural areas, or when performing some psychological acts, such as psychological assessment and rehabilitation practices [62]. Additionally, other challenges might be more difficult to overcome, such as the sense that an adequate therapeutic setting is lacking. This aspect has been particularly exacerbated by the situation of mandatory lockdown that has brought together all who live in the same physical space, namely risking privacy.

Regarding the correlations between the professionals' characteristics (i.e., age and years of professional experience) and the use of ICTs in professional practice, the results showed that were the professionals with more professional experience who presented greater maintenance of psychological support services, but less frequently. However, because it was also the professionals with more professional experience who presented greater maintenance of psychological support services, the decrease in the frequency of the sessions reported by them might have been an intentional procedure to help their own and their clients' adaptation to the new format.

The results failed to show a correlation between age and the use of ICTs, except for frequency and duration of the therapeutic sessions, which was significantly shorter for the oldest than for the youngest psychologists. The decrease in these aspects in the group of older psychologists from the pre- to the during-lockdown period could be possibly explained by the greater discomfort that these professionals experienced with the use of ICTs. The influence of the personal characteristics of the professionals in their attitude towards online psychological counseling was also reported in another study [65], with the psychotherapists who had previous experience with online psychotherapy, who thought that the patients they attend to had positive experiences in this modality, that adopted cognitive behavioral therapy in their practices (in comparison to psychodynamic therapists), and that lives in North America (in comparison to Europe) exhibiting a more positive attitude towards online psychotherapy.

This work has some limitations, namely the sample size and the use of a questionnaire that has not been previously validated to study the attitudes of psychologists toward ICTs (namely toward web-based interventions). However, the data collection took place during the period of absolutely unique and exceptional sanitary measures to prevent the pandemic dispersion of the coronavirus SARS-CoV-2, which causes COVID-19. To understand the impact of these circumstances on professionals' practice is of the utmost relevance, despite the fact that these same circumstances have limited the time to conduct the data collection and the availability of participants in the study. Still, the collaboration of the OPP in this scenario, advertising the study and making the questionnaire available to all its members, contributed to ensure national representation of the participants. The process of adapting an existing instrument, namely obtaining the respective authorizations, would require an extended period of time that would risk missing this window of opportunity. Instead, the questionnaire was adapted from an instrument that was previously used by the authors and that was tested in a pilot-study. Future studies could focus on exploring the reasons that seem to be interfering either negatively or positively with clients' adherence to, and satisfaction with, ICT sessions, so that personalized healthcare services can be provided and tailored to the specificities of each case.

5. Conclusions

It is widely known that the COVID-19 pandemic and associated restrictive measures of physical contact have significantly changed many professional activities. The current work has contributed to our understanding of that impact in the practice of psychology and psychotherapy, in close relation with the use of ICTs. Awareness of these changes can guide future professional practice by allowing the replication of the best practices and experiences shared by the psychologists during the period of maximum lockdown. It can also help to overcome the main difficulties and limitations experienced, for example, by guiding future training in this area, stimulating the creation of guidelines for ICT-based professional practice in different countries, and of measures to promote knowledge of and adherence to these guidelines that are becoming increasingly available.

Author Contributions: Conceptualization, A.R.D. and F.B.; methodology, A.R.D. and A.G.; formal analysis, A.G.; investigation, A.R.D. and A.G.; resources, A.R.D.; data curation, A.R.D.; writing—original draft preparation, A.R.D. and A.G.; writing—review and editing, I.P.C.; visualization, A.R.D. and A.G.; supervision, F.B.; project administration, A.R.D. and F.B.; funding acquisition, A.R.D. All authors have read and agreed to the published version of the manuscript.

Acknowledgments: The authors wish to thank Ordem dos Psicólogos Portugueses (T.N: the Portuguese Psychologists Association) for advertising the present study to its members.

Appendix A

The Use of New Digital Information and Communication Technologies in Psychological Counseling during the COVID-19 Pandemic

This project is conducted by researchers at the Center for Rehabilitation Research of the School of Health, Polytechnic Institute of Porto, and at the Laboratory of Neuropsychophysiology of the Faculty of Psychology and Education Sciences, University of Porto. Its main goal is to study the use of digital technologies in psychological counseling during the COVID-19 pandemic (SARS-CoV-2) in Portugal. To attain this goal, a questionnaire has been developed, targeting psychologists who are effective members of the Portuguese Psychologists Association.

Although the completion of the questionnaire is anonymous, some socio-demographic and professional data will be requested, as well as answers to closed- and open-ended questions. These questions focus on the use of digital technologies in psychological counseling. Please read each question carefully. It is important that your answers are sincere.

If you accept to participate in this study, please click on "Next" to proceed to the informed consent.

Informed Consent

All data will be collected and processed in an anonymous and confidential way, so you will never be asked for your name, professional number, or other personal data that could identify you. The data will be used for research purposes and will never be analysed at the individual level. Your participation is completely voluntary, and your contribution is very important for us, to better understand the role of digital technologies in confinement situations like the one we are going through now. Although you can quit answering the survey at any time without any consequences, we really appreciate your collaboration.

If you want to clarify any question or if you need more information, please contact: Andreia Geraldo (andreiageraldo.psic@gmail.com).

We appreciate your cooperation.

Andreia Geraldo, researcher

Artemisa R Dores, responsible for the project

If you intend to participate in this study, select the option below to proceed to the survey.

I declare that I have read the information above, have become aware of the research aims, and agree to participate in this study.

Socio-demographic and professional data

1. Gender:

    Man
    Woman
    Other

2. Age (years):
3. Education:

    Graduation
    Master's
    PhD

4. Year of completion of the course [please consider the first degree that have allowed you to practice Psychology in Portugal (e.g., Pre-Bologna graduation; Post-Bologna Master's Degree)]:
5. Number of years of professional experience [please count from the moment you started the practice of Psychology services]:
6. Distrit(s) in which you practice Psychology:

    Aveiro
    Beja
    Braga
    Bragança
    Castelo Branco
    Coimbra
    Évora
    Faro
    Guarda
    Leiria
    Lisboa
    Portalegre
    Porto
    Santarém
    Setúbal
    Viana do Castelo
    Vila Real
    Viseu

7. Are you a specialist in Clinical and Health Psychology accredited by the Portuguese Psychologists Association?

   Yes
   No (Note: In case the answer above is Yes, the next question appears)
   Do you have an advanced specialty recognized by the Portuguese Psychologists Association?
   Yes
   No
   If yes, which one(s) of them? (you can choose several)
   Neuropsychology
   Psychogerontology
   Justice Psychology
   Sports Psychology
   Psychotherapy
   Sexology
   Other

8. Select the age group(s) of the population your work with most often (you can choose several):

   Children
   Adolescents
   Adults
   Elderly

9. Indicate which psychological disorders you assess and intervene most often (you can choose several):

   Neurodevelopment disorders
   Mood disorders
   Anxiety disorders
   Personality disorders
   Substance-related disorders and addictive behaviours
   Sleep disorders
   Neurocognitive disorders
   Other(s): (please specify)

   Use of Digital Technologies in Psychological Counselling We ask you to consider your entire professional career as a psychologist, prior to the confinement measures imposed by the declaration of the State of Emergency in Portugal, to answer the following questions.

10. Have you used digital tools to conduct at-distance psychological counselling?

   Never
   Rarely
   Sometimes
   Often
   Always

   (Note: If the previous answer was Never or Rarely, the next question appears. If the answer is no, after responding to 10.1, the participants go directly to question no. 15)

10.1. Which are the main reasons for you having never or rarely used this kind of tools?

I don't know how to apply them in my work
I don't consider them efficient (i.e., the adequate use of the necessary resources for the intervention/treatment)
I don't consider them effective (i.e., the ability of a given program to produce benefit when applied under ideal conditions)
I find them very impersonal
I don't consider them safe enough
I don't consider them ethical enough
I find them very expensive
Other(s): (please specify)

11. Which tool(s) have you already used in at-distance psychological counselling?

E-mail
Audio-conference (e.g., Skype, Facetime, Zoom)
Videoconference (e.g., Skype, Facetime, Zoom)
Online platforms
Online forum
Chat
Social networks (e.g., Facebook, Twitter, WhatsApp, Instagram, LinkedIn)
Smartphone and tablet apps
Virtual rooms (e.g., Second Life)
Telephone calls
Other(s): (please specify)

12. Which device(s) have you already used to maintain at-distance psychological counselling?

Computer
Tablet
Telephone/smartphone
Other(s): (please specify)

13. How do you rate your experience using this type of tools for conducting at-distance psychological counselling before the imposition of confinement measures by the declaration of the national state of emergency?

Very negative
Negative
Neither negative nor positive
Positive
Very positive

14. How do you rate your clients' involvement in therapeutic activities that use this kind of tools before the imposition of confinement measures by the declaration of the national state of emergency?

Very low
Low
Moderate
High
Very high

15. What are the advantages that you have already benefited from, or that you consider you could have benefited from, by using this type of tools in psychological counselling, before the imposition of confinement measures by the declaration of the national state of emergency? Geographic flexibility, both for professionals and clients (i.e., they can interact from any location)

    Time flexibility
    Cost-benefit ratio
    To be able to reach new groups of people in need of psychological counselling
    Easy access to some target groups (e.g., people with anxiety, people with disabilities, refugees)
    New business areas
    None
    Other(s): (please specify)

16. Which are the challenges that you have faced or feared to face with the use of this kind of tools in psychological counselling processes before the imposition of the confinement measures by the declaration of the national state of emergency?

    Reduced therapeutic adherence
    Difficulty in establishing or maintaining the therapeutic relationship
    Significant decrease or increase in the frequency of the sessions
    Temporal management of the sessions
    Setting boundaries
    Interruption of the sessions
    Less client involvement in and commitment to the session
    Lack of non-verbal communication
    (Possible) misunderstandings
    Difficulty in therapeutically approaching a problem/topic
    Lack of security
    Reduced privacy
    Ethical concerns
    None
    Other(s): (please specify)

    Considering the challenges imposed to all psychologists by the COVID-19 pandemic situation (SARS-CoV-2), we ask you to answer the following questions according to your current professional practices.

17. Have you continued to provide psychological counselling to your clients regularly?

    Yes
    No

    (Note: If the answer to the previous question is no, the next question appears, and the participant has finished his/her questionnaire)

    17.1. Which are the reasons that have led you to suspend your professional activity?

18. Have you consulted any supporting documents or guidelines for at-distance psychological counselling or psychological counselling in crisis and catastrophe situations?

    Yes
    No

    (Note: If the answer to the previous question is yes, the next question appears)

18.1. Please insert the name and/or link of the document(s) you consulted.

19. Currently, which percentage of your clients do you continue to monitor regularly when compared to the period before the declaration of the state of emergency in Portugal?

    Between 0% and 25%
    Between 26% and 50%
    Between 51% and 75%
    Between 76% and 100%

20. If there was a significant reduction in the percentage of clients that you regularly monitor, which are the main reasons that you identify for this to have happened?
21. The frequency of the psychological counselling sessions with each client that you continue to monitor

    Diminished a lot
    Diminished
    Remained the same
    Increased
    Increased a lot

22. The duration of the psychological counselling with each client that you continue to monitor

    Diminished a lot
    Diminished
    Remained the same
    Increased
    Increased a lot

23. Which tool(s) do you use to provide regular at-distance psychological counselling to your clients?

    E-mail
    Audio-conference (e.g., Skype, Facetime, Zoom)
    Video-conference (e.g., Skype, Facetime, Zoom)
    Online platforms
    Online forum
    Chat
    Social networks (e.g., Facebook, Twitter, WhatsApp, Instagram, LinkedIn)
    Smartphone and tablet apps
    Virtual rooms (e.g., Second Life)
    Telephone calls
    Other(s): (please specify)

24. Which device(s) have you already used to maintain at-distance psychological counselling?

    Computer
    Tablet
    Telephone/smartphone
    Other(s): (please specify)

25. How do you rate the therapeutic adherence of your clients currently, when compared to in-presence sessions?

    Much smaller

Smaller
More or less the same
Greater
Much greater

26. How do you rate the therapeutic relationship with your clients currently, when compared to in-presence sessions?

Much worse
Worse
More or less the same
Better
Much better

27. How do you rate the results of each therapeutic session currently, when compared to in-presence sessions?

Much worse
Worse
More or less the same
Better
Much better

28. How do you rate the feedback of your clients, when compared to in-presence sessions?

Much worse
Worse
More or less the same
Better
Much better

29. In case you consider that you have adopted some additional precautions in at-distance psychological counselling, when compared to those you adopt in relation to the use of digital technologies in the context of your social relationships, please indicate them.
30. What are the advantages that you identify in at-distance psychological counselling? Geographic flexibility, both for professionals and clients (i.e., they can interact from any location)

Time flexibility
Cost-benefit ratio
To be able to reach new groups of people in need of psychological counselling
Easy access to some target groups (e.g., people with anxiety, people with disabilities, refugees)
New business areas
Other(s): (please specify)

31. Which are the difficulties that you face in promoting at-distance psychological counselling sessions?

Reduced therapeutic adherence
Difficulty in establishing or maintaining the therapeutic relationship
Significant changes in the frequency of the sessions
Temporal management of the sessions
Setting boundaries
Interruption of the sessions

Less client involvement in and commitment to the session
Lack of non-verbal communication
(Possible) misunderstandings
Difficulty in therapeutically approaching a problem/topic
Lack of security
Reduced privacy
Ethical concerns
Other(s): (please specify)

32. What are the difficulties that are reported by your clients in relation to maintaining at-distance psychological counselling?

Thank you for your collaboration.

References

1. An Early View of the Economic Impact of the Pandemic in 5 Charts. International Monetary Fund IMFBlog. Available online: https://blogs.imf.org/2020/04/06/an-early-view-of-the-economic-impact-of-the-pandemic-in-5-charts/ (accessed on 2 May 2020).
2. How the Economy Will Look after the Coronavirus Pandemic: The Pandemic Will Change the Economic and Financial Order Forever. Available online: https://foreignpolicy.com/2020/04/15/how-the-economy-will-look-after-the-coronavirus-pandemic/ (accessed on 2 May 2020).
3. Mühleisen, M. The long and short of the digital revolution. *Financ Dev.* **2018**, *55*, 5–8.
4. Diário da República Eletrónico. (DRE; 18 March 2020). Decreto do Presidente da República n.º 14-A/2020. Available online: https://dre.pt/web/guest/home/-/dre/130399862/details/maximized (accessed on 12 June 2020).
5. WHO. *Fifty-Eighth World Health Assembly: Resolutions and Decisions Annex*; WHO: Geneva, Switzerland, 2005; pp. 108–109.
6. Mendes-Santos, C.; Weiderpass, E.; Santana, R.; Andersson, G. Portuguese Psychologists' attitudes towards internet interventions: An exploratory cross-sectional study. *JMIR Ment. Health* **2020**, *7*, e16817. [CrossRef] [PubMed]
7. Andersson, G. Internet-delivered psychological treatments. *Annu. Rev. Clin. Psychol.* **2016**, *12*, 157–179. [CrossRef] [PubMed]
8. Andersson, G.; Titov, N. Advantages and limitations of Internet-based interventions for common mental disorders. *World Psychiatry* **2014**, *13*, 4–11. [CrossRef] [PubMed]
9. Carlbring, P.; Andersson, G. Internet and psychological treatment. How well can they be combined? *Comput. Hum. Behav.* **2006**, *22*, 545–553. [CrossRef]
10. Schröder, J.; Berger, T.; Westermann, S.; Klein, J.P.; Moritz, S. Internet interventions for depression: New developments. *Dialogues Clin. Neurosci.* **2016**, *18*, 203–212.
11. Wolvers, M.; Bruggeman-Everts, F.Z.; Van der Lee, M.L.; Van de Schoot, R.; Vollenbroek-Hutten, M.M. Effectiveness, mediators, and effect predictors of internet interventions for chronic cancer-related fatigue: The design and an analysis plan of a 3-armed randomized controlled trial. *JMIR Res. Protoc.* **2015**, *4*, e77. [CrossRef]
12. OPP. Parecer 21/CEOPP/2015 da Ordem dos Psicólogos Portugueses (OPP). [Document 21/CEOPP/2015 of the OPP]. Available online: https://www.ordemdospsicologos.pt/ficheiros/documentos/p_21_intervena_aao_aa_disntaancia.pdf (accessed on 3 May 2020).
13. OPP. Linhas de Orientação para a Prática Profissional OPP: Prestação de Serviços de Psicologia Mediados por Tecnologias da Informação e da Comunicação (TIC). [Guidelines for Professional Practice OPP: Provision of Psychology Services Mediated by Information and Communication Technologies (ICT)]. Available online: https://www.ordemdospsicologos.pt/ficheiros/documentos/linhasorientacao_prestacaoservicos_opp_1.pdf (accessed on 15 May 2020).
14. Dores, A.R.; Barbosa, F.; Silva, R. Chegar mais perto dos que estão longe: Therapy 2.0 [Getting Closer to Those Who Are Far: Therapy 2.0]. *Rev. Estud. Investig. Psicol. Educ.* **2017**. [CrossRef]

15. Drda-Kühn, K.; Dores, A.R.; Schlenk, E. Online interventions: Counteracting the exclusion of young people in counselling and therapy. In *Digital Diversity Bildung und Lernen im Kontext Gesellschaftlicher Transformationen*; Angenent, A., Heidkamp, B., Kergel, D., Eds.; Springer: Wiesbaden, Germany, 2019; pp. 321–330. [CrossRef]
16. Andersson, G.; Cuijpers, P. Internet-based and other computerized psychological treatments for adult depression: A meta-analysis. *Cogn. Behav. Ther.* **2009**, *38*. [CrossRef]
17. Barak, A.; Hen, L.; Boniel-Nissim, M.; Shapira, N.A. A comprehensive review and a meta-analysis of the effectiveness of internet-based psychotherapeutic interventions. *J. Technol. Hum. Serv.* **2008**, *26*, 109–160. [CrossRef]
18. Dowling, M.; Rickwood, D. Online counseling and therapy formental health problems: A systematic review of individual synchronous interventions using chat. *J. Technol. Hum. Serv.* **2013**, *31*, 1–21. [CrossRef]
19. Olthuis, J.V.; Watt, M.C.; Bailey, K.; Hayden, J.A.; Stewart, S.H. Therapist-supported internet cognitive behavioural therapy for anxiety disorders in adults. *Cochrane Database Syst. Rev.* **2016**, *3*. [CrossRef] [PubMed]
20. Richards, D.; Richardson, T. Computer-based psychological treatments for depression: A systematic review and meta-analysis. *Clin. Psychol. Rev.* **2012**, *32*, 329–342. [CrossRef]
21. Richards, D.; Viganó, N. Online counseling: A narrative and critical review of the. Literature. *J. Clin. Psychol.* **2013**, *69*, 994–1011. [CrossRef] [PubMed]
22. Topooco, N.; Riper, H.; Araya, R.; Berking, M.; Brunn, M.; Chevreul, K.; Kleiboer, A. Attitudes towards digital treatment for depression: A European stakeholder survey. *Internet Interven.* **2017**, *8*, 1–9. [CrossRef] [PubMed]
23. Schuster, R.; Pokorny, R.; Berger, T.; Topooco, N.; Laireiter, A.R. The advantages and disadvantages of online and blended therapy: Survey study amongst licensed psychotherapists in Austria. *J. Med. Internet Res.* **2018**, *20*, e11007. [CrossRef]
24. Mora, L.; Jeffrey, N.; Chaplin, W. Psychologist treatment recommendations for Internetbased therapeutic interventions. *Comput. Hum. Behav.* **2008**, *24*, 3052–3062. [CrossRef]
25. Wangberg, S.C.; Gammon, D.; Spitznogle, K. In the eyes of the beholder: Exploring psychologists' attitudes towards and use of e-therapy in Norway. *Cyberpsychol. Behav.* **2007**, *10*, 418–423. [CrossRef] [PubMed]
26. Perle, J.G.; Langsam, L.C.; Randel, A.; Lutchman, S.; Levine, A.B.; Odland, A.P.; Marker, C.D. Attitudes toward psychological telehealth: Current and future clinical psychologists' opinions of internet-based interventions. *J. Clin. Psychol.* **2013**, *69*, 100–113. [CrossRef]
27. Vigerland, S.; Ljótsson, B.; Gustafsson, F.B.; Hagert, S.; Thulin, U.; Andersson, G.; Serlachius, E. Attitudes towards the use of computerized cognitive behavior therapy (cCBT) with children and adolescents: A survey among Swedish mental health professionals. *Internet Interv.* **2014**, *1*, 111–117. [CrossRef]
28. Schröder, J.; Berger, T.; Meyer, B.; Lutz, W.; Hautzinger, M.; Späth, C.; Moritz, S. Attitudes towards internet interventions among psychotherapists and individuals with mild to moderate depression symptoms. *Cognit. Ther. Res.* **2017**, *41*, 745–756. [CrossRef]
29. Lamela, D.; Neves, F.R.P. O Efeito da Prática Profissional Baseada na Evidência Nas Atitudes dos Psicólogos Face à Intervenção Psicológica Eletrónica. Master's Thesis, Universidade Lusófona, Porto, Portugal, 2017.
30. Simms, D.; Gibson, K.; O'Donnell, S. To Use or Not to Use: Clinicians' Perceptions of Telemental Health. *Can. Psychol. Psychol. Can.* **2011**, *52*, 41–51. [CrossRef]
31. Bruno, R.; Abbott, J.-A.M. Australian health professionals' attitudes toward and frequency of use of internet supported psychological interventions. *Int. J. Ment. Health* **2015**, *44*, 107–123. [CrossRef]
32. Hadjiconstantinou, M.; Byrne, J.; Bodicoat, D.H.; Robertson, N.; Eborall, H.; Khunti, K.; Davies, M.J. Do web-based interventions improve well-being in type 2 diabetes? A systematic review and meta-analysis. *J. Med. Internet Res.* **2016**, *18*, e270. [CrossRef]
33. Agboola, S.O.; Ju, W.; Elfiky, A.; Kvedar, J.C.; Jethwani, K. The Effect of technology-based interventions on pain, depression, and quality of life in patients with cancer: A systematic review of randomized controlled trials. *J. Med. Internet Res.* **2015**, *17*, e65. [CrossRef] [PubMed]
34. Kuijpers, W.; Groen, W.G.; Aaronson, N.K.; van Harten, W.H. A systematic review of web-based interventions for patient empowerment and physical activity in chronic diseases: Relevance for cancer survivors. *J. Med. Internet Res.* **2013**, *15*, e37. [CrossRef] [PubMed]

35. Loucas, C.E.; Fairburn, C.G.; Whittington, C.; Pennant, M.E.; Stockton, S.; Kendall, T. E-therapy in the treatment and prevention of eating disorders: A systematic review and meta-analysis. *Behav. Res. Ther.* **2014**, *63*, 122–131. [CrossRef] [PubMed]
36. Andersson, G.; Paxling, B.; Roch-Norlund, P.; Östman, G.; Norgren, A.; Almlöv, J.; Carlbring, P. Internet-based psychodynamic versus cognitive behavioral guided self-help for generalized anxiety disorder: A randomized controlled trial. *Psychother. Psychosom.* **2012**, *81*, 344–355. [CrossRef]
37. Hedman, E.; Ljótsson, B.; Rück, C.; Bergström, J.; Andersson, G.; Kaldo, V.; El Alaoui, S. Effectiveness of Internet-based cognitive behaviour therapy for panic disorder in routine psychiatric care. *Acta Psychiatr. Scand.* **2013**, *128*, 457–467. [CrossRef]
38. Mansson, K.N.T.; Frick, A.; Boraxbekk, C.J.; Marquand, A.F.; Williams, S.C.R.; Carlbring, P.; Furmark, T. Predicting long-term outcome of internet-delivered cognitive behavior therapy for social anxiety disorder using fMRI and support vector machine learning. *Transl. Psychiatry* **2015**, *5*, e530. [CrossRef]
39. Carlbring, P.; Gunnarsdóttir, M.; Hedensjö, L.; Andersson, G.; Ekselius, L.; Furmark, T. Treatment of social phobia: Randomised trial of internet-delivered cognitive-behavioural therapy with telephone support. *Br. J. Psychiatry* **2007**, *190*, 120–138. [CrossRef] [PubMed]
40. Paxling, B.; Almlov, J.; Dahlin, M.; Carlbring, P.; Breitholtz, E.; Eriksson, T.; Andersson, G. Guided internet-de¬livered cognitive behavior therapy for generalized anxiety disorder: A randomized controlled trial. *Cogn. Behav. Ther.* **2011**, *40*, 159–173. [CrossRef] [PubMed]
41. Carlbring, P.; Maurin, L.; Törngren, C.; Linna, E.; Eriksson, T.; Sparthan, E.; Andersson, G. Individually-tailored, Internet-based treatment for anxiety disorders: A randomized controlled trial. *Behav. Res. Ther.* **2011**, *49*, 18–24. [CrossRef] [PubMed]
42. Spence, J.; Titov, N.; Dear, B.F.; Johnston, L.; Solley, K.; Lorian, C.; Schwenke, G. Randomized controlled trial of Internet-delivered cognitive behavioral therapy for posttraumatic stress disorder. *Depress. Anxiety* **2011**, *28*, 541–550. [CrossRef]
43. Andersson, G.; Hesser, H.; Veilord, A.; Svedling, L.; Andersson, F.; Sleman, O.; Lamminen, M. Randomised controlled non-inferiority trial with 3-year follow-up of internet-delivered versus face-to-face group cognitive behavioural therapy for depression. *J. Affect. Disord.* **2013**, *151*, 986–994. [CrossRef]
44. Berger, T.; Hämmerli, K.; Gubser, N.; Andersson, G.; Caspar, F. Internet-based treatment of depression: A randomized controlled trial comparing guided with unguided self-help. *Cogn. Behav. Ther.* **2011**, *40*, 251–266. [CrossRef]
45. Carlbring, P.; Hägglund, M.; Luthström, A.; Dahlin, M.; Kadowaki, Å.; Vernmark, K.; Andersson, G. Internet-based behavioral activation and acceptance-based treatment for depression: A randomized controlled trial. *J. Affect. Disord.* **2013**, *148*, 331–337. [CrossRef]
46. Ly, K.H.; Carlbring, P.; Andersson, G. Behavioral activation-based guided self-help treatment administered through a smartphone application: Study protocol for a randomized controlled trial. *Trials* **2012**, *13*. [CrossRef]
47. Mohr, D.C.; Duffecy, J.; Ho, J.; Kwasny, M.; Cai, X.; Burns, M.N.; Begale, M. A randomized controlled trial evaluating a manualized TeleCoaching protocol for improving adherence to a web-based intervention for the treatment of depression. *PLoS ONE* **2013**, *8*, e70086. [CrossRef]
48. O'Mahen, H.A.; Richards, D.A.; Woodford, J.; Wilkinson, E.; McGinley, J.; Taylor, R.S.; Warren, F.C. Netmums: A phase II randomized controlled trial of a guided Internet behavioural activation treatment for postpartum depression. *Psychol. Med.* **2014**, *44*, 1675–1689. [CrossRef]
49. Perini, S.; Titov, N.; Andrews, G. Clinician-assisted Internet-based treatment is effective for depression: Randomized controlled trial. *Aust. N. Z. J. Psychiatry* **2009**, *43*, 571–578. [CrossRef] [PubMed]
50. Ruwaard, J.; Schrieken, B.; Schrijver, M.; Broeksteeg, J.; Dekker, J.; Vermeulen, H.; Lange, A. Standardized web-based cognitive behavioural therapy of mild to moderate depression: A randomized controlled trial with a long-term follow-up. *Cogn. Behav. Ther.* **2009**, *38*, 206–221. [CrossRef] [PubMed]
51. Vernmark, K.; Lenndin, J.; Bjarehed, J.; Carlsson, M.; Karlsson, J.; Öberg, J.; Andersson, G. Internet administered guided self-help versus individualized e-mail therapy: A randomized trial of two versions of CBT for major depression. *Behav. Res. Ther.* **2010**, *48*, 368–376. [CrossRef] [PubMed]
52. Wagner, B.; Horn, A.B.; Maercker, A. Internet-based versus face-to-face cognitive-behavioral intervention for depression: A randomized controlled non-inferiority trial. *J. Affect. Disord.* **2014**, *152–154*, 113–121. [CrossRef]

53. Ly, K.H.; Asplund, K.; Andersson, G. Stress management for middle managers via an acceptance and com¬mitment-based smartphone application: A randomized controlled trial. *Internet Interv.* **2014**, *1*, 95–101. [CrossRef]
54. Zetterqvist, K.; Maanmies, J.; Strom, L.; Andersson, G. Randomized controlled trial of internet-based stress management. *Cogn. Behav. Ther.* **2003**, *32*, 151–160. [CrossRef]
55. Feijt, M.A.; de Kort, Y.A.; Bongers, I.M.; IJsselsteijn, W.A. Perceived Drivers and Barriers to the Adoption of eMental Health by Psychologists: The Construction of the Levels of Adoption of eMental Health Model. *J. Med. Internet Res.* **2018**, *20*, e153. [CrossRef]
56. Glueckauf, R.L.; Maheu, M.M.; Drude, K.P.; Wells, B.A.; Wang, Y.; Gustafson, D.J.; Nelson, E.L. Survey of psychologists' telebehavioral health practices: Technology use, ethical issues, and training needs. *Prof. Psychol. Res. Pract.* **2018**, *49*, 205–219. [CrossRef]
57. Evans, D.J. South African psychologists' use of the Internet in their practices. *S. Afr. J. Psychol.* **2014**, *44*, 162–169. [CrossRef]
58. Cipolletta, S.; Mocellin, D. Online counseling: An exploratory survey of Italian psychologists' attitudes towards new ways of interaction. *Psychother. Res.* **2018**, *28*, 909–924. [CrossRef]
59. OPP. Os Números da Associação. Censo dos Membros Efectivos da OPP [Association Numbers. Census of Effective Members of the OPP]. Available online: https://issuu.com/ordemdospsicologos/docs/dossier-censo-web (accessed on 14 June 2020).
60. LimesurveyGmbH. *LimeSurvey: An Open Source Survey Tool*; LimeSurvey GmbH: Hamburg, Germany, 2019.
61. IBMCorp. *IBM SPSS Statistics for Windows 25*; IBM Corp: Armonk, NY, USA, 2017.
62. Pierce, B.S.; Perrin, P.B.; Tyler, C.M.; McKee, G.B.; Watson, J.D. The COVID-19 telepsychology revolution: A national study of pandemic-based changes in U.S. mental health delivery. *Am. Psychol.* **2020**. [CrossRef] [PubMed]
63. Helou, S.; Helou, E.E.; Abou-Khalil, V.; Wakim, J.; Helou, J.E.; Daher, A.; Hachem, C.E. The effect of the COVID-19 pandemic on physicians' use and perception of telehealth: The case of Lebanon. *Int. J. Environ. Res. Public Health* **2020**, *17*, 4866. [CrossRef] [PubMed]
64. Uscher-Pines, L.; Sousa, J.L.; Raja, P.; Mehrotra, A.; Barnett, M.L.; Huskamp, H.A. Suddenly becoming a "virtual doctor": Experiences of psychiatrists transitioning to telemedicine during the COVID-19 pandemic. *Psychiat. Serv.* **2020**. [CrossRef]
65. Békés, V.; Doorn, K.A. Psychotherapists' attitudes toward online therapy during the COVID-19 pandemic. *J. Psychother. Integr.* **2020**, *30*, 238–247. [CrossRef]

8

Designing ICTs for Users with Mild Cognitive Impairment: A Usability Study

Diana Castilla [1,2,*], Carlos Suso-Ribera [3], Irene Zaragoza [2], Azucena Garcia-Palacios [3] and Cristina Botella [3]

1 Department of Personality, Evaluation and Psychological Treatment, University of Valencia, 46010 Valencia, Spain
2 CIBER of Physiopathology of Obesity and Nutrition (CIBEROBN), ISCIII CB06/03/0052 Instituto Salud Carlos III, 28029 Madrid, Spain; izaragoz@uji.es
3 Department of Basic Psychology, Clinical Psychology and Psychobiology, Universitat Jaume I, 12071 Castellón, Spain; susor@uji.es (C.S.-R.); azucena@uji.es (A.G.-P.); botella@uji.es (C.B.)
* Correspondence: Diana.Castilla@uv.es

Abstract: Background: Research has supported the cost-effectiveness of cognitive training tools enhanced by information and communication technologies (ICT) in several populations, including individuals with mild cognitive impairment (MCI) and age-related cognitive decline. The implementation of ICTs in this population, however, is sometimes challenging to their cognitive and age characteristics. Ultimately, this might compromise the effectiveness of ICT-enhanced therapies in this population. The aim of this study is to test the usability and acceptability of a European project prototype for elderly care, in an attempt to explore the ICT design needs of users with MCI. Methods: Participants were 28 individuals aged 58–95 years and with a diagnosis of MCI. Results: The results showed a low perception of peripheral elements and the need to place main interaction elements in the centre of the screen. The correlation between the general level of autonomy (daily life activities) and the ICT autonomy level was significant and positive. The speed of audio help had a significant impact on performance. Conclusion: The present work contributes to the literature on ICT usability needs of users with MCI. Some usability recommendations for designing interfaces for this type of user are provided in the text.

Keywords: usability; speech interfaces; cognitive impairment; ICT; elderly; cognitive decline

1. Introduction

1.1. Demographic Changes and Mild Cognitive Impairment

The age profile is expected to change globally in the coming decades. According to the U.S. Census Bureau's latest ageing report, the population will be much older in 2050. Specifically, in the next 35 years it is expected that the increase in the number of older individuals will be considerably greater than that of the younger population [1]. Consequently, with the ageing of the population, the possibility of an increase in the number of cognitively impaired individuals will also rise.

According to a World Health Organization report dementia and cognitive impairment lead the list of chronic diseases contributing to disability and dependence among older people worldwide. Forty-seven million people suffered from dementia in the world in 2015, and due to the ageing of the population globally, this number is expected to be tripled by 2050. These demographic changes not only have a strong impact on the daily lives of patients and their relatives, but also they have substantial consequences for public finances. Specifically, the estimated global cost of dementia care in 2010 was US$604 billion, and it is projected that its worldwide cost in 2030 could be US$1.2 trillion or more [2].

In the previous paragraph, we have presented the global impact of dementia, which is often characterized by an important cognitive impairment. However, dementia and its associated cognitive impairment do not start abruptly. Conversely, dementia is a dimensional construct that begins with small changes in the brain and symptomatology. In this sense, mild cognitive impairment (MCI) is the clinical syndrome that describes the transitional zone between normal cognitive status and dementia and it is estimated that approximately 10% to 15% of individuals with MCI will develop dementia [3]. Therefore, an important societal goal is to delay the transition between MCI and dementia or at least to reduce the speed of the cognitive decline in patients with MCI. Cognitive training is the most frequently reported form of cognition-focused intervention. It contains sessions involving practice on tasks that target aspects of cognition such as attention, memory, and language [4]. There is now sufficient support for the effectiveness of such training in individuals with MCI [5,6]. However, traditional face-to-face interventions may not always be accessible to the older individuals on a large scale because of accessibility reasons (e.g., having to travel long distances to specialized treatment centres) and limited public economic resources. For this reason, interest in the development of technological applications for the cognitive treatment in older adults is increasing [7]. Several studies have provided evidence about the efficiency of cognitive training tools based on information and communication technologies (ICT) when applied as an adjunct therapy for recovering or improving performance on cognitive skills and self-confidence, as well as for an early intervention in individuals with MCI and age-related cognitive decline [8–12].

In particular, reminiscence therapy appears to be an important therapy in MCI and Alzheimer's disease. Reminiscence therapy is a non-pharmacological intervention used to prompt past memories with music and old photographs, which also facilitates social interactions and increases self-esteem. The use of ICT seems to be particularly appropriate in this kind of intervention. For example, some studies demonstrate the feasibility of using readily available technology (digital video, images, and music) to produce personalized multimedia biographies that hold special meaning for individuals with Alzheimer's disease and MCI and their families [13–16].

1.2. Information and Communication Technologies (ICTs) and Cognitive Decline

Rapid technological advances offer an excellent opportunity to face the challenge of promoting independence, strengthening social connectedness, and preventing isolation in older individuals [17,18]. Furthermore, a recent meta-analysis that using computers for leisure produced an overall significant reduction in the risk of dementia [19].

In addition to its recreational role, a systematic review of technology-supported reminiscence therapy also supported the benefits of using technology in the elderly, this time for therapeutic purposes [20]. Some of these benefits include access to rich and engaging multimedia reminiscence materials, opportunities for people with dementia to participate in social interactions and take ownership of conversations, and a reduction in barriers due to motor deficits during interactions with media. Reminiscence therapy interventions based on ICT have also showed their efficacy in depression treatment in the elderly [21]. This is important because several studies have pointed out that depression, social isolation, and loneliness can negatively impact cognitive impairment [22–26]. In a similar line of supporting the benefits of using technology in the elderly, another study suggested that interventions with tailored social networks and social contacts are also needed to increase social contact in the elderly and to help them to delay and cope with cognitive impairment [23].

Cognitive decline in capabilities, such as memory, attention, perceptual speed, or spatial abilities, is part of normal ageing [27], and for this reason, the new age demography brings new challenges related to the way to improve the independence and quality of life of elderly people and, especially, promote their well-being in different ways [28]. New technologies can help to face these challenges, but their utilization in the elderly and specifically in persons with MCI might have some associated challenges. Although technology is increasingly present in everyday life, the elderly usually face usability problems related to the unsuitable design of central features, such as the graphic user interface

The final sample consisted of 28 participants with a MCI diagnosis from two nursing homes: 50% men and 50% women, aged between 58 and 95 years, with an average of 76.98 years ($SD = 9.56$).

The literacy level was mostly very basic because 84.6% of the sample only went to school up to the age of 14 (see Table A1). The average age when the sample left school was 11.27 ($SD = 5.07$), with a mean of 5.92 years of school attendance ($SD = 3.67$). Three participants never attended school, even though they could all read and write because they learned at home. Two participants did not recall going to school. This educational level (low or none) is representative of people from 65 to 85 years of age in small cities or towns in rural areas, given that the country had great economic difficulties during the 1940s and 1950s as a result of the Spanish civil war (1936 to 1939). At that moment, most of them left school and went to work at an early age to help their families.

Regarding their previous experience using ICTs, 82.1% had never used a personal computer or a tablet before this study, and only 7.1% of them had used a personal computer or a tablet more than 10 times.

The participants were randomly divided into four groups of seven participants each in order to test the system in four iterations.

Apart from the end-users, three professional caregivers (working at the recruitment centres) took part in the experiment as observers.

2.3. Materials

2.3.1. Main Software

The first ehcoBUTLER [58] functional prototype was the main software used for the study. The prototype was developed following all the usability characteristics of the BUTLER system, an emotional and social platform designed for elderly people with low digital literacy skills that has proven its usability and acceptability with elderly people without cognitive impairment [21,46,59,65].

The most important design feature of ehcoBUTLER is the navigation system, which follows a linear structure (i.e., like a step-by-step system) [46]. First, in the main menu, the user selects the application to use. Then, on each step, a human-looking avatar explains where they are and what they can do next. The avatar is "the butler" and its goal is to help them to decide what to do in every step of the system. The avatar is represented graphically as a young man and provides the help through audio (a synthetic voice) and text. The buttons have different colors depending on the type of action they allow: green is for buttons whose actions allow the user to continue with a task; red allows to interrupt a task (i.e., delete data or undo a concluded step); and orange represents secondary actions. Because all the system applications follow the same design principles, the email application was selected for the usability test. A complete description of the email task will be facilitated in the procedure section.

2.3.2. Variables and Measuring Instruments

As we described in more detail below, the assessment protocol consisted of three parts, namely user information (collected before the task), an evaluation of task-related information (performance and user's opinion), and effectiveness of the task as reported by professional caregivers.

User Profile

The user profile data were collected before the usability test. It included demographic data such as sex and educational level. In addition, we evaluated the user's experience with computers and the Internet, as well as whether the user had an e-mail account and had taken any computer training courses previously.

The level of autonomy in daily life activities was measured based on the professional's clinical judgement after an interview with the participant. The following item was then responded: "The user can perform his/her daily routines entirely unassisted" with a 5-point Likert scale with response labels: (0) strongly disagree, (1) somewhat disagree, (2) neither disagree nor agree, (3) somewhat agree, and (4) strongly agree.

Measures Based on User Performance

Success rate. The success rate was determined in absolute values: 0 (did not successfully perform the task); 1 (successfully performed the task).

Assistance received. The experimenter was not allowed to help the user solve the task. However, participants could be reminded that they could review the avatar's help, which counted as a new attempt. They could also be reminded about the name of the email recipient or on how to find a letter on the keyboard. Any help was annotated.

Number of attempts. The number of attempts was recorded, based on the number of times the experimenter had to show the user how to review the avatar instructions to find out how to continue.

Instruments Measuring the User's Opinion

Post-test questionnaire for the user: face scales [66] can help to evaluate the mood state in patients with cognitive impairment [67,68]. This questionnaire assesses the user's opinion of the system, with all the items using a 5-point face scale, rated from left to right with the following labels: strongly disagree, disagree, neither agree nor disagree, agree, and strongly agree. The variables measured were perceived ease of use, learnability and controllability, self-efficacy, flexibility, clear and easy to understand, usefulness, and intention to use.

Finally, a single item using a 5-point face scale to explore the feelings during the test was rated from left to right with the following labels: very bad, bad, neither bad nor good, good, very good.

All the items were obtained from a previous usability study with elderly users (see [32]).

Measures Regarding Professional's Judgment

The NASA Task Load Index–TLX [69] was filled in by the professional caregivers to evaluate the perceived workload. This is done to obtain a measure of the effectiveness of a task. This questionnaire provides an overall workload score based on six subscales: mental demand, physical demand, temporal demand, performance, effort, and frustration. Each scale is divided into 21 degrees from very low to very high. The experimenter trained the professional caregivers before the user test on how to fill in the NASA-TLX properly.

2.3.3. Hardware

Two set-ups were tested for this study. First, a 10"tablet (*Samsung Galaxy tablet Tab2*) was used because this was originally expected to be a suitable set-up due to its portability and affordable price. However, this was ruled out at the beginning of the study due to additional usability difficulties resulting from the use of the logical keyboard of the device, which hides half the screen during typing processes (see Figure A1). The second set-up which was finally used in the study, was a personal computer with a touch screen and physical keyboard, big keys in ABC order, and a normal keyboard with QWERTY order (*all in one MSI Model AE222-274 G3250 4GB 1TB W10 21.5* inches). A videocamera with a tripod was used to record the sessions.

In addition to the experimenter, the professional caregivers also assessed indicators of performance on the task (whether the user completed the task or not, the number of attempts, the degree of assistance needed during the test, and the technology used). They also reported their clinical judgment about the difficulty of the task, feelings observed in the user, together with suggestions and recommended improvements in the system. Finally, the professional assessed the ability of the user to use the system in an autonomous way (i.e., without any kind of support), using a 5-point Likert scale with response labels 0 = strongly disagree, 1 = somewhat disagree, 2 = neither disagree nor agree, 3 = somewhat agree, and 4 = strongly agree.

2.3.4. Statistical Software

For data analysis, IBM SPSS 22.0 (IBM Corp., Armonk, NY, USA) was used. Descriptive statistics were performed to explore the frequency and percentage of responses for all the variables and a Spearman correlation analysis was conducted to explore the relationship between the user's level of general autonomy and the number of attempts, as well as the relationship between the user's level of general autonomy and the extent to which the user could use the system autonomously in the future. A contingency table was created to explore the relationship between the user's performance and feelings during the task. This was done to explore whether the user's feelings were related to performance. To investigate whether the non-verbal language displayed by the users matched with their reported feelings, we asked the professionals to rate the observed user's feelings. Then both ratings were correlated by Spearman analysis. Then, results were graphically represented with Microsoft Excel (Microsoft Corporation, Redmond, WA, USA).

2.4. Procedure

To carry out this study, several nursing homes and socio-health organizations dedicated to elderly care in the region of Valencia (Spain) were contacted. We debriefed the managers of the organizations about the objective of the project and the need to test the system with people with MCI diagnosed by a physician (neurologist or geriatrician).

Two collaboration agreements were finally signed between the Jaume I University and two nursing homes from the Health Department of the Valencian Community (Spain). It took two months for the study to be conducted, including the development phases.

The medical staff of both nursing homes selected users with MCI as candidates for the study. Due to the candidates' cognitive state, the nursing homes contacted their families to obtain their informed consent to participate and permission to video-tape the sessions. For users under the tutelage of the local government (Health Counsel of the Valencian Community), an additional permit was required to carry out the study. The research was conducted following the American Psychological Association's ethical principles and code of conduct [70]. The study was approved by the Ethics Committee of the Gestión Sociosanitaria del Mediterráneo (GESMED, Socio-Sanitary Management of the Mediterranean; REC number: CD643566/2017). The participants' data confidentiality and anonymity were ensured. Forty-six users were asked to participate in this study voluntarily. Of these, 33 agreed to participate and 28 met the inclusion criteria and signed the data and recording confidentiality agreement. The experimental session consisted of a usability test [60], where a task analysis was carried out [61]. The experimenter took all the necessary hardware to be used in the study to the nursing homes. The rooms used in the centres were big enough to place the equipment and facilitate the movement of people with reduced mobility.

The centre's psychologists (the professional caregiver) accompanied the participants while the expert in usability (the experimenter) conducted the tests. Next, the experimenter presented the task and administered the pre-test assessment protocol (demographic data and previous experience with computers and the Internet). Once the questionnaires were completed, the experimenter explained the task to the user, gave them the instructions for the task on paper, and asked if they would prefer to use a physical or a logical keyboard.

The main task involved writing an email to a specific contact already registered in the address book and attaching a specific picture using the ehcoBUTLER system. The user had the instructions on paper, with the name of the contact in red, the text of the email, and the image to be attached, so that they could follow the instructions as easily as possible and could effectively perform the task. Therefore, the user did not have to memorize the instructions. The secondary task required the evaluation of the avatar and the help voice from a qualitative point of view. We also asked the participants to explain the reasons for their preferences. In order to obtain reliable data on task performance, the sessions were video-taped. A usability expert reviewed the sessions.

The role of the experimenter was to encourage the users to perform the task autonomously, without providing additional instructions. If the users required assistance, the experimenter encouraged them to interact with the avatar. Success meant that the user could complete the task without the help of the experimenter. If any kind of help was needed to complete the task, this was noted as failure. The number of attempts was recorded according to the number of times the experimenter had to show the user how to review the avatar instructions to find out how to continue. The experimenter stood next to the users throughout the usability test (see Figure A2).

In accordance with the Iterative User Interface Design [60], the study was divided into four iterative cycles. This began with the first functional prototype of the system and included seven new users in every iteration. Usability issues were found in each iteration and the proposals for improvement were implemented by the development team. In each iteration the usability issues found were fixed, and after tested again, until arriving to iteration 4, where no usability problems were found. Finally, a re-test was carried out with the users from iteration 1 (see Figure A3). Finally, after finalizing the test, the post-test questionnaires were answered by the users with the experimenter's support (their opinion about the system and how they felt during the test). The professional's clinical judgment was also recorded at this stage. As noted earlier, this included whether the user completed the task, the number of attempts, the assistance received, the opinion about the system and the technology used, the workload experienced, and suggestions and recommended changes.

3. Results

3.1. Main Usability Findings

3.1.1. Solved through Behavior Program Changes

An important problem was related to the way in which users pressed on the screen. The users performed very long pulsations (an average of 3–4 s pressing), which led to the following problems: instead of clicking on the main button (e.g., continue), the secondary button (e.g., copy) was activated. Thus, the text label button was copied, as shown in Figure 1, as opposed to following to the next action.

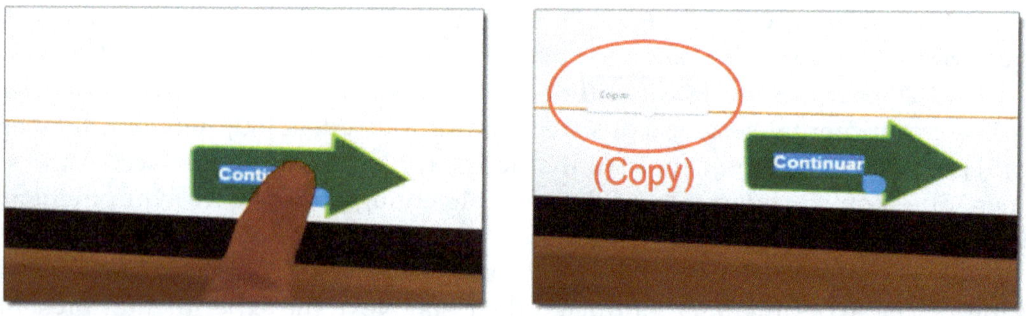

(a) (b)

Figure 1. Troubles found due to very long pulsations. (**a**) Text label button selected due to very long pulsation. (**b**) Secondary button activated (copy) instead clicking on the main action button (the green arrow).

This problem was solved by writing a piece of code that overrides the behaviour in the web browsers related to the right-click mouse events by converting these events to left-click mouse events.

Another usability issue observed was the user's need to see what they are pressing while interacting with the touch screen. As a result of this, they clicked outside buttons. To solve this problem, we programmed an interaction area higher than the visual button only, thus preventing missclicking for this reason.

Regarding the help audio facilitated by the avatar voice (a synthetic voice), we found problems with standard speech speed (around 3 words per second). Some participants had problems following the instructions because these were too fast for them. The speed was changed to 2 words per second, adding 8 spaces (2 s) between sentences in order to clearly separate the concepts in the instructions. For example: "You are now viewing your letter (2 s of silence). If you like it (2 s of silence), press the green button that says: Send letter". After changing the voice speed, 92% of the users informed that they liked the voice and that it was easy to understand.

3.1.2. Solved through Graphical Changes

The main usability finding we encountered related to the cognitive state and mental model of this type of user had to do with their attentional capacity. A large number of users did not see the interaction buttons during the first usability iteration. Our first hypothesis was that maybe they suffer some cognitive blindness to bottom elements, which might be caused by the dark grey colour of the graphic user interface (GUI). This is shown in Figure 2a. Because we anticipated that some users might perceive that the dark grey band was an external element, the graphic user interface was redesigned and the dark grey colour was replaced by an orange line, following the upper design as in Figure 2b.

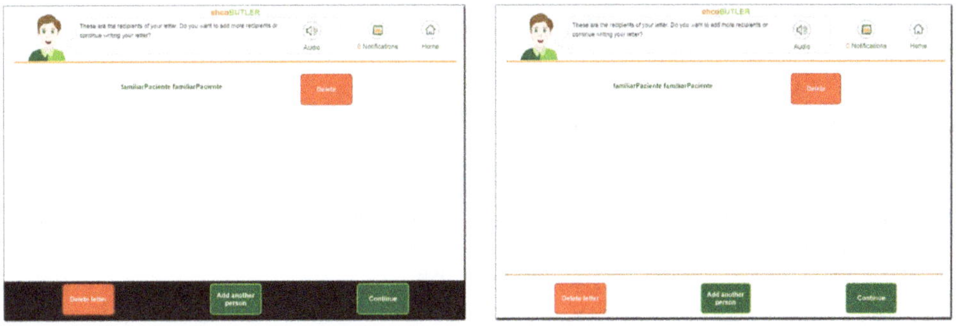

(a) (b)

Figure 2. Graphic user interface (GUI) colour change in bottom interaction area. (**a**) Original design. (**b**) Modified design.

Despite this change, users still did not see the elements at the bottom. The study of the sessions revealed that the less autonomous users presented a very acute attentional focus towards the centre of the screen, to the detriment of the interaction elements placed at the bottom or sides of the screen. In order to solve this problem, the graphic user interface was redesigned again, placing the main interaction elements in the central area, that is, within the attentional focus of these users (see Figure 3). With this change, the interaction issues were fully resolved.

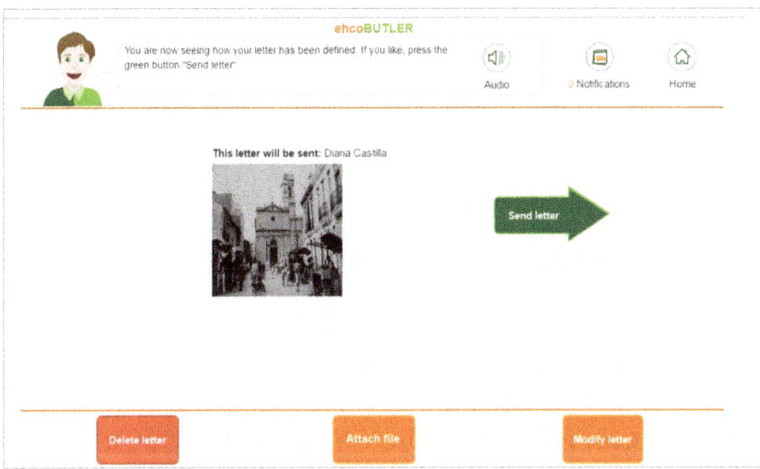

Figure 3. Final graphic user interface.

3.2. *Quantitative Results*

3.2.1. Task Performance

Good results were obtained on task performance. Specifically, 89% of the participants successfully completed the task (even though the majority of them had no previous ICT experience).

3.2.2. Number of Attempts

The number of attempts to complete the task varied across participants (range 1 to 6). However, 50% of the users managed to complete it in just 1 or 2 attempts (median = 2.50, *SD* = 1.59). Comparing the sum of attempts during the study, we observed that there was a higher number of attempts at the beginning of the study due to usability problems related to the touch interaction (long pulsations that activate selecting text or the contextual menu). We conducted a Spearman correlation analysis between the user's general level of autonomy, rated by the professional caregivers, and the number of attempts. The correlation was not significant ($r_s = 0.17$, $p = 0.396$).

3.2.3. Workload NASA Task Work Load Index)

The workload during the task was low or very low on all subscales (see Figure 4), achieving a general mean of 4.55 (*SD* = 5.65) and means on all scales below the central point of 11 (range 0 to 21, Very low demand = 0; Very high demand = 21).

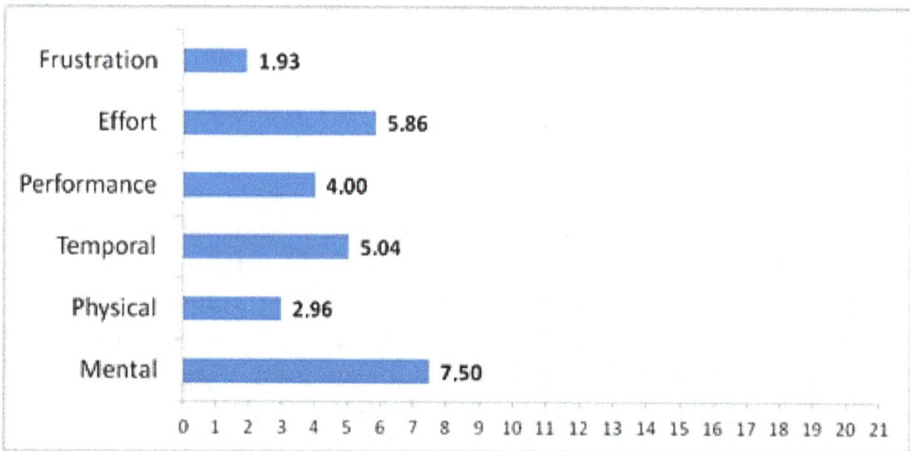

Figure 4. NASA task work load index results.

3.3. *Quantitative Results*

3.3.1. Usability Variables and User Opinion

In general, the users' opinion was good, as all the usability variables were scored on the positive side of the scale exceeding the midpoint (i.e., exceeding 2 points on a scale ranging from 0 to 4). Specifically, the users found the system easy to use and useful for their lives, they felt confident while using it, felt that they had control over the system, found the button size large enough to see it and interact with it, and reported that they would like to use the system in the future (see Figure 5).

The variable with the highest average score was ease of use, with 3.07 (*SD* = 0.98), followed by useful with 3.00 (*SD* = 1.19).

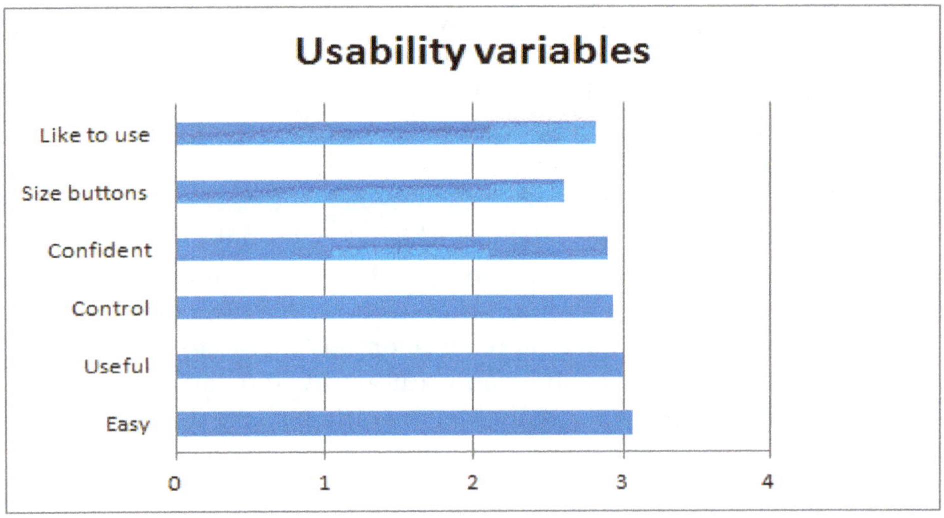

Figure 5. Average of usability variables.

Regarding their feelings during the test, 79% of the users felt from normal to very good. A contingency table was created to explore the relationship between user performance and feelings during the task (see Table 1).

Table 1. User performance vs. feelings during the task: contingency table.

		Task Performance		Total
		Fail	Success	
User Felt	Very bad	0	0	0
	Bad	2	1	3
	Neutral	1	4	5
	Good	0	15	15
	Very good	0	5	5
Total		3	25	28

Only three users (10%) referred to feeling bad during the experiment. They indicated that they felt nervous because of the test conditions (people looking at them and assessing what they were doing). The number of users who felt bad or failed the task were too low to perform a Chi-square analysis.

3.3.2. Intention to Use

Regarding the intention to use the system in the future, 82% of the users expressed that they would like to use it often in the future (21% strongly agree; 61% somewhat agree; 7% neither disagree nor agree; 0% somewhat disagree, 11% strongly disagree).

3.3.3. Preferences about Avatar Appearance and Voice

From a graphic point of view, users indicated that they liked the age of the avatar (young), estimating that it was about 30 years old. Regarding the voice, none of the participants perceived that it was a synthetic voice. Adjectives such as "nice", "polite", or "kind" were used the most to describe it.

3.4. Professional Opinion

3.4.1. Ability to Use the System in an Autonomous Way

Before the experiment, the professional caregivers rated the level of autonomy the users had in their everyday lives while performing any kind of task.

After the usability task, the professional caregivers also rated their clinical judgment about the level of user autonomy using the system, revealing that 46% of the users would be able to autonomously use the system in the future without any kind of support. Only in 14% of the cases did the professional caregivers describe that the users would need frequent support, but they felt that 39% of the sample would always need support.

We conducted a Spearman correlation analysis between the user's general level of autonomy, rated by the professional caregivers and the extent to which they thought the user could use the system autonomously. The correlation was significant and positive ($r_s = 0.45$; $p = 0.016$). This correlation indicates that the professional caregivers thought that users with a high degree of autonomy in their everyday lives could also use the system in a more autonomous way in the future, whereas users with low autonomy in their routines would also have low autonomy in using the system. It seems logical that if the user is not autonomous in his/her daily life, it would be very difficult for him/her to use the system without assistance.

3.4.2. Sessions Needed to Learn to Use the System in an Unassisted Manner

The following analysis evaluates to which extent the professionals believed that the users would be able to use the system on their own with some training. According to the professionals' opinion, 39% of users would always need support to use the system. The also indicated that 36% of users would need more than 10 training sessions to use the system on their own. Finally, they reported that 14% of them would need between 5 and 10 training sessions to use the system autonomously and 11% of them would only need 2 to 4 training sessions (see Figure 6).

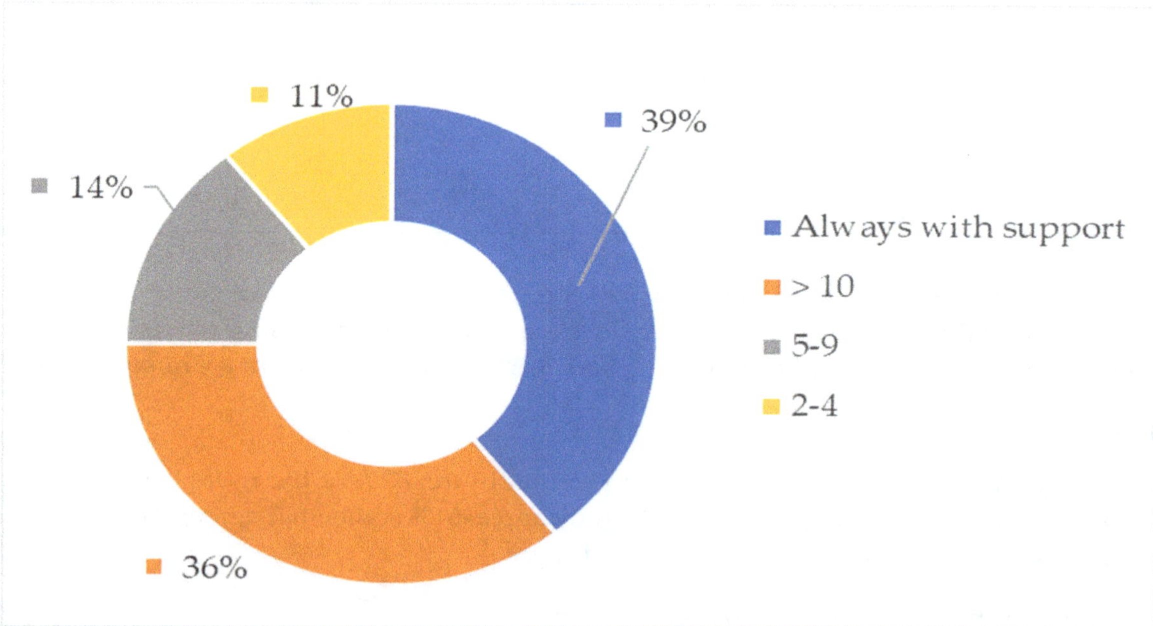

Figure 6. Estimated number of training sessions to use the system in an autonomous way.

3.4.3. Professional Opinion about the Users' Feelings

The professionals also rated how they thought the users felt during the test. We conducted a Spearman correlation analysis between feeling scores given by the user and those given by the professional. The correlation was significant and positive ($r_s = 0.59$; $p = 0.001$), indicating a large agreement between the experienced user feeling and the professional caregiver's impression about the user's feeling.

4. Discussion

The present study aimed to test the usability of a prototype system designed for users with MCI and make adaptations to it based on the results. For this purpose, a functional prototype email system was designed based on the usability design principles of the Butler system (i.e., the design followed the National Institute on Aging checklist [71] and added linear navigation and audio and text help through an avatar) [59]. The system was tested in two nursing homes of the Health Council of the Valencian Community (Spain). The results showed differences between the present study and the findings obtained from previous research with the same web design but a different population (i.e., people without cognitive impairment) [32,46]. The main usability issues revealed in the present study compared with those of users without MCI were the following:

- *Related to spatial abilities and attention.* The results showed a low perception of peripheral elements and the need to place the main interaction elements (e.g., continue the action in the step-by-step navigation) in the center of the screen because less autonomous users showed an attentional focus on this central part of the screen and attentional blindness to the peripheral graphical elements.
- *Related programming interaction.* Given that users expect a real time change in buttons (such as sinking down when pressed), the interaction with the buttons was performed by pressing them for a long time, causing an unexpected interaction result (copying text or activating the secondary browser menu). On the other hand, we observed the user's need to see what they were pressing while touching the buttons. This explains why they clicked outside the buttons.
- *Related audio help.* The standard speed of synthetic speech (3 words per second) was too fast, and most of the users were not able to follow the instructions.

Our findings raise some novel questions about the design of interfaces for MCI users. For example, several studies point out that the use of audio and text support can benefit both novel and experienced older users [72]. However, audio interfaces also could represent a new usability barrier because they force the user to work with memory and mental agility. These new interfaces allow us to avoid the keyboard and present a user interface with less text, but the audio interface adds other difficulties such as having to understand and retain information while making interaction decisions. It is well known that, because speech is linearized, audio instructions as a unimodal strategy impose difficulties in the elderly [73]. In the case of cognitively impaired users, this effort could become another step in the technological barrier stairway. If we take into account that one of the handicaps in MCI is memory loss and a decrease in mental agility, we could encounter a real barrier that goes beyond usability and could become a serious accessibility problem for this kind of user.

Regarding the audio interface to support the interaction, previous studies with elderly users without cognitive impairment suggest that speed adjustment is not necessary [72]. However, our findings showed that it is likely to be necessary to adjust the speed of the speech, as well to add a short time separation between phrases for users with MCI, probably because they need more time to process information. Our study revealed positive results from adjusting the speech speed to 2 words per second and adding 2 s of silence between short sentences, which was done to clearly separate the concepts of the instructions and to give the user time to understand them. At this point, we think it is important to differentiate between input and output audios. Our study only explores this feature as an output of an application, that is, when the user receives information passively (in our case as a complement of the text help). We cannot extrapolate our conclusions to audio inputs, that is, when the user gives audio instructions to the system.

In addition to the findings with the audio interface, our results showed usability difficulties related to the graphic design. A metaphor in this context is how we represent an interaction with the system in an understandable way. For example, a metaphor in a graphic interface could be represented by the buttons and other visual elements like the avatar or the space to write. The commonly used metaphors represented in the technology do not correspond to the previous experience of users with a low technological profile and according literature this can be a barrier [59,74]. This might be the reason why the users in our study made long pulsations while waiting for a change of state in the buttons. These results support the idea that assistive technologies should introduce graphic elements that match the users' previous experience. This opens an avenue for a new dimension that should be considered in the design of this type of technology. Following this need to adapt ICTs to the mental model of the elderly, it could be advisable to represent objects and object behaviours that users could be familiar with. For example, if we represent a button in an application, the feedback when pressing it could be seeing the button sink.

Previous literature highlights the negative effects of age on spatial abilities, memory, attention, and perceptual speed [19,27,75]. Thus, because navigation is one of the greatest difficulties for older users, linear navigation can be useful for improving usability results with elderly users [46,76,77]. Experiencing MCI considerably increases these cognitive and motor difficulties, which adds new challenges in designing webs for this kind of user. Some studies propose linear navigation to avoid spatial disorientation when using websites [75]. However, cognitive impairment influences spatial orientation and, consequently, makes this usability problem even greater. The linear navigation solution cannot fix this because, for users with MCI, spatial orientation might not be limited to navigation among the different parts of the system. The problem could be that, on each screen, the user must make an effort that requires attention and guidance. This idea seems somewhat aligned with the change blindness concept [55] because the users could not find the changes between different screens, and so there was disorientation beyond navigation. A possible solution is to combine different strategies to maintain the attention on interaction effortlessly. For example, one option could be combining the linear navigation with audio and help text and a design in which the main interactions (to continue the task) are placed in the centre of the screen.

Also in relation to cognitive performance, research has evidenced that, when the user is familiar with the learning object, the memory and learning processes are faster [78]. However, cognitive impairments such as memory loss or disorientation could increase the difficulties in recognizing or memorizing objects. Natural interfaces such as speech mode try to replicate a natural and user-friendly interaction. Audio outputs (from the system to the user) can be useful for users who receive help and instructions in real time [72], but audio inputs (from the user to the system) require other mental processes that demand the specific use of memory, such as remembering specific words from the instructions or predicting (or remembering) what step will be next. In this regard, a recent study [39] evidenced significant difficulties in speech recognition in patients with MCI even when embodied conversational agents were successfully implemented. Our study only explored audio outputs, and the results showed that the speech speed could be an important factor in designing audio interfaces.

Another finding was that a positive and significant correlation between the general level of autonomy and the ICT autonomy level was obtained. This result could indicate that the level of autonomy in everyday activities could be a good predictor of the level of user autonomy in the use of assistive technologies, which might have some clinical implications. For example, this could be used as guiding information when having to select the type of interface or amount of support that is provided to users (e.g., those with less daily autonomy should be offered more help or easier interfaces).

From a qualitative point of view, the results of our study showed that users did not perceive the difference between a synthetic voice and a human voice during the testing. These results are important as they suggest that this system can be effectively used in the elderly, which is in line with past literature [72]. This finding supports the idea that the use of mechanical audio interfaces, which are cheaper to develop than audios recorded directly by humans, are suitable for this kind of population. Given that this was perceived like a human voice and did not eliminate emotional qualities, this procedure is promising in this field.

The present study has a number of limitations. First, although the sample size is large enough to obtain usability conclusions, the number of users limits the statistical analysis that can be performed with the data. Additionally, the fact that they all belonged to the same country limits the cultural generalization of the findings. Furthermore, the experimental design limits our conclusions to the specific task of "composing" an email and attaching a picture. Other tasks and interfaces should be used to test our usability recommendations for MCI users. An additional limitation refers to the existence of a single professional rater of the patient's performance. Even though this is the usual practice in clinical settings, the existence of a second evaluator is always preferable for reliability purposes. Finally, this work did not explore in-depth the impact of physical or logical keyboards on performance.

5. Conclusions

In spite of the limitations of this study, the findings resulted in a number of recommendations for the use of ICT in persons with MCI and open the door to exploring new dimensions of spatial orientation on graphic user interfaces. New technologies can help to improve the wellbeing and quality of life of users with MCI or early dementia. However, due to their cognitive impairment, such individuals suffer from a lack of orientation, not only when navigating between screens, but when interacting with a single screen. Simplifying technologies for MCI users should be an important societal goal. The use of linear navigation could be a key element in this direction, but it is not the only one. Designers have a new challenge of "designing interaction in the middle" because the main area of attention for these users was the centre of the screen. Another recommendation is to design the interaction area bigger than the visual button. This should be done because there is a general tendency to press the buttons outside the image in an attempt to see what they are pressing. In addition, the results suggested that natural interfaces, such as audio interfaces, might be useful for these users if the speed is adapted to their cognitive needs. In this sense, text-to-speech technology can be a suitable and cost-effective alternative because users do not distinguish the human voice from a bot. Therefore, based on our findings one recommendable speech speed for similar users and purposes would be 2 words per second and adding 2 s of silence between short sentences. Ultimately, the utility of the results lies in the fact that achieving design interfaces that give MCI users independence could help to prolong the time they live independently at home and might help improve their quality of life. One way of doing this, for instance, would be providing them with a number of alternative care possibilities, such as a cognitive rehabilitation program that they can perform at home autonomously. The main contribution of this study consists of exploring the usability needs of users with MCI on ICT systems and providing some usability recommendations for designing interfaces for this kind of user.

Author Contributions: Conceptualization, D.C., A.G.-P. and C.B.; methodology, D.C. and A.G.-P.; validation, D.C. and I.Z.; formal analysis, D.C. and C.S.-R.; investigation, D.C., C.B., A.G.-P., I.Z. and C.S.-R.; resources, D.C., C.B. and A.G.-P.; data curation, D.C.; writing—original draft preparation, D.C. and I.Z.; writing—review and editing, A.G.-P., C.S.-R. and C.B.; visualization, D.C.; supervision, C.B. and A.G.-P.; project administration, D.C.; funding acquisition, C.B. All authors have read and agreed to the published version of the manuscript.

Acknowledgments: We would like to give special thanks for their interest and professional support to the technical team in charge of ehcoBUTLER programming and development: Rafael Ordóñez, Juan Antonio Grande and Sergio Barrera. Also, we would like to thanks for their involvement and professional support to the staff of the nursing homes that participated in this research: "Residencia de la Tercera Edad y Centro de día "La Vila" (Almussafes, Valencia, Spain) and "Residencia y centro de día de personas mayores dependientes de Chiva" (Chiva, Spain).

Appendix A

Table A1. Summary of sociodemographic characteristics of the sample.

ID	Number of Iteration	Cognitive Diagnosis	Age	Sex	School-Leaving Age	PC Experience
1	1	MCI	73	M	12	Never
2	1	MCI	83	F	10	Never
3	1	MCI	85	M	Didn't remember	Never
4	1	MCI	71	F	14	Never
5	1	MCI	94	M	14	Never
6	1	MCI	88	M	10	Never
7	1	MCI	95	F	10	Never
8	2	MCI	67	M	14	Never
9	2	MCI	58	M	13	Once
10	2	MCI	89	F	8	Never
11	2	MCI	90	F	14	Never
12	2	MCI	86	F	Didn't go to school	Never
13	2	MCI	89	M	Didn't go to school	Never
14	2	MCI	85	F	Didn't go to school	Never
15	3	MCI	76	F	8	Never
16	3	MCI	70	M	14	Never
17	3	MCI	85	M	7	Never
18	3	MCI	71	F	13	Never
19	3	MCI	69	M	15	Never
20	3	MCI	75	M	Didn't remember	More than 10
21	3	MCI	76	M	14	From 1 to 10
22	4	MCI	81	M	12	Never
23	4	MCI	70	F	16	More than 10
24	4	MCI	88	F	12	Never
25	4	MCI	67	M	20	From 1 to 10
26	4	MCI	81	F	18	Never
27	4	MCI	91	F	11	Never
28	4	MCI	78	F	14	Never

Notes: MCI: Mild Cognitive Impairment. PC experience: number of times that the person used a personal computer before this study. Sex: M = Male, F = Female.

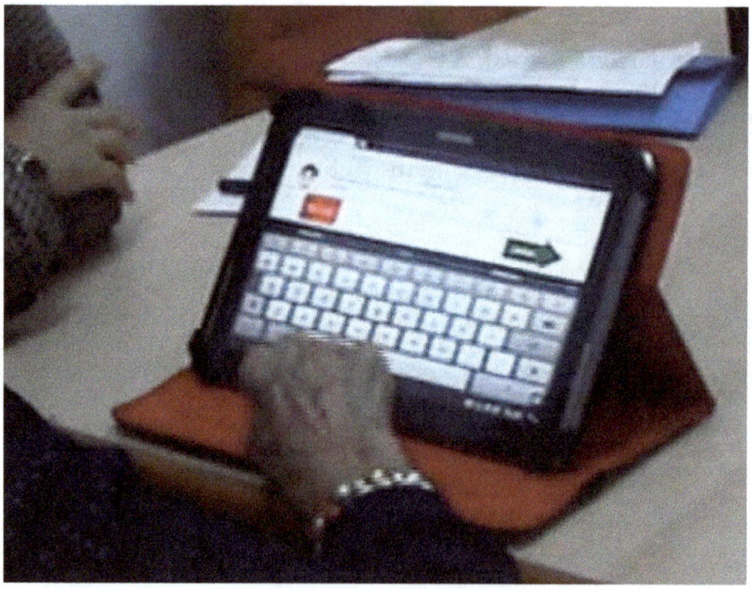

Figure A1. Usability problem on tablets due logic keyboard.

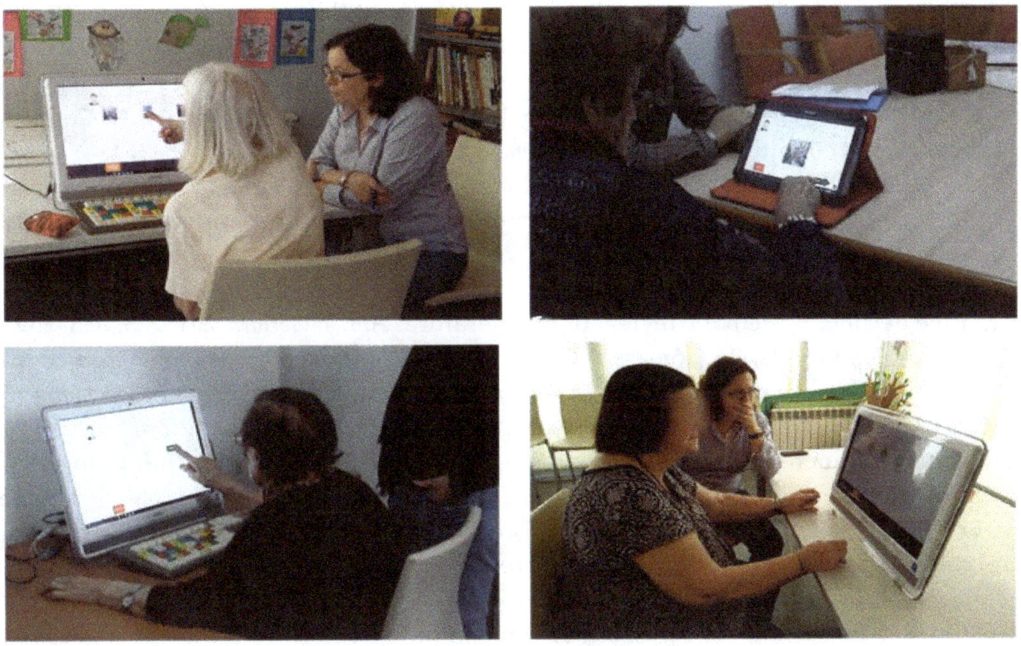

Figure A2. Set-up during usability testing.

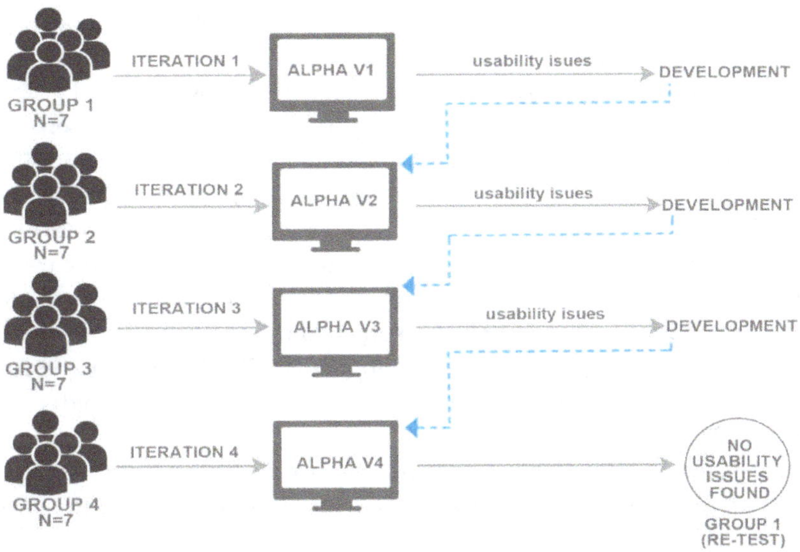

Figure A3. Diagram of iterative cycles performed in the usability test.

References

1. He, W.; Goodkind, D.; Kowal, P. An Aging World: 2015 International Population Reports. In *U.S. Census Bureau, International Population Reports, P95/16-1, An Aging World 2015*; US Government Printing Office: Washington, DC, USA, 2016; p. 204.
2. WHO. Governments Commit to Advancements in Dementia Research and Care. Geneva. Available online: http://www.who.int/mediacentre/news/releases/2015/action-on-dementia/en/ (accessed on 25 November 2017).
3. Fischer, P.; Jungwirth, S.; Zehetmayer, S.; Weissgram, S.; Hoenigschnabl, S.; Gelpi, E.; Tragl, K.H. Conversion from subtypes of mild cognitive impairment to Alzheimer dementia. *Neurology* **2007**, *68*, 288–291. [CrossRef] [PubMed]
4. Martin, M.; Clare, L.; Altgassen, A.M.; Cameron, M.H.; Zehnder, F. Cognition-based interventions for healthy older people and people with mild cognitive impairment. *Cochrane Database Syst. Rev.* **2011**, *19*, CD006220. [CrossRef] [PubMed]

5. Brum, P.S.; Forlenza, O.V.; Yassuda, M.S. Treino cognitivo em idosos com Comprometimento Cognitivo Leve: Impacto no desempenho cognitivo e funcional. *Dement. e Neuropsychol.* **2009**, *3*, 124–131. [CrossRef] [PubMed]
6. Liu, X.Y.; Li, L.; Xiao, J.Q.; He, C.Z.; Lyu, X.L.; Gao, L.; Yang, X.W.; Cui, X.G.; Fan, L.H. Cognitive training in older adults with mild cognitive impairment. *Biomed. Environ. Sci.* **2016**, *29*, 356–364.
7. Zhang, H.; Huntley, J.; Bhome, R.; Holmes, B.; Cahill, J.; Gould, R.L.; Wang, H.; Yu, X.; Howard, R. Effect of computerised cognitive training on cognitive outcomes in mild cognitive impairment: A systematic review and meta-analysis. *BMJ Open* **2019**, *9*, e027062. [CrossRef]
8. Coyle, H.; Traynor, V.; Solowij, N. Computerized and virtual reality cognitive training for individuals at high risk of cognitive decline: Systematic review of the literature. *Am. J. Geriatr.* **2015**, *23*, 335–359. [CrossRef]
9. Franco, M.; Jones, K.; Woods, B.; Gómez, P. Gradior: A personalized computer-based cognitive training programme for early intervention in dementia. In *Early Psychosocial Interventions in Dementia. Evidence-Based Practice*; Moniz-Cook, E., Manthorpe, J., Eds.; Jessica Kingsley Publishers: London, UK, 2009.
10. García-Betances, R.I.; Jiménez-Mixco, V.; Arredondo, M.T.; Cabrera-Umpiérrez, M.F. Using virtual reality for cognitive training of the elderly. *Am. J. Alzheimers Dis. Other Demen.* **2015**, *30*, 49–54. [CrossRef]
11. Palau, F.; Franco, M.; Bamidis, P.; Losada, R.; Parra, E.; Papageorgiou, S.; Vivas, A.B. The effects of a computer-based cognitive and physical training program in a healthy and mildly cognitive impaired aging sample. *Aging Ment. Health* **2014**, *18*, 838–846. [CrossRef]
12. Shuchat, J.; Ouellet, É.; Moffat, N.; Belleville, S. Opportunities for virtual reality in cognitive training with persons with mild cognitive impairment or Alzheimer's disease. *Nonpharmacol. Ther. Dement.* **2012**, *3*, 35.
13. Baecker, R.M.; Marziali, E.; Chatland, S.; Easley, K.; Crete, M.; Yeung, M. Multimedia biographies for individuals with Alzheimer's disease and their families. In Proceedings of the World Congress on Internet in Medicine, Toronto, ON, Canada, 14–19 October 2006.
14. Barban, F.; Annicchiarico, R.; Pantelopoulos, S.; Federici, A.; Perri, R.; Fadda, L.; Carlesimo, G.A.; Ricci, C.; Giuli, S.; Scalici, F.; et al. Protecting cognition from aging and Alzheimer's disease: A computerized cognitive training combined with reminiscence therapy. *Int. J. Geriatr. Psychiatry* **2015**, *31*, 340–348. [CrossRef]
15. Damianakis, T.; Crete-Nishihata, M.; Smith, K.L.; Baecker, R.M.; Marziali, E. The psychosocial impacts of multimedia biographies on persons with cognitive impairments. *Gerontologist* **2010**, *50*, 23–35. [CrossRef]
16. Pino, M.; Boulay, M.; Jouen, F.; Rigaud, A.S. "Are we ready for robots that care for us?" Attitudes and opinions of older adults toward socially assistive robots. *Front. Aging Neurosci.* **2015**, *7*, 1–15. [CrossRef]
17. Cornejo, R.; Tentori, M.; Favela, J. Enriching in-person encounters through social media: A study on family connectedness for the elderly. *Int. J. Hum. Comput. Stud.* **2013**, *71*, 889–899. [CrossRef]
18. Khosravi, P.; Rezvani, A.; Wiewiora, A. The impact of technology on older adults' social isolation. *Comput. Hum. Behav.* **2016**, *63*, 594–603. [CrossRef]
19. Yates, L.A.; Ziser, S.; Spector, A.; Orrell, M. Cognitive leisure activities and future risk of cognitive impairment and dementia: Systematic review and meta-analysis. *Int. Psychogeriatr.* **2016**, *28*, 1791–1806. [CrossRef] [PubMed]
20. Lazar, A.; Thompson, H.; Demiris, G. A systematic review of the use of technology for reminiscence therapy. *Health Educ. Behav.* **2014**, *41*, 51S–61S. [CrossRef] [PubMed]
21. Preschl, B.; Maercker, A.; Wagner, B.; Forstmeier, S.; Baños, R.M.; Alcañiz, M.; Castilla, D.; Botella, C. Life-review therapy with computer supplements for depression in the elderly: A randomized controlled trial. *Aging Ment. Health* **2012**, *16*, 964–974. [CrossRef]
22. Shankar, A.; Hamer, M.; McMunn, A.; Steptoe, A. Social isolation and loneliness: Relationships with cognitive function during 4 years of follow-up in the English Longitudinal Study of Ageing. *Psychosom. Med.* **2013**, *75*, 161–170. [CrossRef]
23. Wang, B.; He, P.; Dong, B. Associations between social networks, social contacts, and cognitive function among Chinese nonagenarians/centenarians. *Arch. Gerontol. Geriatr.* **2015**, *60*, 522–527. [CrossRef]
24. Wilson, R.S.; Boyle, P.A.; James, B.D.; Leurgans, S.E.; Buchman, A.S.; Bennett, D.A. Negative social interactions and risk of mild cognitive impairment in old age. *Neuropsychology* **2015**, *29*, 561–570. [CrossRef]
25. Wilson, R.S.; Krueger, K.R.; Arnold, S.E.; Schneider, J.A.; Kelly, J.F.; Barnes, L.L.; Tang, Y.; Bennett, D.A. Loneliness and Risk of Alzheimer Disease. *Arch. Gen. Psychiatry* **2007**, *64*, 234. [CrossRef] [PubMed]

26. Windsor, T.D.; Gerstorf, D.; Pearson, E.; Ryan, L.H.; Anstey, K.J. Positive and negative social exchanges and cognitive aging in young-old adults: Differential associations across family, friend, and spouse domains. *Psychol. Aging* **2014**, *29*, 28–43. [CrossRef]
27. Boutet, I.; Milgram, N.W.; Freedman, M. Cognitive decline and human (Homo sapiens) aging: An investigation using a comparative neuropsychological approach. *J. Comp. Psychol.* **2007**, *121*, 270–281. [CrossRef] [PubMed]
28. National Collaborating Centre for Mental Health (UK). *Dementia: A NICE-SCIE Guideline on Supporting People with Dementia and Their Carers in Health and Social Care*; British Psychological Society: Leicester, UK, 2007.
29. Sonderegger, A.; Schmutz, S.; Sauer, J. The influence of age in usability testing. *Appl. Ergon.* **2016**, *52*, 291–300. [CrossRef]
30. Wagner, N.; Hassanein, K.; Head, M. The impact of age on website usability. *Comput. Hum. Behav.* **2014**, *37*, 270–282. [CrossRef]
31. Zhou, J.; Rau, P.-L.P.; Salvendy, G. Use and Design of Handheld Computers for Older Adults: A Review and Appraisal. *Int. J. Hum. Comput. Interact.* **2012**, *28*, 799–826. [CrossRef]
32. Castilla, D.; Botella, C.; Miralles, I.; Bretón-lópez, J.; Dragomir-davis, A.; Zaragoza, I.; Garcia-palacios, A. Teaching digital literacy skills to the elderly using a social network with linear navigation: A case study in a rural area. *Int. J. Hum. Comput. Stud.* **2018**, *118*, 24–37. [CrossRef]
33. Dunn, T. Usability for Older Web Users. Available online: https://www.webcredible.com/blog/usability-older-web-users/ (accessed on 25 March 2019).
34. Hogan, M. Age Differences in Technophobia: An Irish Study. In *Information Systems Development*; Springer: Boston, MA, USA, 2009; pp. 117–130.
35. Chua, S.L.; Chen, D.-T.; Wong, A.F.L. Computer anxiety and its correlates: A meta-analysis. *Comput. Hum. Behav.* **1999**, *15*, 609–623. [CrossRef]
36. Wang, C.; Chen, J. Overcoming technophobia in poorly-educated elderly—The HELPS-seniors service learning program. *Int. J. Autom. Smart Technol.* **2015**, *5*, 173–182.
37. Friemel, T.N. The digital divide has grown old: Determinants of a digital divide among seniors. *New Media Soc.* **2016**, *18*, 313–331. [CrossRef]
38. Vroman, K.G.; Arthanat, S.; Lysack, C. "Who over 65 is online?" Older adults' dispositions toward information communication technology. *Comput. Hum. Behav.* **2015**, *43*, 156–166. [CrossRef]
39. Wargnier, P.; Benveniste, S.; Jouvelot, P.; Rigaud, A.S. Usability assessment of interaction management support in LOUISE, an ECA-based user interface for elders with cognitive impairment. *Technol. Disabil.* **2018**, *30*, 105–126. [CrossRef]
40. Campoverde-Molina, M.; Lujan-Mora, S.; Garcia, L.V. Empirical Studies on Web Accessibility of Educational Websites: A Systematic Literature Review. *IEEE Access* **2020**, *8*, 91676–91700. [CrossRef]
41. European Commission Web Accessibility | Shaping Europe's Digital Future. Available online: https://ec.europa.eu/digital-single-market/en/web-accessibility (accessed on 7 July 2020).
42. European Commission. Directive (EU) 2016/2102 of the European Parliament and of the Council of 26 October 2016 on the accessibility of the websites and mobile applications of public. Document 32016L2102 sector bodies. *Off. J. Eur. Union.* **2016**, *L327*, 1–15.
43. W3C Web Accessibility Initiative WAI. Web Content Accessibility Guidelines (WCAG) Overview. Available online: https://www.w3.org/WAI/standards-guidelines/wcag/ (accessed on 7 July 2020).
44. W3C Web Accessibility Initiative WAI. Overview of "Web Accessibility for Older Users: A Literature Review". Available online: https://www.w3.org/WAI/older-users/literature/ (accessed on 6 July 2020).
45. W3C Web Accessibility Initiative WAI. Cognitive Accessibility at W3C | Web Accessibility Initiative (WAI) | W3C. Available online: https://www.w3.org/WAI/cognitive/ (accessed on 6 July 2020).
46. Castilla, D.; Garcia-Palacios, A.; Miralles, I.; Breton-Lopez, J.; Parra, E.; Rodriguez-Berges, S.; Botella, C. Effect of Web navigation style in elderly users. *Comput. Hum. Behav.* **2016**, *55*, 909–920. [CrossRef]
47. Arthanat, S. Promoting Information Communication Technology Adoption and Acceptance for Aging-in-Place: A Randomized Controlled Trial. *J. Appl. Gerontol.* **2019**. Available online: https://pubmed.ncbi.nlm.nih.gov/31782347/ (accessed on 6 April 2020).
48. Fernando, S.; Money, A.; Elliman, T.; Lines, L. Developing assistive web-base technologies for adults with age-related cognitive impairments. *Transform. Gov. People Process Policy* **2009**, *3*, 131–143. [CrossRef]
49. Haesner, M.; Steinert, A.; O'Sullivan, J.L.; Steinhagen-Thiessen, E. Evaluating an accessible web interface for older adults—The impact of mild cognitive impairment (MCI). *J. Assist. Technol.* **2015**, *9*, 219–232. [CrossRef]

50. Lauriks, S.; Reinersmann, A.; Van der Roest, H.G.; Meiland, F.J.; Davies, R.J.; Moelaert, F.; Mulvenna, M.D.; Nugent, C.D.; Dröes, R.M. Review of ICT-based services for identified unmet needs in people with dementia. *Ageing Res. Rev.* **2007**, *6*, 223–246. [CrossRef]
51. Jackson, G.R.; Owsley, C. Visual dysfunction, neurodegenerative diseases, and aging. *Neurol. Clin.* **2003**, *21*, 709–728. [CrossRef]
52. Rizzo, M.; Anderson, S.W.; Dawson, J.; Nawrot, M. Vision and cognition in Alzheimer's disease. *Neuropsychologia* **2000**, *38*, 1157–1169. [CrossRef]
53. Rizzo, M.; Sparks, J.; McEvoy, S.; Viamonte, S.; Kellison, I.; Vecera, S.P. Change blindness, aging, and cognition. *J. Clin. Exp. Neuropsychol.* **2009**, *31*, 245–256. [CrossRef]
54. Caird, J.K.; Edwards, C.J.; Creaser, J.I.; Horrey, W.J. Older Driver Failures of Attention at Intersections: Using Change Blindness Methods to Assess Turn Decision Accuracy. *Hum. Factors J. Hum. Factors Ergon. Soc.* **2005**, *47*, 235–249. [CrossRef] [PubMed]
55. Whitenton, K. Change Blindness Causes People to Ignore What Designers Expect Them to See. Available online: https://www.nngroup.com/articles/change-blindness/ (accessed on 25 March 2019).
56. García-Betances, R.I.; Cabrera-Umpiérrez, M.F.; Ottaviano, M.; Pastorino, M.; Arredondo, M.T. Parametric Cognitive Modeling of Information and Computer Technology Usage by People with Aging- and Disability-Derived Functional Impairments. *Sensors* **2016**, *16*, 266. [CrossRef] [PubMed]
57. Contreras-Somoza, L.M.; Irazoki, E.; Castilla, D.; Cristina, B.; Toribio-guzmán, J.M.; Parra-Vidales, E.; Suso-Ribera, C.; Suárez-López, P.; Perea-Bartolomé, M.V.; Franco-Martín, M.Á. Study on the acceptability of an ICT platform for older adults with mild cognitive impairment. *J. Med. Syst.* **2020**, *44*, 120. [CrossRef]
58. European Commission. ehcoBUTLER. A Global Ecosystem for the Independent and Healty Living of Elder People with Mild Cognitive Impairments. | Projects | H2020 | CORDIS | Grant Agreement ID: 643566. 2018. Available online: https://cordis.europa.eu/project/rcn/194077/factsheet/en (accessed on 25 March 2019).
59. Castilla, D.; Garcia-Palacios, A.; Bretón-López, J.; Miralles, I.; Baños, R.M.; Etchemendy, E.; Farfallini, L.; Botella, C. Process of design and usability evaluation of a telepsychology web and virtual reality system for the elderly: Butler. *Int. J. Hum. Comput. Stud.* **2013**, *71*, 350–362. [CrossRef]
60. Nielsen, J. *Usability Engineering*; Academic Press: Boston, MA, USA, 1993.
61. Dumas, J.S.; Redish, J. *A Practical Guide to Usability Testing*; Intellect Books: Exeter, UK, 1999.
62. Mateos, R.; Franco, M.; Sanchez, M. Care for dementia in Spain: The need for a nationwide strategy. *Int. J. Geriatr. Psychiatry* **2010**, *25*, 881–884. [CrossRef]
63. Europe, A. Spain—National Dementia Strategies—Policy in Practice. Available online: https://www.alzheimer-europe.org/Policy-in-Practice2/National-Dementia-Strategies/Spain (accessed on 29 March 2019).
64. Arriola, E.; Carnero, C.; Freire, A.; López-Mogil, R.; López-Trigo, J.A.; Manzano, S.; Olazarán, J. *Deterioro Cognitivo Leve en el Adulto Mayor. Documento de Consenso*; Sociedad Española de Geriatría y Gerontología, Ed.; Sociedad Española de Geriatría y Gerontología: Madrid, Spain, 2017.
65. Botella, C.; Etchemendy, E.; Castilla, D.; Baños, R.M.; García-Palacios, A.; Quero, S.; Alcañiz, M.; Lozano, J.A. An e-health system for the elderly (Butler Project): A pilot study on acceptance and satisfaction. *Cyberpsychol. Behav.* **2009**, *12*, 255–262. [CrossRef] [PubMed]
66. Lorish, C.D.; Maisiak, R. The face scale: A brief, nonverbal method for assessing patient mood. *Arthritis Rheum.* **1986**, *29*, 906–909. [CrossRef]
67. Stern, R.A.; Arruda, J.E.; Hooper, C.R.; Wolfner, G.D.; Morey, C.E. Visual analogue mood scales to measure internal mood state in neurologically impaired patients: Description and initial validity evidence. *Aphasiology* **1997**, *11*, 59–71. [CrossRef]
68. Yang, F.; Dawes, P.; Leroi, I.; Gannon, B. Measurement tools of resource use and quality of life in clinical trials for dementia or cognitive impairment interventions: A systematically conducted narrative review. *Int. J. Geriatr. Psychiatry* **2017**, *33*, 1–11. [CrossRef]
69. Hart, S.; Staveland, L. Development of NASA-TLX (Task Load Index): Results of empirical and theoretical research. In *Human Mental Workload*; Hancock, P., Meshkati, N., Eds.; North Holland Press: Amsterdam, The Netherlands, 1988; pp. 139–183.
70. American Psychological Association. Ethical Principles of Psychologists and Code of Conduct. Available online: https://www.apa.org/ethics/code/ (accessed on 3 February 2020).
71. National Institute on Aging. Making Your Web Site Senior Friendly: A Checklist. Available online: https://www.hsdl.org/?view&did=770661 (accessed on 14 June 2020).

72. Christopher Mayer, C.; Morandell, M.; Gira, M.; Fagel, S. *AAL Joint Programme Ambient Assisted Living User Interfaces AALuis i Project Identification Ambient Assisted Living User Interfaces*; European Commission: Brusels, Belgium, 2011.
73. Freiherr, J.; Lundström, J.N.; Habel, U.; Reetz, K. Multisensory integration mechanisms during aging. *Front. Hum. Neurosci.* **2013**, *7*, 1–6. [CrossRef] [PubMed]
74. Kim, H.; Hirtle, S.C. Spatial metaphors and disorientation in hypertext browsing. *Behav. Inf. Technol.* **1995**, *14*, 239–250. [CrossRef]
75. Techentin, C.; Voyer, D.; Voyer, S.D. Spatial Abilities and Aging: A Meta-Analysis. *Exp. Aging Res.* **2014**, *40*, 395–425. [CrossRef]
76. Barnard, Y.; Bradley, M.D.; Hodgson, F.; Lloyd, A.D. Learning to use new technologies by older adults: Perceived difficulties, experimentation behaviour and usability. *Comput. Hum. Behav.* **2013**, *29*, 1715–1724. [CrossRef]
77. Graf, P.; Mandler, G. Activation makes words more accessible, but not necessarily more retrievable. *J. Verbal Learn. Verbal Behav.* **1984**, *23*, 553–568. [CrossRef]
78. Mandler, G. Recognizing: The judgment of previous occurrence. *Psychol. Rev.* **1980**, *87*, 252–271. [CrossRef]

9

Using the Personalized Advantage Index for Individual Treatment Allocation to Blended Treatment or Treatment as Usual for Depression in Secondary Care

Nadine Friedl [1,*], Tobias Krieger [1], Karine Chevreul [2], Jean Baptiste Hazo [3], Jérôme Holtzmann [4], Mark Hoogendoorn [5], Annet Kleiboer [6], Kim Mathiasen [7,8], Antoine Urech [9], Heleen Riper [10,11,12] and Thomas Berger [1]

1 Department of Clinical Psychology, University of Bern, 3012 Bern, Switzerland
2 URC Eco Ile-de-France (AP-HP), Hotel Dieu, 1, Place du Parvis Notre Dame, 75004 Paris, France
3 Eceve, Unit 1123, Inserm, University of Paris, Health Economics Research Unit, Assistance Publique-Hôpitaux de Paris, 75004 Paris, France
4 University Hospital Grenoble Alpes, Mood Disorders and Emotional Pathologies Unit, Pôle de Psychiatrie, Neurologie et Rééducation Neurologique, 38043 Grenoble, France
5 Department of Computer Science, VU University Amsterdam Faculty of Sciences, De Boelelaan 1081m, 1081 HV Amsterdam, The Netherlands
6 Section Clinical Psychology, Faculty of Behavioural and Movement Sciences, Vrije Universiteit Amsterdam and EMGO+ Institute for Health Care and Research, Van der Boechorststraat 1, 1081 BT Amsterdam, The Netherlands
7 Department of Psychology, Faculty of Health Sciences, University of Southern Denmark, 5230 Odense M, Denmark
8 Center of Telepsychiatry, University of Southern Denmark, 5000 Odense, Denmark
9 INSELSPITAL, University Hospital Bern, University Clinic for Neurology, University Acute-Neurorehabilitation Center, 3010 Bern, Switzerland
10 Department of Psychiatry and the Amsterdam Public Health Research Institute, GGZ inGeest/Amsterdam UMC, Vrije Universiteit, de Boelelaan 1117, 1081 HV Amsterdam, The Netherlands
11 Department of Research and Innovation, GGZ inGeest Specialized Mental Health Care, Oldenaller 1, 1081 HJ Amsterdam, The Netherlands
12 Department of Clinical, Neuro-and Developmental Psychology and the Amsterdam Public Health Research Institute, Vrije Universiteit Amsterdam, van der Boechorststraat 7, 1081 BT Amsterdam, The Netherlands
* Correspondence: nadine.friedl@psy.unibe.ch

Abstract: A variety of effective psychotherapies for depression are available, but patients who suffer from depression vary in their treatment response. Combining face-to-face therapies with internet-based elements in the sense of blended treatment is a new approach to treatment for depression. The goal of this study was to answer the following research questions: (1) What are the most important predictors determining optimal treatment allocation to treatment as usual or blended treatment? and (2) Would model-determined treatment allocation using this predictive information and the personalized advantage index (PAI)-approach result in better treatment outcomes? Bayesian model averaging (BMA) was applied to the data of a randomized controlled trial (RCT) comparing the efficacy of treatment as usual and blended treatment in depressive outpatients. Pre-treatment symptomatology and treatment expectancy predicted outcomes irrespective of treatment condition, whereas different prescriptive predictors were found. A PAI of 2.33 PHQ-9 points was found, meaning that patients who would have received the treatment that is optimal for them would have had a post-treatment PHQ-9 score that is two points lower than if they had received the treatment that is suboptimal for them. For 29% of the sample, the PAI was five or greater, which means that a substantial difference between the two treatments was predicted. The use of the PAI approach for clinical practice must be further confirmed in prospective research; the current study supports the identification of specific interventions favorable for specific patients.

Keywords: personalized advantage index; depression; blended treatment; CBT; treatment selection; Bayesian model averaging

1. Introduction

Globally, 300 million people of all ages suffer from depression [1]. Depression is one of the most common problems seen in clinical practice, and it is associated with high societal costs, as well as great suffering [2]. Given this burden, the need for improved access to efficacious and cost-effective treatments is essential [3]. In the last decades, research has focused on examining different treatment options for depression. Especially, cognitive behavior therapy (CBT) and interpersonal therapy (IPT) can be seen as first-line treatments [4,5]. Moreover, current studies are aimed at scaling up treatments for depression. One way to do so is through internet-based therapies [5]. Whereas the most dominant format in which treatment is delivered is through face-to-face contact, internet-based therapies have received much attention in recent years [6]. The efficacy and cost-effectiveness of the latter have been supported by a growing number of research [7–9]. Even though only a few studies have directly compared internet-based with face-to-face CBT for depression, results suggest it to have similar overall effects [6].

A newer approach to depression treatment is to combine web-based technologies with face-to-face therapy, called blended treatment. Blended treatment includes any combination of face-to-face therapy and internet-based interventions, e.g., web-based components are used as an adjunctive intervention or are integrated during face-to-face therapy [10]. Although research that investigates the efficacy of blended treatment formats is still scarce, preliminary results suggest their feasibility and their efficacy in reducing symptoms of depression [11–15]. For example, a randomized controlled trial by Berger and colleagues [16] showed the superiority of blended treatment, consisting of an internet-based intervention as an adjunct to face-to-face psychotherapy, in comparison to regular face-to-face psychotherapy in a pragmatic randomized controlled study in patients with a unipolar affective disorder in routine care. Another recent study showed the noninferiority of blended treatment to conventional CBT for patients with depression and found blended treatment to be cost-effective [17]. Moreover, the blended treatment has also been evaluated in an inpatient setting where patients suffering from depression that received an online self-help program in addition to inpatient psychotherapy improved significantly more than patients who received online information about depression in addition to inpatient psychotherapy [18]. Furthermore, a recent systematic review showed that, compared to face-to-face therapy, a blended treatment may help maintaining initially achieved changes within psychotherapy in the long-term [19].

Potential benefits of blending treatments may be a greater reduction in depressive symptoms and increased cost-effectiveness [20], as well as an improvement of patients' adherence to the treatment program [21]. Furthermore, an asset of a blended treatment may be that it combines the advantages of both treatment forms [3,14,22,23]. For example, the face-to-face contact enables clinicians to individualize or tailor the treatment and to react in crisis situations, while providing online modules between sessions could promote patient engagement and enhance the translation of treatment into daily life (e.g., [24]). On the other hand, when online components are not used by the patients in blended treatments, reductions in the number of face-to-face sessions may lead to worse treatment outcomes [25]. Furthermore, therapists may raise concerns of overburdening depressed patients [18]. So far, it is not clear for which patients blended treatment may be a feasible option and for which patients a conventional treatment should be favored.

Patients with depression may differ substantially from each other, and evidence suggests that the diagnostic categories leave room for great diversity [26,27]. This results in differences with regard to patients' illness courses and individual treatment responses [28]. Research suggests that individual patient characteristics may moderate the efficacy of different treatments at an individual level [29]. It is, therefore, important to recognize that no single treatment is likely to be the best for everyone, even though, on a group level, it is efficacious for patients suffering from depression [26,30]. This is why more and more researchers move away from investigating treatment efficacy on a group level and instead focus on custom-tailoring the treatment to the individual patient [30,31]. In this sense, it may be a solution to increase the overall treatment response rates [32].

Precision medicine tries to tailor treatments to the specific needs of the patient [33]. More recently, in clinical psychology and psychotherapy, algorithms are used that predict from which treatment a patient benefits the most [34]. As an example, Becker and colleagues [35] introduce a conceptual framework that helps classifying applications of predictive modeling in mental health research. These authors try to bridge the gap between psychologists and predictive modelers with providing a common language for classifying predictive modeling mental health research. They suggest that e-mental health researchers should focus more on the validity of model predictions instead of solely focusing on identifying predictors. Another example is the personalized advantage index PAI) approach, which identifies patients with a certain disorder (e.g., major depression) who benefit more from one treatment than another [30]. Using the personalized advantage index (PAI), it is possible to identify the treatment that predicts a better treatment outcome for a given patient if there are two comparably effective treatments to choose from [36]. The PAI estimates how much a specific treatment is better for an individual patient than another, and its feasibility and relevance have been shown in several studies on the treatment of depression [36–40]. Baseline patient characteristics can be divided into two types of predictors: a prognostic variable predicts treatment outcome irrespective of treatment condition, whereas a prescriptive variable predicts a differential treatment response to two or more treatment modalities [29,30]. Up to today, different treatments have been compared using the PAI, and its values range from 1.4 when comparing CBT to CBT with integrated exposure and emotion-focused elements [38] up to 8.9 when comparing cognitive therapy to IPT [40]. Higher absolute values of the PAI stand for stronger predicted benefits of one treatment over another. Being able to identify the best treatment for an individual with depression is essential, because it may make health care delivery more efficient [32]. Even though predictive modeling is still very young in the field of e-mental health [41], Bremer and colleagues [42] were able to predict clinical outcomes and costs of patients with depression prior to starting blended psychotherapy in a subsample of the current study using machine learning techniques.

In the current study, treatment as usual (TAU), i.e., regular face-to-face psychotherapy, was compared to blended treatment for patients with major depressive disorder (MDD) in secondary care. The present study set out to answer the following research questions: (1) What are the most important predictors determining optimal treatment allocation to TAU or blended treatment? and (2) Would model-determined treatment allocation using this predictive information and the PAI-approach result in better treatment outcomes? To the best of our knowledge, this is the first study comparing different treatment delivering formats, i.e., traditional face-to-face CBT versus blended CBT, by using the PAI-approach.

2. Materials and Methods

Data used in the present study was drawn from the European project "European COMPARative effectiveness research on blended depression treatment" (E-COMPARED, February 2018) [43]. The E-COMPARED project included a randomized, controlled, noninferiority trial that examined the clinical and cost-effectiveness of blended treatment compared to treatment as usual in routine care in nine European countries. Adult patients diagnosed with MDD were recruited in primary or in specialized mental health care. The current study uses the data of the four countries that recruited patients in specialized mental health care (France, the Netherlands, Switzerland, and Denmark). The following inclusion criteria were met by participants: (1) being 18 years of age or older, (2) meeting Diagnostic and Statistical Manual of Mental Disorders (DSM-IV) diagnostic criteria for MDD as confirmed by a telephone-administered MINI international neuropsychiatric interview (M.I.N.I.) version 5.0 [44], and (3) minimal to severe symptoms of depression based on a score of 5 or above on the patient health questionnaire-9 (PHQ-9) [45]. Exclusion criteria for participating in the study were: (1) high risk for suicide according to the M.I.N.I.; (2) psychiatric comorbidity such as substance dependence, bipolar affective disorder, psychotic illness, or obsessive compulsive disorder; (3) currently receiving another psychological treatment for depression; (4) being unable to comprehend the spoken and written language of the country where the study is conducted; (5) not having access to a computer with fast internet connection; and (6) not having a smartphone that is compatible with the mobile component of the intervention that is offered. Patients were randomized to blended treatment or TAU using an allocation scheme with a computerized random number generator at an allocation ratio of 1:1 and between 8 and 14 allocations per block. Details about the study design are described elsewhere [43]. For Switzerland, this study was approved by the cantonal ethics committees Bern and Zurich (registration number: 001/15; date: 18 March 2015); for Denmark, the study was approved by the Ethics Committee of the Region of Southern Denmark (registration number S-20150150; date: 18 November 2015); for France, the study was approved by the "Comité de protection des personnes", Ile de France V (registration number 15033-*n*° 2015-A00565-44; date: 2 June 2015); and, for the Netherlands, the study was approved by the METC VUMC (registration number 2015.078; date: 8 May 2015). Furthermore, all participants provided written informed consent and gave permission to all E-COMPARED partners to use their anonymized data.

2.1. Sample

The current study has a sample size of n = 251. The sample consists of 83 participants from the Netherlands (33.9%), 79 participants from France (32.2%), 44 from Switzerland (18.0%), and 39 participants from Denmark (15.9%). The mean age at baseline was 41.0 years (SD = 13.7), and 68.2% of the participants were female. The majority were either single (33.5%) or married (31.8%), and 21.2% of participants were living together and 12.8% were divorced. In the TAU condition, 57.9% of the sample suffered from a recurrent depression, 45.2% from a current melancholic depressive episode, 7.9% from a comorbid dysthymia, and 46.8% from a comorbid anxiety disorder. The number of patients are taking antidepressant medication at the time of the baseline measurement was 53.2%. In the blended treatment condition, 53.8% of the participants suffered from a recurrent depression, 34.5% from a current melancholic depressive episode, 5.9% from a comorbid dysthymia, and 61.3% had a comorbid anxiety disorder. Half of the participants (49.6%) were taking antidepressant medication at baseline.

2.2. Interventions

Individual face-to-face CBT was combined with internet-based CBT elements delivered through a platform for blended treatment. Three different online platforms were used across the participating countries. Switzerland used "Deprexis" [46], whereas Denmark used NoDep [47] and France and the Netherlands used the platform "Moodbuster" [3]. The most important components of the treatment were cognitive restructuring, behavioral activation, psychoeducation, and relapse prevention, which were delivered over 11–20 sessions. In the blended treatment, a smaller number of face-to-face sessions is offered, and some sessions are replaced by online modules. Treatment was provided by CBT therapists who received special training on how to deliver the blended treatment. In Switzerland and the Netherlands, the therapists were either licensed CBT therapists or CBT therapists who were supervised by an experienced licensed CBT therapist. In Denmark, the treatment was delivered by either licensed psychologists or psychologists under supervision of licensed psychologists. In France, the blended treatment was provided by licensed psychotherapists [43].

The TAU treatment was defined as the routine care that patients received in specialized mental health care when they were diagnosed with depression. In practice, this meant that the TAU group received regular fact-to-face CBT.

2.3. Measures

2.3.1. Primary Outcome

The primary outcome measure for this study was the PHQ-9 [45] assessed after 12 weeks. The PHQ-9 consists of nine questions which are based upon the DSM-IV criteria for the diagnosis of depressive disorders. It is used as a diagnostic instrument and as a severity measure for depression. A 5-point difference in PHQ-9 scores is seen as clinically significant [48]. The validity and sensitivity to change of the PHQ-9 were satisfactory in previous studies [49,50]. Cronbach's alpha in the present study was 0.78.

2.3.2. Predictor Variables

We used an exploratory approach and included a total of 28 potential predictors measured at baseline in the analysis. All variables of the baseline assessment that did not exceed a number of acceptable missing values (<50%) were included. We classified the variables into four categories: (1) sociodemographic variables, (2) symptomatology and quality of life, (3) healthcare utilization, and (4) patient expectancy.

The sociodemographic variables included age, marital status, education, gender, and country and were assessed with single item questions. Variables related to symptomatology and treatment history were recurrent depression, therapy preference, dysthymia, melancholic depressive episodes, comorbid anxiety, and current use of antidepressants. Quality of life was measured with the EQ-5D [51]. Healthcare utilization was assessed with the TiC-P [52]. The TiC-P examines healthcare consumption and productivity losses as a consequence of a mental disorder via a self-report questionnaire. The questions include contacts within the healthcare sector and the use of medication. All the questions aim at the period of the last four months before the start of the treatment (see Table 1 for the items of the TiC-P that have been included). Patient expectancy was measured by the credibility and expectancy questionnaire (CEQ; [53]).

Table 1. TiC-P items included in the analysis.

"How many times did you consult a general practitioner?" "How many times did you consult a psychologist?" "How many times did you consult a psychotherapist?", "How many times did you consult a psychiatrist?", and "How many times did you consult a professional from an ambulatory mental health institution?" "How many times did you consult a professional from a clinic for alcohol or drugs?" and "How many times did you consult self-help groups?"	"How many days did you spend in a day-time treatment program in a regular hospital?" "How many days did you spend in a day-time treatment program in a psychiatric hospital?" and "How many days did you use outpatient psychotherapeutic services in addition to your psychotherapy?"	"How many admissions to a regular hospital did you have?" and "How many admissions to a psychiatric hospital did you have?" "How many admissions to a rehabilitation clinic did you have?" "Do you have a paid job?" "Did health problems oblige you to call in sick from work at any time?"

2.4. Data Analytical Strategy

Regarding the predictor variables, a bottom-up approach was followed, which means that even though some variables might have a particular relevance to one treatment or the other, the predictors are treated equally in the data analysis.

2.4.1. Missing Data

In line with previous research using the PAI approach, we included those participants for which PHQ-9 scores after 12 weeks were available [36,38,40]. This left us with n = 245, representing 97.6% of the total sample. Distributed over the two conditions, there were 126 patients in the TAU condition and

119 patients in the blended treatment condition. With regard to the baseline measures, missing values were found in the dimensions credibility and expectancy of the CEQ (3.7% respectively 4.1%), the EQ-5D (1.6%), antidepressants (1.2%), prior psychotherapy (40.4%), comorbid melancholic episodes (14.3%), comorbid dysthymia (5.3%), comorbid anxiety (2.4%), and some items of the TiC-P (2.0–40.8%). We imputed these missings in the baseline measures with the R *missForest* [54]. Here, missing values are predicted on the basis of a random forest approach, trained on observed values of the available data. An advantage of *missForest* is that it imputes categorical and continuous variables simultaneously [55]. It has been shown to be highly accurate and to outperform other imputation methods due to its small imputation error [56]. The imputed data set is the basis for all analyses that follow.

2.4.2. Bayesian Model Averaging (BMA)

There are different data analysis approaches that can be used to identify baseline variables that predict outcome in one treatment versus another. Data analysis approaches that rely on one model only can only include a limited number of baseline measures that could be predictors. In that case, the most common rule that is used states that at least 10 observations per predictor are necessary to not exceed a level of bias which is acceptable [57,58]. If we had followed this approach, we could have only included a small number of predictors. Furthermore, the problem with relying upon a single selected model is that it may result in overconfidence in the conclusions drawn regarding quantified associations. The problem is that there may be alternative models that have different subsets of predictors that fit the data just as well as the one selected model [59,60]. Overfitted models cause uncertainty regarding the actual value of findings, because they may not replicate in future samples [61]. Bayesian model averaging (BMA) is a method that can account for model uncertainty while providing a better predictive ability. The BMA method has two advantages. First, it results in predictions that are less risky and. second, BMA provides simpler model choice criteria, because it uses the Bayesian inference for model prediction and selection [62]. With BMA, a posterior probability is estimated on the basis that each considered model is the correct one. This included the aforementioned model uncertainty in the estimates for the parameter and inferences. That means that BMA averages over all possible predictor sets and delivers model choice criteria that help to identify the most probable model. With using BMA, sharper predictions can be derived from the data, especially in cases with many possible predictors but a limited sample size. Several studies have supported BMA's predictive performance [60,63–66].

The data frame was divided into two subsets: the TAU condition and the blended treatment condition. Using the R package *BAS*, for each condition, a separate linear regression model was computed [67]. Then, Bayesian adaptive sampling (BAS) without replacement for variable selection in linear models using the function *bas.lm* with treatment outcome was applied (PHQ-9 score after 12 weeks) as the dependent variable. The relative importance of each variable was evaluated using the posterior probabilities that were calculated for each potential predictor. The marginal posterior inclusion probabilities functioned as the criteria for determining the importance of the potential predictors. Values above 0.5 point out that the predictor has been incorporated in more than half the models; thus, in the present study, in over 15,000 models. The nominal variables were split into their different categories, which enabled a precise interpretation of the results. The model performance was further evaluated using posterior probabilities. The appropriate *bas.lm* function was chosen based on the following considerations: a Laplace approximation to the Jeffreys-Zellner-Siow (JZS) prior for the integration of alpha = 1 was used as the criterion for the priors, which is called the "ZS-null". The JZS prior uses the Zellner-Siow Cauchy prior on the coefficients and the Jeffreys prior on sigma. The squared scale of the prior, where the default is alpha = 1, can be controlled using the optional parameter "alpha" [38,67]. Marginal inclusion probabilities were calculated with the "MCMC+BAS" method, which runs an initial Markov chain Monte Carlo (MCMC) algorithm and then samples without replacement, as in BAS. Compared to the BAS alone, the "MCMC+BAS" method is the preferred option, because it provides estimates with low bias [68]. The number of models was set to 30,000 assuming that each additional model would add only a small increment to the cumulative probability, i.e., not leading to essential differences in posterior distributions. Due to the limited sample size, the models have been built and tested in the same dataset.

2.4.3. Personalized Advantage Index (PAI)

When predicting the therapy outcome for each patient, applying a leave-one-out approach ("jackknife") to estimate regression models is an essential beginning step in generating the PAI [36,38,69]. In this procedure, overfitting can be avoided by excluding each target patient for whom the PAI prediction is estimated from the model. For each patient, two regression models were built using the treatment-specific predictors identified with BMA. For each patient, a factual prediction (PHQ-9 score at 12 weeks of the treatment the patient has received) and a counterfactual prediction (PHQ-9 score at 12 weeks of the intervention the patient did not receive) were estimated. In the next step, those two predictions were compared, and the prediction that resulted in the best outcome for the patient was defined to be the optimal treatment for that patient. When comparing the observed change scores, the size of the predicted difference of receiving the treatment with the greater predicted benefit is ultimately the PAI [36]. The higher the absolute values of the PAI, the stronger is the predicted benefit of one treatment over another. The interpretation of the PAI can be demonstrated with a recent study that used the PHQ-9 as the primary outcome and found a PAI of 2.5 [70]. This means that if patients had received their "optimal" treatment (out of the two), their PHQ-9 score at 12 weeks would have been 2.5 points lower than if they had obtained their nonoptimal treatment.

3. Results

Henceforth, we firstly report the five best models for each treatment condition, and, secondly, we report the PAI results. The best models are defined based on the highest posterior probability and the lowest Bayesian information criterion (BIC).

3.1. Variables Predicting Outcome in TAU

The five best models predicting depression severity at 12 weeks in the TAU condition are displayed in Table 2. The Bayes factor, number of predictors, R^2, log marginal likelihood, and the posterior probabilities are provided for each model. Model 1 has the largest Bayes factor and the largest posterior probability (0.02) and, thus, seems to fit the data best. As a result, Model 1 was selected as our final predictive model of the PHQ-9 score at 12 weeks in the TAU condition.

Table 2. Five best models for treatment as usual (TAU).

Fit Indices	Model 1	Model 2	Model 3	Model 4	Model 5
Bayes Factor	1	0.934	0.597	0.572	0.510
Number of Variables	6	6	6	5	6
R^2	0.428	0.445	0.441	0.440	0.439
Log Marginal Likelihood	22.729	22.659	22.213	22.170	22.056
Posterior Probabilities	0.021	0.019	0.012	0.012	0.011

While the selected model includes six variables in total, the strongest predictors of the PHQ-9 score at 12 weeks in the TAU condition included the pretreatment PHQ-9 score (Prob = 100%), CEQ expectancy (Prob = 97%), "How many days did you use outpatient psychotherapeutic services in addition to your psychotherapy?" (Prob = 95%), "How many times did you consult a psychiatrist?" (Prob = 64%), Denmark (Prob = 58%), and "How many days did you attend a day-time treatment program in a psychiatric hospital?" (Prob = 51%). A higher pretreatment score, more consultations with a psychiatrist, and more days in a day-time treatment program in a psychiatric hospital prior to treatment predicted a higher PHQ-9 score at 12 weeks. Higher expectancy scores, receiving TAU in Denmark, and more days using outpatient psychotherapeutic services in addition to the psychotherapy prior to treatment predicted lower PHQ-9 scores at 12 weeks. The effects of other variables appeared minimal due to their small posterior probabilities. See Appendix 1 in the Supplemental Online Material for the complete list of variables and their inclusion probabilities.

3.2. *Variables Predicting Outcome in the Nlended Treatment*

Table 3 gives an overview of the five best models to predict treatment outcome in the blended treatment condition. Based on the posterior probabilities and the Bayes factor, Model 1 was rated the best model. Thus, Model 1 was selected as the final predictive model for the blended treatment condition.

Table 3. Five best models for the blended treatment condition.

Fit Indices	Model 1	Model 2	Model 3	Model 4	Model 5
Bayes Factor	1	0.887	0.577	0.525	0.516
Number of Variables	6	5	4	6	6
R^2	0.398	0.416	0.392	0.429	0.446
Log Marginal Likelihood	19.852	19.731	19.301	19.207	19.190
Posterior Probabilities	0.012	0.011	0.007	0.006	0.006

Based on the posterior probabilities, the most important predictors for treatment outcome in the blended treatment were the pretreatment PHQ-9 score (Prob = 99.9%), regular hospital admissions (Prob = 99.9%), EQ-5D quality of life (Prob = 74.6%), CEQ expectancy (Prob = 72.3%), consulting self-help groups (Prob = 70.0%), and being widowed (Prob = 49.7%). CEQ credibility reached a posterior probability of 42.9%. A higher pretreatment PHQ-9 score, being widowed, more hospital admissions, and consulting self-help groups predicted higher PHQ-9 scores at 12 weeks. A higher expectancy for improvement and a higher quality of life predicted lower PHQ-9 scores after 12 weeks. See Appendix 2 in the Supplemental Online Material for the posterior probabilities of all variables measured at baseline.

3.3. *Personalized Advantage Index*

Using the treatment specific predictors described above, the prediction of a patient's PHQ-9 score after 12 weeks was computed separately for each treatment condition. The true error of the PHQ-9 score predictions at 12 weeks was 4.16, representing the average absolute difference between the predicted and actual, observed scores across all patients. Patients who were categorized as having received their optimal treatment had a mean PHQ-9 score of 9.67 (n = 124) at 12 weeks, whereas patients who were classified as having received their suboptimal treatment had a mean PHQ-9 score of 12.00 (n = 121). Figure 1 shows the frequency of predicted PHQ-9 scores at 12 weeks for every patient in both the optimal and suboptimal treatments.

In the first step, an individual PAI was calculated for each patient. Secondly, the average PAI was calculated as the mean difference in PHQ-9 scores between the optimal and the suboptimal treatments for each patient. The average PAI of the current study was 2.33. The PAI can be read as follows: if patients had received the treatment that is "optimal" for them, their PHQ-9 score at 12 weeks would have been 2.33 points lower than if they had received the treatment that is suboptimal for them. In Figure 2, the frequencies of the individual PAIs are shown. A PAI that is five or greater would mean that a substantial difference was predicted between the two treatments, because 5 points on the PHQ-9 stands for a minimal clinically meaningful difference for individual change [71]. This was the case for 29% of the patients in this sample.

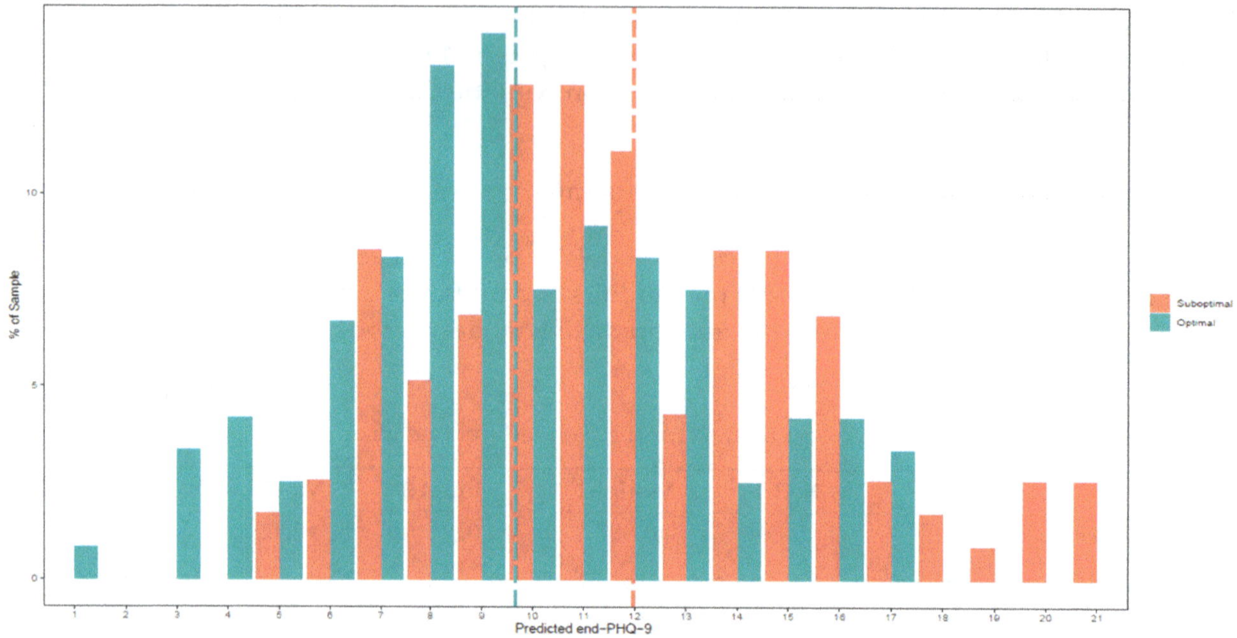

Figure 1. Frequency of predicted PHQ-9 scores at 12 weeks.

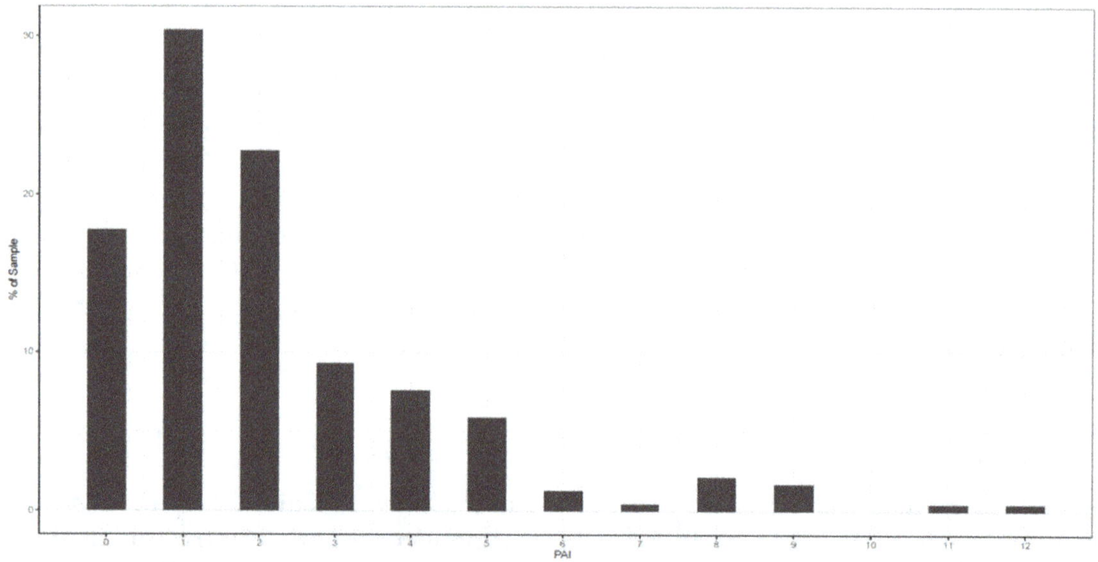

Figure 2. Frequencies of individual personalized advantage indexes (PAIs).

4. Discussion

Regarding the predictors of treatment outcome at 12 weeks in each of the interventions, different relevant predictors were identified for TAU and the blended treatment, respectively. In the TAU condition, a lower pretreatment PHQ-9 score, less consultations with a psychiatrist and less days in a day-time treatment program in a psychiatric hospital, higher expectancy, receiving TAU in Denmark, and more days using outpatient psychotherapeutic services in the four months prior to the study predicted a better treatment outcome, i.e., a lower PHQ-9 score (at 12 weeks). In contrast, in the blended treatment condition, a lower pretreatment PHQ-9 score, not being widowed, less hospital admissions and consulting self-help, a higher expectancy for improvement, and a higher EQ-5D score predicted lower scores at 12 weeks; thus, a better treatment outcome.

To offer an initial interpretation of our findings, the distinction between prescriptive and prognostic predictors is used. Prognostic variables predict treatment outcomes regardless of treatment conditions [30,38]. In contrast, prescriptive variables may support differential indications by predicting whether a patient will benefit more from one treatment in comparison to another. In the present study, the pretreatment depressive symptomatology and treatment expectancy are the only prognostic predictors, i.e., the only variables that predict treatment outcome in both conditions. This is in line with previous research that has found pretreatment symptomatology and expectancy to be important predictors of treatment outcome, in the sense that higher symptomatology before treatment predicts worse end-state symptomatology [30,34,36,38,72,73] and higher expectancy for improvement predicts better treatment outcome [74,75]. Interestingly, for internet-based treatments, higher baseline symptomatology is not necessarily a negative predictor of treatment outcome. More often the opposite is found, i.e., that higher depressive symptomatology pretreatment predicts better treatment outcomes [76–78]. This might be partly explained by the efficacy nature of previous randomized controlled trials (RCTs) in comparison to the routine care and effectiveness nature of the current study.

Regarding the prescriptive predictors, our findings partly corroborate findings from previous studies predicting treatment outcomes for patients with depression. With regard to prescriptive predictors of the blended treatment condition, a lower quality of life and being widowed predicted worse treatment outcomes. In contrast to the present result, the study by Huibers and colleagues [40] found a higher quality of life to be a prognostic predictor, i.e., to predict favorable outcomes irrespective of treatment conditions.

For the TAU condition, more consultations with a psychiatrist and more days in a day-time treatment program in a psychiatric hospital predicted worse treatment outcomes. This could mean that patients' symptomatology and patients' general functioning is too severe to be able to profit from TAU. Furthermore, to our knowledge, there are no international studies regarding psychotherapy of depression, indicating country as a relevant predictor of outcome.

Healthcare utilization within the four months prior starting treatment was found to be a prescriptive predictor in both conditions. Healthcare uptake may be a proxy for a higher somatic or mental burden and/or may represent a more severe symptomatology of depression. In previous studies, more complex cases (e.g., with chronic symptoms and psychiatric comorbidities) or more severe depressive symptomatology predicted a worse therapy outcome [29,38,79–81]. Interestingly, more hospital admissions only predicted worse treatment outcomes in the blended treatment condition. A possible interpretation of this finding is the fact that the online modules in the blended treatment protocol are highly standardized to target depressive symptomatology. As a result, they may have not sufficiently addressed comorbid symptoms. Somatic comorbidities in patients with depression are not a scarcity and have an influence on individual treatment response and illness course, because they can complicate treatment [81]. Furthermore, the number of hospital admissions may also be a proxy for case complexity and higher mental burden, which in turn may have a negative impact on treatment outcome.

This study's results demonstrate that BMA makes it possible to use a limited set of baseline variables to predict treatment outcome. This is in line with a recent study by Bremer and colleagues [42] that showed the feasibility of providing personalized treatment recommendations at baseline regarding clinical and cost-effectiveness using a subsample of the current study by evaluating various machine learning techniques. Moreover, the present study showed that despite sharing the same diagnosis, patients might benefit more from different treatments. The current study found a PAI of 2.33, indicating that patients could have a PHQ-9 score at 12 weeks that is, on average, more than two points lower if they receive their model-determined optimal treatment in comparison to the suboptimal treatment. This value is in the range of other studies that have found PAIs ranging from 1.35 [38] up to 8.9 [40]. Importantly, for almost one-third (29%) of the patients in the present study, a substantial difference was predicted between the two treatment modalities as the individual PAI was 5 or greater. This result is in line with increasing evidence suggesting that differential treatment responses are not rare and might play an important role for an individual patient and the health care system [30].

The current study has several limitations. First of all, the relatively small sample size did not allow us to build and test the models in separate samples. Using the same sample for testing and building the model might lead to a potential risk of overconfidence. Nevertheless, if studies are designed to develop and validate prescriptive prediction scores that can be tested in future hypothesis-driven confirmatory studies, a smaller sample size might be legitimate [82]. Secondly, the results are based solely on self-reports, and future studies should also include observer ratings. Third, the restricted set of baseline measures is another limitation. Constructs such as personality traits or the familiarity with computers have not been assessed but may have influenced engagement with the online component. Relatedly, people with a low socioeconomic status or senior citizens may not have been well represented in the present study sample. Such groups may not have the opportunity to benefit from the blended treatment, because they may not have access to a computer or a smartphone and/or lack the knowledge to use them. As a consequence, the restricted sample in the present study limits the generalizability of the results. Furthermore, the current study predicts treatment outcome after 12 weeks. Future studies should predict long-term treatment outcome [83]. Finally, we have followed a data-driven approach instead of a theory-driven approach. Although the two methods should be considered complementary [84], a disadvantage of data-driven research is that it is not experiential, and relying on the data alone might not capture the whole picture. Relatedly, the predictors found in the current study need to be validated and replicated in future hypothesis-driven studies.

In spite of the limitations above, the current study is promising to contribute to the further understanding of treatment for depression, because it investigates implications for the use of the blended treatment for patients with depression. Clinical practice should consider factors found to play a role in the treatment and processes of change to provide the optimal treatment for each individual. For example, the quality of life should be taken into account, as these patients may need a more intense treatment protocol that integrates face-to-face interventions with web-based technologies. This interpretation is in line with the notion that more severely depressed patients see the availability of an online program between face-to-face sessions as an advantage of the blended treatment [85]. Furthermore, healthcare utilization should be evaluated prior to treatment selection, because it can give valuable information about the patients' needs, treatment history, and course of illness. In addition, the predictors found to be important in this study and in previous studies could be taken into account to make an informed treatment recommendation in clinical practice. However, future studies with larger samples and more advanced techniques are necessary to validate the current findings, and the identified predictors have to be tested within clinical routine treatment settings. Moreover, prospective studies need to integrate the PAI in the diagnostics process at the beginning of a treatment.

5. Conclusions

To conclude, with the first aim of the study, two prognostic predictors, namely, pretreatment symptomatology and treatment expectancy, were found. Furthermore, several prescriptive predictors were found, predicting the treatment outcome respective of each of the two conditions. Some of our findings are in line with previous research, but other variables, such as baseline healthcare utilization, have not been investigated in this context. The interpretations regarding the prognostic and prescriptive predictors need to be tested empirically, because they are somewhat speculative. Furthermore, this study showed an advantage of model-determined treatment allocation to the TAU or blended treatment, as one-third of the participants had a PAI larger than 5, which means they would have improved significantly if they had received their "optimal" treatment. Although the results need to be validated in future hypothesis-driven studies, the predictors found to be important in the current study should be taken into account to make an informed treatment recommendation in clinical practice.

Author Contributions: N.F. analyzed the data and wrote the manuscript under the supervision of T.B. All authors critically revised the manuscript and contributed substantially to this work. All authors have read and agreed to the published version of the manuscript.

References

1. World Health Organization. Depression. 2018. Available online: https://www.who.int/news-room/fact-sheets/detail/depression (accessed on 21 November 2019).
2. World Health Organization. The Global Burden of Disease: 2004 Update. 2008. Available online: https://www.who.int/healthinfo/global_burden_disease/2004_report_update/en/ (accessed on 3 October 2019).
3. Kemmeren, L.; Van Schaik, D.J.; Riper, H.; Kleiboer, A.M.; Bosmans, J.E.; Smit, J.H. Effectiveness of blended depression treatment for adults in specialised mental healthcare: Study protocol for a randomised controlled trial. *BMC Psychiatry* **2016**, *16*, 113. [CrossRef] [PubMed]
4. Karasu, T.B.; Gelenberg, A.; Merriam, A.; Wang, P. Treatment of patients with major depressive disorder. In *American Psychiatric Association Practice Guidelines for the Treatment of Psychiatric Disorders Compendium*; American Psychiatric Publishing: Washington, DC, USA, 2000; pp. 413–495.
5. Cuijpers, P. Psychotherapies for adult depression: Recent developments. *Curr. Opin. Psychiatry* **2015**, *28*, 24–29. [CrossRef] [PubMed]
6. Carlbring, P.; Andersson, G.; Cuijpers, P.; Riper, H.; Hedman-Lagerlöf, E. Internet-based vs. face-to-face cognitive behavior therapy for psychiatric and somatic disorders: An updated systematic review and meta-analysis. *Cognit. Behav. Ther.* **2018**, *47*, 1–18. [CrossRef]
7. Arnberg, F.K.; Linton, S.J.; Hultcrantz, M.; Heintz, E.; Jonsson, U. Internet-delivered psychological treatments for mood and anxiety disorders: A systematic review of their efficacy, safety, and cost-effectiveness. *PLoS ONE* **2014**, *9*, e98118. [CrossRef]
8. Gerhards, S.; De Graaf, L.; Jacobs, L.; Severens, J.; Huibers, M.; Arntz, A.; Riper, H.; Widdershoven, G.; Metsemakers, J.F.M.; Evers, S.M.A.A. Economic evaluation of online computerised cognitive–behavioural therapy without support for depression in primary care: Randomised trial. *Br. J. Psychiatry* **2010**, *196*, 310–318. [CrossRef]
9. Richards, D.; Richardson, T. Computer-based psychological treatments for depression: A systematic review and meta-analysis. *Clin. Psychol. Rev.* **2012**, *32*, 329–342. [CrossRef]
10. Krieger, T.; Meyer, B.; Sude, K.; Urech, A.; Maercker, A.; Berger, T. Evaluating an e-mental health program ("deprexis") as adjunctive treatment tool in psychotherapy for depression: Design of a pragmatic randomized controlled trial. *BMC Psychiatry* **2014**, *14*, 285. [CrossRef]
11. Hickie, I.B.; Davenport, T.A.; Luscombe, G.M.; Moore, M.; Griffiths, K.M.; Christensen, H. Practitioner-supported delivery of internet-based cognitive behaviour therapy: Evaluation of the feasibility of conducting a cluster randomised trial. *Med. J. Aust.* **2010**, *192*, S31–S35. [CrossRef]
12. Høifødt, R.S.; Lillevoll, K.R.; Griffiths, K.M.; Wilsgaard, T.; Eisenmann, M.; Waterloo, K.; Kolstrup, N. The clinical effectiveness of web-based cognitive behavioral therapy with face-to-face therapist support for depressed primary care patients: Randomized controlled trial. *J. Med. Int. Res.* **2013**, *15*, e153.
13. Kessler, D.; Lewis, G.; Kaur, S.; Wiles, N.; King, M.; Weich, S.; Sharp, D.J.; Araya, R.; Hollinghurst, S.; Peters, T.J. Therapist-delivered Internet psychotherapy for depression in primary care: A randomised controlled trial. *Lancet* **2009**, *374*, 628–634. [CrossRef]
14. Kooistra, L.C.; Wiersma, J.E.; Ruwaard, J.; van Oppen, P.; Smit, F.; Lokkerbol, J.; Cuijpers, P.; Riper, H. Blended vs. face-to-face cognitive behavioural treatment for major depression in specialized mental health care: Study protocol of a randomized controlled cost-effectiveness trial. *BMC Psychiatry* **2014**, *14*, 290. [CrossRef]
15. Robertson, L.; Smith, M.; Castle, D.; Tannenbaum, D. Using the Internet to enhance the treatment of depression. *Aust. Psychiatry* **2006**, *14*, 413–417. [CrossRef]
16. Berger, T.; Krieger, T.; Sude, K.; Meyer, B.; Maercker, A. Evaluating an e-mental health program ("deprexis") as adjunctive treatment tool in psychotherapy for depression: Results of a pragmatic randomized controlled trial. *J. Affect. Disord.* **2018**, *227*, 455–462. [CrossRef] [PubMed]
17. Thase, M.E.; Wright, J.H.; Eells, T.D.; Barrett, M.S.; Wisniewski, S.R.; Balasubramani, G.K.; McCrone, P.; Brown, G.K. Improving the efficiency of psychotherapy for depression: Computer-assisted versus standard CBT. *Am. J. Psychiatry* **2017**, *175*, 242–250. [CrossRef] [PubMed]

18. Zwerenz, R.; Becker, J.; Knickenberg, R.J.; Siepmann, M.; Hagen, K.; Beutel, M.E. Online Self-Help as an Add-On to Inpatient Psychotherapy: Efficacy of a New Blended Treatment Approach. *Psychother. Psychosom.* **2017**, *86*, 341–350. [CrossRef] [PubMed]
19. Erbe, D.; Eichert, H.-C.; Riper, H.; Ebert, D.D. Blending face-to-face and internet-based interventions for the treatment of mental disorders in adults: Systematic review. *J. Med. Int. Res.* **2017**, *19*, e306. [CrossRef] [PubMed]
20. Wright, J.H.; Wright, A.S.; Albano, A.M.; Basco, M.R.; Goldsmith, L.J.; Raffield, T.; Otto, M.W. Computer-assisted cognitive therapy for depression: Maintaining efficacy while reducing therapist time. *Am. J. Psychiatry* **2005**, *162*, 1158–1164. [CrossRef]
21. Clough, B.A.; Casey, L.M. Technological adjuncts to increase adherence to therapy: A review. *Clin. Psychol. Rev.* **2011**, *31*, 697–710. [CrossRef]
22. Riper, H.; Van Ballegooijen, W.; Kooistra, L.; De Wit, J.; Donker, T. *Preventie & eMental-Health-Prevention & eMental-Health*; Vrije Universiteit Commissioned by ZonMw: Amsterdam, The Netherlands, 2013.
23. Van der Vaart, R.; Witting, M.; Riper, H.; Kooistra, L.; Bohlmeijer, E.T.; van Gemert-Pijnen, L.J. Blending online therapy into regular face-to-face therapy for depression: Content, ratio and preconditions according to patients and therapists using a Delphi study. *BMC Psychiatry* **2014**, *14*, 355. [CrossRef]
24. Wentzel, J.; van der Vaart, R.; Bohlmeijer, E.T.; van Gemert-Pijnen, J.E. Mixing online and face-to-face therapy: How to benefit from blended care in mental health care. *JMIR Mental Health* **2016**, *3*, e9. [CrossRef]
25. Ruwaard, J.; Kok, R. Wild West eHealth: Time to hold our horses? *Eur. Health Psychol.* **2015**, *17*, 45–49.
26. Zilcha-Mano, S. Major developments in methods addressing for whom psychotherapy may work and why. *Psychother. Res.* **2018**, *29*, 693–708. [CrossRef] [PubMed]
27. Kazdin, A.E. Evidence-based treatment and practice: New opportunities to bridge clinical research and practice, enhance the knowledge base, and improve patient care. *Am. Psychol.* **2008**, *63*, 146. [CrossRef] [PubMed]
28. Cuijpers, P.; Van Straten, A.; Bohlmeijer, E.; Hollon, S.D.; Andersson, G. The effects of psychotherapy for adult depression are overestimated: A meta-analysis of study quality and effect size. *Psychol. Med.* **2010**, *40*, 211–223. [CrossRef]
29. Fournier, J.C.; DeRubeis, R.J.; Shelton, R.C.; Hollon, S.D.; Amsterdam, J.D.; Gallop, R. Prediction of response to medication and cognitive therapy in the treatment of moderate to severe depression. *J. Consult. Clin. Psychol.* **2009**, *77*, 775. [CrossRef]
30. Cohen, Z.D.; DeRubeis, R.J. Treatment selection in depression. *Ann. Rev. Clin. Psychol.* **2018**, *14*, 209–236. [CrossRef]
31. Fisher, A.J.; Boswell, J.F. Enhancing the personalization of psychotherapy with dynamic assessment and modeling. *Assessment* **2016**, *23*, 496–506. [CrossRef]
32. Hollon, S.D.; Cohne, Z.D.; Singla, D.R.; Andrews, P. Recent Developments in the Treatment of Depression. *Behav. Ther.* **2019**, *50*, 257–269. [CrossRef]
33. Hamburg, M.A.; Collins, F.S. The path to personalized medicine. *N. Engl. J. Med.* **2010**, *363*, 301–304. [CrossRef]
34. Van Bronswijk, S.C.; Lemmens, L.H.; Keefe, J.R.; Huibers, M.J.; DeRubeis, R.J.; Peeters, F.P. A prognostic index for long-term outcome after successful acute phase cognitive therapy and interpersonal psychotherapy for major depressive disorder. *Depress. Anxiety* **2018**, *36*, 252–261. [CrossRef]
35. Becker, D.; van Breda, W.; Funk, B.; Hoogendoorn, M.; Ruwaard, J.; Riper, H. Predictive modeling in e-mental health: A common language framework. *Internet Interv.* **2018**, *12*, 57–67. [CrossRef] [PubMed]
36. DeRubeis, R.J.; Cohen, Z.D.; Forand, N.R.; Fournier, J.C.; Gelfand, L.A.; Lorenzo-Luaces, L. The Personalized Advantage Index: Translating research on prediction into individualized treatment recommendations. A demonstration. *PLoS ONE* **2014**, *9*, e83875. [CrossRef] [PubMed]
37. Cohen, Z.D.; Kim, T.; Van, H.; Dekker, J.; Driessen, E. Recommending Cognitive-Behavioral Versus Psychodynamic Therapy for Mild to Moderate Adult Depression. *Psychother. Res.* **2017**, *30*, 137–150. [CrossRef] [PubMed]
38. Friedl, N.; Berger, T.; Krieger, T.; Caspar, F.; Grosse Holtforth, M. Using the Personalized Advantage Index for individual treatment allocation to cognitive behavioral therapy (CBT) or a CBT with integrated exposure and emotion-focused elements (CBT-EE). *Psychother. Res.* **2019**. [CrossRef]

39. DeRubeis, R.J.; Hollon, S.D.; Amsterdam, J.D.; Shelton, R.C.; Young, P.R.; Salomon, R.M.; O'Reardon, J.P.; Lovett, M.L.; Gladis, M.M.; Brown, L.L. Cognitive therapy vs. medications in the treatment of moderate to severe depression. *Arch. Gen. Psychiatry* **2005**, *62*, 409–416. [CrossRef]
40. Huibers, M.J.; Cohen, Z.D.; Lemmens, L.H.; Arntz, A.; Peeters, F.P.; Cuijpers, P.; DeRubeis, R.J. Predicting optimal outcomes in cognitive therapy or interpersonal psychotherapy for depressed individuals using the personalized advantage index approach. *PLoS ONE* **2015**, *10*, e0140771. [CrossRef]
41. Van Breda, W.; Bremer, V.; Becker, D.; Hoogendoorn, M.; Funk, B.; Ruwaard, J.; Riper, H. Predicting therapy success for treatment as usual and blended treatment in the domain of depression. *Internet Interv.* **2018**, *12*, 100–104. [CrossRef]
42. Bremer, V.; Becker, D.; Kolovos, S.; Funk, B.; Van Breda, W.; Hoogendoorn, M.; Riper, H. Predicting therapy success and costs for personalized treatment recommendations using baseline characteristics: Data-driven analysis. *J. Med. Internet Res.* **2018**, *20*, e10275. [CrossRef]
43. Kleiboer, A.; Smit, J.; Bosmans, J.; Ruwaard, J.; Andersson, G.; Topooco, N.; Berger, T.; Krieger, T.; Botella, C.; Banos, R. European COMPARative Effectiveness research on blended Depression treatment versus treatment-as-usual (E-COMPARED): Study protocol for a randomized controlled, non-inferiority trial in eight European countries. *Trials* **2016**, *17*, 387. [CrossRef]
44. Sheehan, D.V.; Lecrubier, Y.; Sheehan, K.H.; Amorim, P.; Janavs, J.; Weiller, E.; Hergueta, T.; Baker, R.; Dunbar, G.C. The Mini-International Neuropsychiatric Interview (MINI): The development and validation of a structured diagnostic psychiatric interview for DSM-IV and ICD-10. *J. Clin. Psychiatry* **1998**, *59*, 22–33.
45. Kroenke, K.; Spitzer, R.L.; Williams, J.B. The PHQ-9: Validity of a brief depression severity measure. *J. Gen. Intern. Med.* **2001**, *16*, 606–613. [CrossRef] [PubMed]
46. Meyer, B.; Berger, T.; Caspar, F.; Beevers, C.G.; Andersson, G.; Weiss, M. Effectiveness of a Novel Integrative Online Treatment for Depression (Deprexis): Randomized Controlled Trial. *J. Med. Internet Res.* **2009**, *11*, e15. [CrossRef] [PubMed]
47. Mathiasen, K.; Andersen, T.E.; Riper, H.; Kleiboer, A.A.; Roessler, K.K. Blended CBT versus face-to-face CBT: A randomised non-inferiority trial. *BMC Psychiatry* **2016**, *16*, 432. [CrossRef] [PubMed]
48. Kroenke, K. Enhancing the clinical utility of depression screening. *CMAJ Can. Med. Assoc. J.* **2012**, *184*, 281–282. [CrossRef] [PubMed]
49. Kroenke, K.; Spitzer, R.L. The PHQ-9: A new depression diagnostic and severity measure. *Psychiatr. Ann.* **2002**, *32*, 509–515. [CrossRef]
50. Manea, L.; Gilbody, S.; McMillan, D. Optimal cut-off score for diagnosing depression with the Patient Health Questionnaire (PHQ-9): A meta-analysis. *Can. Med. Assoc. J.* **2012**, *184*, E191–E196. [CrossRef]
51. EuroQol. EuroQol—A new facility for the measurement of health-related quality of life. *Health Policy* **1990**, *16*, 199–208.
52. Bouwmans, C.; De Jong, K.; Timman, R.; Zijlstra-Vlasveld, M.; Van der Feltz-Cornelis, C.; Tan, S.S.; Hakkaart-van Roijen, L. Feasibility, reliability and validity of a questionnaire on healthcare consumption and productivity loss in patients with a psychiatric disorder (TiC-P). *BMC Health Serv. Res.* **2013**, *13*, 217. [CrossRef] [PubMed]
53. Devilly, G.J.; Borkovec, T.D. Psychometric properties of the credibility/expectancy questionnaire. *J. Behav. Ther. Exp. Psychiatry* **2000**, *31*, 73–86. [CrossRef]
54. Stekhoven, D.J. *Missforest: Nonparametric Missing Value Imputation Using Random Forest*; R Package Version, 1; Astrophysics Source Code Library: Leicester, UK, 2013.
55. Stekhoven, D.J.; Buhlmann, P. MissForest: Non-parametric missing value imputation for mixed-type data. *Bioinformatics* **2012**, *28*, 112–118. [CrossRef]
56. Waljee, A.K.; Mukherjee, A.; Singal, A.G.; Zhang, Y.; Warren, J.; Balis, U.; Marrero, J.; Zhu, J.; Higgins, P.D. Comparison of imputation methods for missing laboratory data in medicine. *BMJ Open* **2013**, *3*, e002847. [CrossRef]
57. Peduzzi, P.; Concato, J.; Feinstein, A.R.; Holford, T.R. Importance of events per independent variable in proportional hazards regression analysis II. Accuracy and precision of regression estimates. *J. Clin. Epidemiol.* **1995**, *48*, 1503–1510. [CrossRef]
58. Vittinghoff, E.; McCulloch, C.E. Relaxing the rule of ten events per variable in logistic and Cox regression. *Am. J. Epidemiol.* **2007**, *165*, 710–718. [CrossRef] [PubMed]

59. Raftery, A.E.; Madigan, D.; Hoeting, J.A. Bayesian model averaging for linear regression models. *J. Am. Stat. Assoc.* **1997**, *92*, 179–191. [CrossRef]
60. Stock, E.M.; Kimbrel, N.A.; Meyer, E.C.; Copeland, L.A.; Monte, R.; Zeber, J.E.; Gulliver, S.B.; Morissette, S.B. A Bayesian model averaging approach to examining changes in quality of life among returning Iraq and Afghanistan Veterans. *Int. J. Methods Psychiatry Res.* **2014**, *23*, 345–358. [CrossRef] [PubMed]
61. Babyak, M.A. What you see may not be what you get: A brief, nontechnical introduction to overfitting in regression-type models. *Psychosom. Med.* **2004**, *66*, 411–421.
62. Fragoso, T.M.; Bertoli, W.; Louzada, F. Bayesian model averaging: A systematic review and conceptual classification. *Int. Stat. Rev.* **2018**, *86*, 1–28. [CrossRef]
63. Fernandez, C.; Ley, E.; Steel, M.F. Benchmark priors for Bayesian model averaging. *J. Econom.* **2001**, *100*, 381–427. [CrossRef]
64. Fernandez, C.; Ley, E.; Steel, M.F. Model uncertainty in cross-country growth regressions. *J. Appl. Econom.* **2001**, *16*, 563–576. [CrossRef]
65. Ley, E.; Steel, M.F.J. On the effect of prior assumptions in Bayesian model averaging with applications to growth regression. *J. Appl. Econom.* **2009**, *24*, 651–674. [CrossRef]
66. Steel, M.F. Bayesian model averaging and forecasting. *Bull. Inflat. Macroecon. Anal.* **2011**, *200*, 30–41.
67. Clyde, M.A. BAS: Bayesian Variable Selection and Model Averaging using Bayesian. In *Adaptive Sampling*; 2018; R Package Version 1.5.3; Available online: https://cran.r-project.org/web/packages/BAS/BAS.pdf (accessed on 15 September 2019).
68. Clyde, M.A.; Ghosh, J.; Littman, M.L. Bayesian adaptive sampling for variable selection and model averaging. *J. Comput. Gr. Stat.* **2011**, *20*, 80–101. [CrossRef]
69. Efron, B.; Gong, G. A leisurely look at the bootstrap, the jackknife, and cross-validation. *Am. Stat.* **1983**, *37*, 36–48.
70. Deisenhofer, A.K.; Delgadillo, J.; Rubel, J.A.; Böhnke, J.R.; Zimmermann, D.; Schwartz, B.; Lutz, W. Individual treatment selection for patients with posttraumatic stress disorder. *Depress. Anxiety* **2018**, *35*, 541–550. [CrossRef]
71. Lowe, B.; Unutzer, J.; Callahan, C.M.; Perkins, A.J.; Kroenke, K. Monitoring depression treatment outcomes with the patient health questionnaire-9. *Med. Care* **2004**, *42*, 1194–1201.
72. Dinga, R.; Marquand, A.F.; Veltman, D.J.; Beekman, A.T.F.; Schoevers, R.A.; van Hemert, A.M.; Penninx, B.; Schmaal, L. Predicting the naturalistic course of depression from a wide range of clinical, psychological, and biological data: A machine learning approach. *Transl. Psychiatry* **2018**, *8*, 241. [CrossRef]
73. Hamilton, K.E.; Dobson, K.S. Cognitive therapy of depression: Pretreatment patient predictors of outcome. *Clin. Psychol. Rev.* **2002**, *22*, 875–893. [CrossRef]
74. Constantino, M.J.; Arnkoff, D.B.; Glass, C.R.; Ametrano, R.M.; Smith, J.Z. Expectations. *J. Clin. Psychol.* **2011**, *67*, 184–192. [CrossRef]
75. Greenberg, R.P.; Constantino, M.J.; Bruce, N. Are patient expectations still relevant for psychotherapy process and outcome? *Clin. Psychol. Rev.* **2006**, *26*, 657–678. [CrossRef]
76. Spek, V.; Nyklíček, I.; Cuijpers, P.; Pop, V. Predictors of outcome of group and internet-based cognitive behavior therapy. *J. Affect. Disord.* **2008**, *105*, 137–145. [CrossRef]
77. Andersson, G.; Hedman, E. Effectiveness of guided internet-based cognitive behavior therapy in regular clinical settings. *Verhaltenstherapie* **2013**, *23*, 140–148. [CrossRef]
78. Bower, P.; Kontopantelis, E.; Sutton, A.; Kendrick, T.; Richards, D.A.; Gillbody, S.; Knowles, S.; Cuijpers, P.; Andersson, G.; Christensen, H.; et al. Influence of initial severity of depression on effectiveness of low intensity interventions: Meta-analysis of individual patient data. *BMJ (Clin. Res.)* **2013**, *346*, f540. [CrossRef]
79. Thase, M.E.; Reynolds, C.F.; Frank, E.; Simons, A.D. Response to cognitive-behavioral therapy in chronic depression. *J. Psychother. Pract. Res.* **1994**, *3*, 304–314.
80. Blom, M.B.; Spinhoven, P.; Hoffman, T.; Jonker, K.; Hoencamp, E.; Haffmans, P.J.; van Dyck, R. Severity and duration of depression, not personality factors, predict short term outcome in the treatment of major depression. *J. Affect. Disord.* **2007**, *104*, 119–126. [CrossRef]
81. Delgadillo, J.; Huey, D.; Bennett, H.; McMillan, D. Case complexity as a guide for psychological treatment selection. *J. Consult. Clin. Psychol.* **2017**, *85*, 835–853. [CrossRef]

82. Luedtke, A.; Sadikova, E.; Kessler, R.C. Sample Size Requirements for Multivariate Models to Predict Between-Patient Differences in Best Treatments of Major Depressive Disorder. *Clin. Psychol. Sci.* **2019**, *7*, 445–461. [CrossRef]
83. Van Bronswijk, S.C.; DeRubeis, R.J.; Lemmens, L.H.; Peeters, F.P.; Keefe, J.R.; Cohen, Z.D.; Huibers, M. Precision medicine for long-term depression outcomes using the Personalized Advantage Index approach: Cognitive therapy or interpersonal psychotherapy? *Psychol. Med.* **2019**, 1–11. [CrossRef]
84. Gillan, C.M.; Whelan, D.R. What big data can do for treatment in psychiatry. *Curr. Opin. Behav. Sci.* **2017**, *18*, 34–42. [CrossRef]
85. Urech, A.; Krieger, T.; Möseneder, L.; Biaggi, A.; Vincent, A.; Poppe, C.; Meyer, B.; Riper, H.; Berger, T. A patient post hoc perspective on advantages and disadvantages of blended cognitive behaviour therapy for depression: A qualitative content analysis. *Psychother. Res.* **2019**, *29*, 986–998. [CrossRef]

10

ZIEL: Internet-Based Self-Help for Adjustment Problems: Results of a Randomized Controlled Trial

Christian Moser [1,*], Rahel Bachem [2], Thomas Berger [1] and Andreas Maercker [2]

1 Clinical Psychology and Psychotherapy, University of Bern, 3012 Bern, Switzerland; thomas.berger@psy.unibe.ch
2 Psychopathology and Clinical Intervention, University of Zürich, 8050 Zürich, Switzerland; rahel.bachem@gmail.com (R.B.); maercker@psychologie.uzh.ch (A.M.)
* Correspondence: christian.moser@psy.unibe.ch

Abstract: Adjustment Disorder (AjD) represents a healthcare paradox. On the one hand, it is one of the most diagnosed mental disorders worldwide. On the other hand, AjD and its possible treatment options remain a severely neglected field of research. In this context, we developed a self-guided online intervention for adjustment problems, named ZIEL, and tested its efficacy. It is based on and extends a bibliotherapeutic treatment approach for symptoms of AjD. In our study, a total of 98 individuals who had experienced a life event in the last two years, were randomly assigned to care as usual (CAU) or an online intervention group (CAU + online intervention). The primary endpoint was AjD symptom severity measured by Adjustment Disorder–New Module 20 (ADNM-20). Secondary endpoints were depressive symptoms, quality of life and other variables such as satisfaction and usability. Both the intervention and the control group improved comparably well regarding the severity of adjustment disorder symptoms post-treatment. However, participants in the intervention group showed significantly fewer depressive symptoms and a significantly higher quality of life (Cohen's *d*: 0.89 (BDI) and −0.49 (SF-12)). The intervention was well-received by users with an above average usability rating. Overall, the results suggest that the ZIEL intervention has the promise to contribute to the treatment of AjD and reduce symptom burden by means of a scalable low-barrier approach.

Keywords: adjustment disorder; e-mental health; self-guided intervention; disorders specifically related to stress

---

1. Introduction

"It's really wonderful how much resilience there is in human nature," famous Dracula novelist Stoker stated at the end of the 19th century, against the background of his own adverse experiences [1]

However, there are events in the lives of people that can exceed their psychological resilience. Adjustment Disorder (AjD) marks the transition between normal stress response and impairments with clinically relevant severity or duration [2]. Even if the specific nature of this shift is debated, it does exist [3,4]. What is remarkable, however, is the extent to which the state of clinical practice diverges from the research efforts on AjD. On the one hand, it is one of the most diagnosed mental disorders worldwide [5]. On the other hand, research on AjD and its possible treatment remain a severely neglected field of study [6].

One reason for the gap between practice and research is the lack of diagnostic reliability and validity of AjD, in its ICD-10 and DSM-5 sub-threshold conceptualization [7–9]. However, the evidence base for a full-threshold understanding has been increasing. Amongst others, this includes an equal symptom-severity to e.g., major depression, a lowered quality of life and comparably earlier execution of suicidal ideations [10–13]. Consequently, a re-conceptualization of AjD in the ICD-11 was achieved [4].

It is now being recognized as a full-threshold disorder with the core symptoms of preoccupation with the stressor (e.g., constant rumination) and failure to adapt (e.g., concentration problems) [14].

The importance of this change becomes apparent when looking at the current AjD health care situation. A large proportion of diagnosed individuals do not receive treatment at all [15]. The majority that do, receive it in primary health care settings. Here, AjD is just as likely to be treated with pharmacotherapy like other severe mental disorders; the crucial difference being, that there is no evidence base for this practice with AjD [4,16]. As Strain and Friedman recommend, the first-line of treatment for AjD is psychotherapy, where different general approaches like Cognitive Behavioral Therapy, Eye-Movement Desensitization and Reprocessing, Client-centered Psychotherapy and various brief psychological interventions have been tested with varying success [17–20]. Disorder-specific approaches are rare, but they do exist.

Regarding this scarcity of disorder-specific AjD treatment approaches, there have been various new impulses in the context of Internet-based interventions for AjD in recent years. One of the first digital AjD-specific treatments used Virtual Reality elements to enhance a face-to-face intervention. So-called "EMMA's World", proved to be an effective alternative to traditional treatment and led to significant improvements in areas of depression, relaxation and social interactions for participants [21]. A more recent development of the same group, called TAO, is currently being tested [22]. It combines approaches from cognitive-behavioral therapy (CBT) and Positive Psychology for the guided treatment of AjD. Preliminary findings show good results for both user-friendliness and acceptance for participants [23]. A different approach is pursued with BADI (Brief Adjustment Disorder Intervention), a self-guided intervention for AjD [24]. It combines exercises in relaxation, time management, mindfulness and coping with interpersonal difficulties. Results of a randomized controlled trial show a medium effect size of the intervention on adjustment disorder symptoms [24]. Lastly, there is a new guided online intervention for chronic stress, that explicitly includes AjD. It uses a larger catalog of contemporary CBT techniques, e.g., exposure, sleep management and behavioral activation. A first trial showed moderate to large improvements in terms of perceived stress, as well as in functional impairment and work ability [24].

From a client's point of view, internet-based interventions offer significant advantages, some of which make AjD uniquely suited for this approach [25,26]. First, there is the potential for optimal timing of the intervention. In principle, online interventions could be made available immediately after the occurrence of an adverse life event, for example, via smartphone. This also eliminates the stigma, that would typically be associated with both a strong reaction to a stressor and a visit of a therapist, and usually prevents many individuals from utilizing available help [27]. Finally, the main advantage of self-guided interventions, in particular, is their enormous scalability. It allows not just for consistent availability of services but also ensures economic viability. Both the cost of distribution and the marginal costs added by each new user, converge towards zero with larger numbers of participants.

At the same time, digitalization also opens new possibilities for researchers and practitioners. A central idea is an iterative and incremental approach, as it is part for example, of the agile software development framework [28]. Instead of strictly sequential production, one assumes continuous development of an intervention, driven by constant learning. This has various advantages. Firstly, it allows for rapid iterations of just specific parts of either the content or technology. Scope and functionality can be efficiently expanded based on momentary resources and needs [26]. Secondly, the software allows for detailed analytics of use. With little additional effort, different functionalities or variants of modules can be tested in direct comparison [29]. Thirdly, the translational lag with the transfer of current research findings into clinical practice is significantly shorter than with traditional approaches [30]. Altogether, this bears the potential to significantly improve the quality and availability of care for individuals in need on a long-term basis.

These considerations form the basis of this study and its two objectives: Firstly, the development of a sustainable self-guided intervention for AjD called "Back to your own life (German acronym: ZIEL)." Secondly, to test the efficacy of this intervention, compared to a care as usual control group (CAU). We hypothesized that the active treatment condition would be superior to CAU on measures of AjD symptom severity and that effects would be stable in the three-month follow-up. The goal is to contribute and to expand the growing efforts in the field of AjD research and care.

2. Experimental Section

2.1. *Study Design*

This randomized controlled trial (RCT) compared an immediate intervention group with a CAU-only control group. The program was only accessible during the intervention stage. The participants of the control group got their access after the four-week post-assessment. The immediate intervention group was followed up until three months after randomization to examine the stability of potential gains. The trial was registered with Clinicaltrials.gov and was approved by the Ethics Committee of the School of Arts and Science at the University of Zürich, Switzerland (1 February 2016) [31].

2.2. *Recruitment*

We recruited individuals from the general population from January 2018 until March 2019. For this purpose, we used a study recruitment web page, which was advertised on various websites, forums, and social media. Additionally, we advertised the study at various psychiatric hospitals around Switzerland. The study web page presented general information about adjustment problems and AjD, an outline of the study, a link to 24 h emergency phone numbers, and a registration form.

Individuals who registered received detailed information about the study via e-mail. Individuals who signed informed consent were asked to complete online self-report questionnaires. Based on the answers, the eligibility criteria were assessed. For inclusion, the following criteria had to be met: Minimum age of 18 years, the existence of an emergency address and a life event between two weeks and two years before the participation that still negatively impacts their lives. The latter recorded by means of the Adjustment Disorder-New Module 20 (ADNM-20) stressor list.

The following criteria led to exclusion: Moderate or severe depressive symptoms (BDI > 18), suicidality (BDI suicidality item > 1), a diagnosis of psychotic, bipolar or other serious mental or physical disorders requiring immediate treatment. Individuals who did not meet the criteria were referred to adequate services and had the opportunity to access the intervention outside of the study.

2.3. *Enrollment*

A flowchart of the enrollment sequence is depicted in Figure 1. A total of 421 individuals signed up on the recruitment site, 315 gave informed consent and completed the baseline questionnaires. Out of those, 217 had to be excluded based on the inclusion and exclusion criteria. The remaining 98 participants were randomly assigned to one of the two trial conditions: the CAU plus internet intervention condition or the CAU control condition. Randomization was carried out by an independent researcher at the University of Bern. The independent researcher used anonymized numbers for the allocation, via a pre-produced 1:1 ratio, random sequence [32]. The allocation list was concealed from the investigators and participants. After the randomization, the participants received an email regarding their allocation.

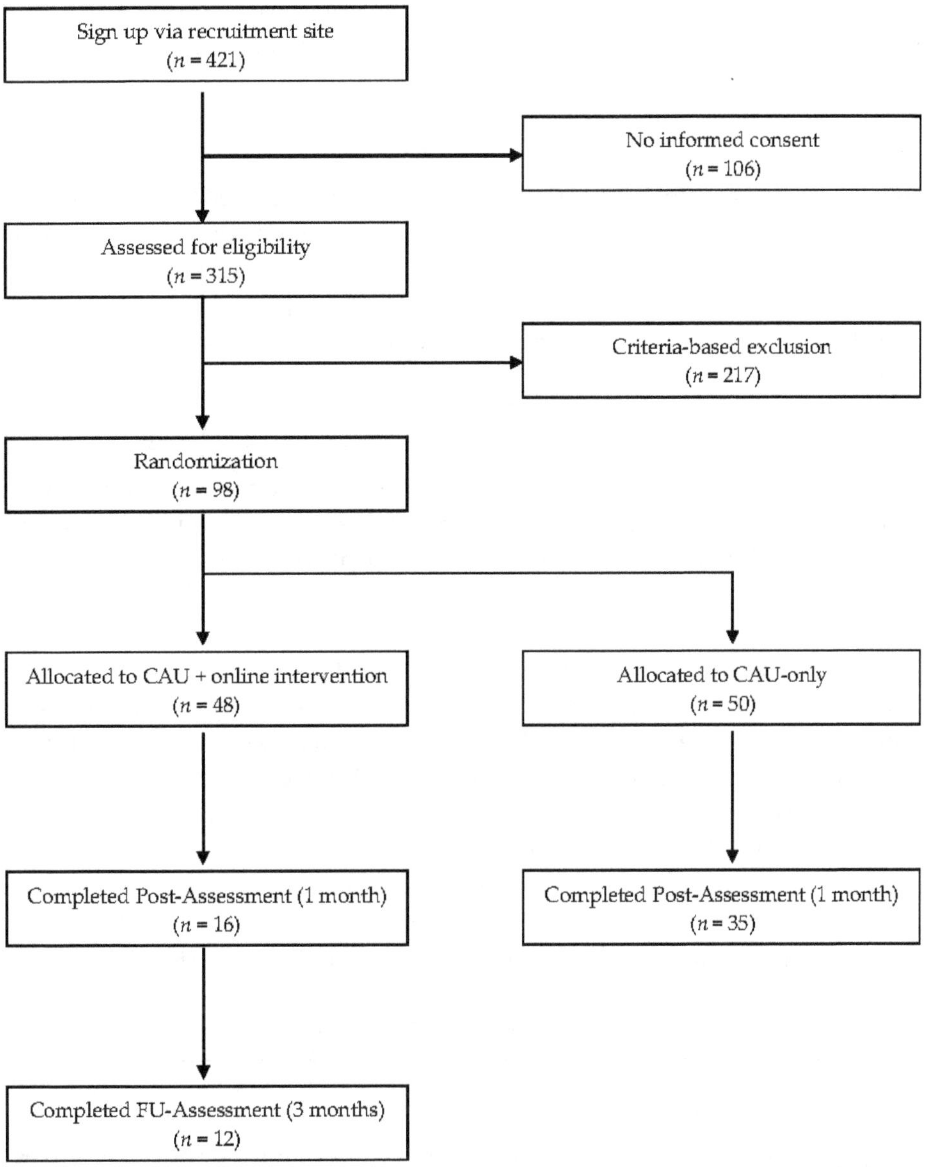

Figure 1. Participant flow.

2.4. *Online Intervention*

2.4.1. Platform

Technologically, we wanted to create the conditions for continuous in-house intervention-development. A platform should enable us to efficiently adapt to advancements in research and on the end-user side. Consequently, we have aimed to implement powerful open source components whenever possible. One example would be the front-end toolkit Bootstrap that we used for mobile-first interface design [33]. In addition to high quality, the use of popular tools provides good accessibility for potential follow-up projects.

Another aim that guided development was a good user experience (UX) throughout the study. One instance of how this goal manifests itself, is the so called reduction of friction. In the context of UX, this is understood to mean that the intervention is used with as little disruption and frustration as possible to prevent users from abandoning their tasks at hand. An example of this would be the registration, as the first entry point to the study. Contrary to a common multi-step procedure, ZIEL-users could enter the registration-process with just one click of a button.

2.4.2. Intervention

The intervention is based on a manual by Bachem and Maercker [34]. This manual is aimed at AjD for burglary victims and has already been successfully tested in a paper-based version [35]. Based on the theoretical model of AjD for the ICD-11, it integrates evidence-based techniques from the areas of post-traumatic stress disorder, anxiety disorders and depression [36]. The intervention is to be carried out over 4 weeks, whereby the content can be freely chosen by the users according to their current needs or symptoms.

In the first part, users are introduced to the concept of AjD and guided to assess their current symptom burden. Building on this, they get support in deciding whether the intervention is appropriate or whether it is better to make use of traditional support services. This is followed by a second part with self-help exercises, modelled along symptoms or symptom clusters as typically experienced by those affected.

In the first section on sense of self, the stress response and previous coping strategies are examined in more detail, also in light of existing risk and protective factors. In the second section on coping, a series of cognitive strategies are introduced in order to learn how to deal better with presenting burdens. These include techniques such as stopping thoughts from ruminating, as well as correcting cognitive biases (i.e., addressing preoccupations). In the third section on activation, the user deals primarily with the utilization of personal resources at various levels. This includes functional goal setting as well as e.g., the initiation of physical activities (i.e., addressing failure to adapt symptoms). Lastly, the section on recovery covers how activity and rest phases can best be kept in balance in the future, as well as a number of relaxation techniques. Table 1 depicts the details of the content sections.

Table 1. Section overview.

Section 1: Introduction	Psychoeducation; learning to evaluate the psychological burden caused by a life event; deciding about the adequacy of the intervention.
Section 2: Sense of self	Analyzing the individual adjustment reaction; learning about risk and protective factors; inspecting individual former coping strategies.
Section 3: Coping	Recognizing and correcting cognitive biases; writing a narrative exposure exercise; managing anxiety and rumination.
Section 4: Activation	Physical exercising; setting realistic positive goals; regaining positive experiences; evaluating milestones of the personal history.
Section 5: Recovery	Learning to balance activity and relaxation; getting to know various approaches to relaxation; improving sleep and imaginative techniques.

The preservation of a self-directed approach resulted from the perspective of a possible scalable implementation in a standard care setting. After a negative life event, there is a time window of about one month in which a possible development of AjD takes place [14]. In order to support affected people to a relevant extent on such short notice, a reliance on skilled workforce would not be feasible regarding availability and organization. Closely related is the decision in favor of a completely anonymous and automated usage scenario. Social barriers to timely care should be eliminated as far as possible. Finally, the content was re-written agnostic of a specific stressor, restructured into shorter text-sections and additionally made available as audio versions. Figure A1 shows illustrative screenshots of the intervention.

2.5. Outcome Measures

2.5.1. Adjustment Disorder Symptom Severity

The Adjustment Disorder-New Module 20 (ADNM-20) is a self-report questionnaire to track life events and identify adjustment issues. In the first part, it records acute and chronic life events by means of a semi-structured stressor list. In the second part, the AjD core symptoms of preoccupation and failure to adapt (4 items each) as well as accessory symptoms of avoidance, depressive mood, anxiety and impulse disturbance (12 items) are measured. All 20 items are measured on a 4-point Likert-type scale (1 = *never*, 4 = *often*) [37]. Additionally, a total sum score indicates the overall symptom burden and allows for the identification of high risk for AjD (score above 47.5) [38]. The scale offers satisfactory psychometric properties as shown in previous studies [36,37]. The internal consistency of the ADNM-20 in the present study was good for the sum score (Cronbach's α 0.85), and acceptable for the subscales preoccupations (Cronbach's α 0.78), failure to adapt (Cronbach's α 0.73) and good for the accessory symptoms (Cronbach's α 0.83).

2.5.2. General Psychopathology

The Brief Symptom Inventory, Short Form (BSI-18) is a self-report questionnaire to assess general psychological distress. Syndromes of somatization, depression, and anxiety are measured by 18 items on a 5-point Likert-type scale (0 = not at all, 4 = very strong) [39]. The BSI-18 exhibits robust psychometric qualities in previous studies [38]. In the present study, Cronbach's α was 0.82.

2.5.3. Depressive Symptoms

The Beck Depression Inventory (BDI) is a self-report questionnaire to assess depressive symptoms. Each of the 21 items is rated on a 4-point Likert-type scale (0 = not at all, 3 = very strong) [40]. The BDI offers sufficient psychometrics properties [41]. In the present study, Cronbach's α was 0.77.

2.5.4. Quality of Life

The Short Form Health Survey–12 (SF-12) is a self-report questionnaire to assess health-related quality of life. Both a physical and a mental health index are measured by 12 items on a 5-point Likert-type scale [42]. The instrument shows robust psychometrics properties [43]. In the present study, Cronbach's α for the mental health subscale was 0.78 and for the physical health subscale, 0.76.

2.5.5. Expectations about Treatment

The Credibility/Expectancy Questionnaire (CEQ) is a self-report questionnaire to assess treatment expectancy and the credibility of its rationale. The subscales of treatment credibility and outcome expectation are measured by six items in total, each on a scale of 1 (not at all) to 9 (very much). The CEQ exhibits robust psychometric qualities [44]. In the present study, Cronbach's α was 0.88.

2.5.6. Usability

The System Usability Scale (SUS) is a self-report questionnaire to assess the usability of a system. Each of the ten items was adapted to the use-case and is measured on a 5-point Likert-type scale (1 = strongly agree, five strongly disagree) [45]. The SUS offers robust psychometric properties [46]. In the present study, Cronbach's α was 0.84.

2.5.7. Adherence

The intervention platform automatically registered various indices of adherence for each anonymized account-ID: Number of logins, individual pageviews, pageviews per login, total and average time spent in the intervention.

2.6. *Power Analysis*

The power analysis was conducted with G*Power 3 to determine the appropriate sample size for the detection of differences between the two groups [47]. We aimed at the detection of a medium effect size of 0.5, based on previous research by Eimontas et al. [22]. Accordingly, a power analysis showed that with an alpha error level of 0.05 and a power of (1-beta) of 0.80 about 128 individuals would be needed.

2.7. *Statistical Analysis*

To test group differences in both demographic data and baseline measures, independent sample *t*-tests, respectively χ^2-tests for nominal data variables were used. Differential outcomes at posttreatment were evaluated according to an intention-to-treat principle using a mixed-model repeated-measures analysis of variance with time (pre-post) as a within-group factor and treatment condition as a between-group factor. This approach was favored as it uses all available data of each subject. Missing values are not substituted; rather parameters of missing values are estimated [48]. Within- and between-group effect sizes (Cohen's d) were calculated based on estimated means and the pooled standard deviation from the observed means. Within-group changes in outcome scores from posttreatment to follow-up were analyzed using paired *t*-tests for people who completed the post and the follow-up-assessment in the intervention group only. To test predictions to the outcome, we calculated linear regression models regressing each adherence measure on the 4-week primary outcome (ADNM-20) controlling for baseline scores in the intervention group. Post hoc tests were Bonferroni corrected for multiple comparisons. All analysis was performed in R and the package lme4 [49,50].

3. Results

3.1. *Pre-Treatment Evaluation*

The conditions in both groups did not differ in terms of AjD symptom burden or demographic characteristics. The incidence of AjD in the intervention group was 71% ($n = 34$) and 72% in the CAU group ($n = 36$). Table 2 provides corresponding details for demographic characteristics. Likewise, the perception of credibility and expectancy of the intervention was the same for participants in both conditions ($p > 0.47$).

3.2. *Dropout Analysis*

Overall, 47 (active, $n = 32$; CAU, $n = 15$) participants (48%) did not complete the posttreatment assessment, even though they had been invited three times in weekly intervals via automated email. The difference in response between the two groups is significant ($p < 0.01$). This can likely be attributed to the fact, that the control group did not gain access to the intervention until after completing the post-assessments. Reasons for dropping out remained unknown since there was no way to reach and question the respective users. As for predictors of dropout, there were no significant differences observed in terms of demographics, pre-treatment or post-treatment scores (all *p*s > 0.21) between those who provided data and those who did not.

3.3. *Treatment Outcomes*

The observed and estimated means for the self-report questionnaires are presented in Table 3. Mixed-model linear regression analysis with group as a fixed factor and time as a repeated factor (pre-post) were conducted for each of the dependent outcome measures.

Table 2. Pre-Treatment Evaluation.

	Intervention Group $n = 48$	**CAU-Only Group** $n = 50$	**Statistic**
Mean age, years (SD)	40.54 (13.0)	40.28 (12.8)	$t(96) = 0.10$ $p = 0.92$
Gender *n* (%)			
Female	40 (83.3)	44 (88.0)	$Chi^2 = 0.44$ $p = 0.51$
Male	8 (16.7)	6 (12.0)	
Marital status, *n* (%)			
Single	11 (22.9)	10 (20.0)	$Chi^2 = 2.06$ $p = 0.72$
Married	28 (37.5)	24 (48.0)	
Living together	10 (20.8)	11 (22.0)	
Divorced	7 (14.6)	4 (8.0)	
Widowed	2 (4.2)	1 (2.0)	
Number of kids, *n* (%)			
None	23 (47.9)	27 (54.0)	$Chi^2 = 3.36$ $p = 0.50$
One	7 (14.6)	11 (22.0)	
Two	13 (27.1)	10 (20.0)	
Three	4 (8.3)	1 (2.0)	
More than three	1 (2.1)	1 (2.0)	
Employment, *n* (%)			
Full-time paid work	13 (27.1)	23 (46.0)	$Chi^2 = 5.60$ $p = 0.35$
Part-time paid work	19 (39.6)	15 (30.0)	
Unemployed	2 (4.2)	2 (4.0)	
At home parent	4 (8.3)	1 (2.0)	
Student	5 (10.4)	3 (6.0)	
Retired	5 (10.4)	6 (12.0)	
Highest education, *n* (%)			
Compulsory school	1 (2.1)	0 (0.0)	$Chi^2 = 5.06$ $p = 0.17$
Apprenticeship	15 (31.3)	8 (16.0)	
College	5 (10.4)	4 (8.0)	
University	27 (56.3)	38 (76.0)	
Current psychological treatment, *n* (%)			
Yes	15 (31.3)	9 (18.0)	$Chi^2 = 2.33$ $p = 0.13$
No	33 (68.8)	41 (82.0)	
Current medications, *n* (%)			
Yes	5 (10.4)	2 (4.0)	$Chi^2 = 1.52$ $p = 0.22$
No	43 (89.6)	43 (86.0)	
Experience with E-Mental Health, *n* (%)			
Yes, good	5 (10.4)	4 (8.0)	$Chi^2 = 0.17$ $p = 0.68$
Yes, bad	0 (0.0)	0 (0.0)	
No	43 (89.6)	46 (92.0)	

Table 3. Treatment Outcomes. Observed and Estimated Means for Primary and Secondary Outcome Measures and Within- and Between-Group effect-sizes.

	Pre-Treatment	Post-Treatment (Observed)		Post-Treatment (Estimated)		Follow-Up (Observed)		Post-Treatment Between-Group Comparisons (Group by Time)	Pre-Post Within-Group Effect Sizes (Estimated, ** for $p \leq 0.01$)	Between-Group Effect Sizes at Post (Est.)	
Measure	*n*	M (SD)	*n*	M (SD)	*n*	M (SE)	*n*	M (SD)	F and df	Cohen's *d* (95% CI)	Cohen's *d* (95% CI)
ADNM-20 Preoccupation											
CAU	50	13.12 (1.79)	35	11.41 (1.99)	50	11.70 (2.01)			$F_{1,96} = 0.03$	0.69 (0.47–0.91)	0.03 (−0.43–0.50)
Intervention	48	12.23 (2.22)	16	11.50 (2.15)	48	11.63 (2.27)	12	10.17 (2.37)		0.27 (0.09–0.45)	
ADNM-20 Failure to adapt											
CAU	50	9.85 (2.73)	35	8.68 (2.30)	50	8.66 (2.29)			$F_{1,96} = 3.13$	0.37 (0.18–0.57)	0.40 (−0.07–0.87)
Intervention	48	9.35 (2.12)	16	7.75 (2.25)	48	7.88 (2.09)	12	7.92 (2.07)		0.74 (0.52–0.93)	
ADNM-20 Accessory symptoms											
CAU	50	31.42 (5.70)	35	28.05 (4.82)	50	28.32 (5.41)			$F_{1,96} = 0.33$	0.55 (0.36–0.75)	0.51 (0.02–1.00)
Intervention	48	28.00 (6.37)	16	25.32 (6.64)	48	25.35 (6.38)	12	22.75 (5.85)		0.41 (0.18–0.63)	
BDI											
CAU	50	11.78 (3.87)	35	9.86 (4.44)	50	11.20 (4.78)			$F_{1,96} = 19.52$ **	0.13 (−0.06–0.31)	0.83 (0.41–1.25)
Intervention	48	10.83 (5.13)	16	9.76 (6.72)	48	10.23 (4.80)	12	4.44 (4.90)		0.72 (0.48–0.97)	
BSI-18											
CAU	50	12.52 (8.87)	35	11.41 (8.67)	50	10.80 (7.72)			$F_{1,96} = 0.49$	0.20 (0.02–0.39)	0.17 (−0.24–0.57)
Intervention	48	14.56 (9.18)	16	11.08 (6.22)	48	12.17 (8.72)	12	5.27 (5.46)		0.27 (0.14–0.39)	
$SF\text{-}12_{PH}$											
CAU	50	14.62 (3.34)	35	14.79 (3.29)	50	14.52 (3.15)			$F_{1,96} = 3.16$	−0.03 (−0.22–0.15)	0.36 (−0.04–0.76)
Intervention	48	14.60 (3.09)	16	15.20 (3.12)	48	15.60 (2.88)	12	18.00 (2.68)		0.33 (0.09–0.58)	
$SF\text{-}12_{MH}$											
CAU	50	15.96 (2.58)	35	15.68 (2.25)	50	15.96 (2.47)			$F_{1,96} = 13.52$ **	0.02 (−0.24–0.27)	0.74 (0.32–1.16)
Intervention	48	16.98 (2.62)	16	17.73 (2.40)	48	17.77 (2.40)	12	18.36 (2.01)		0.31 (0.07–0.55)	

For the primary outcome, the effect of the ADNM-20 was not qualified by significant Group × Time interactions for either the sum score ($F_{1,96} = 2.38$, p = ns), or for the subscales ($F_{1,96} = 0.03$–3.13, p = ns; see Table 3), meaning that the symptom severity did not decrease significantly in the intervention group compared to the control group. Between-group effect sizes based on estimated means, corrected for baseline differences, were small for the sum score ($d = 0.31$) and small to medium sized for the subscales ($d = 0.03$–0.51; see Table 3). Within-group comparisons based on estimated means in the treatment group showed large effect sizes for the sum score ($d = 1.04$) and small to medium effect sizes for the subscales ($d = 0.27$–0.74; see Table 3). Within-group effect sizes in the control group were medium-sized for the sum score ($d = 0.70$) and small to medium-sized as well for the subscales ($d = 0.37$–0.69; see Table 3).

As for secondary outcomes, the effect of the BDI showed significant Group × Time interactions (BDI: $F_{1,96} = 19.5$ $p < 0.01$). At post, between-group effect sizes based on estimated means were $d = 0.89$, meaning that for the intervention group, there was a large effect in terms of depressive symptom decrease compared to the control group. Within-group comparisons based on the estimated means in the treatment group showed large effect sizes (BDI: $d = 0.95$). In contrast, within-group effect sizes in the control group were negligible (BDI: $d = 0.20$). Treatment effects for the intervention group at three-month-follow-up were stable (pre–follow-up, $d = 0.95$) as no significant differences could be detected in comparison to the effects at post ($p > 0.30$).

For the SF-12 mental health subscale, there was a significant Group × Time interaction ($SF\text{-}12_{MH}$: $F_{1,96} = 13.52$, $p < 0.01$). At post, between-group effect sizes based on estimated means were $d = 0.74$, meaning that for the intervention group, there was a medium effect in terms of increased mental health-related quality of life compared to the control group at post. Within-group comparisons based on the estimated means in the treatment group showed small effect sized at post ($SF\text{-}12_{MH\_post}$: $d = 0.31$) and significantly improved to medium effect size at follow-up ($SF\text{-}12_{MH\_fu}$: $d = 0.68$, $p < 0.01$). In contrast, within-group effect sizes in the control group were negligible at post ($SF\text{-}12_{MH}$: $d = 0.02$). For the SF-12 physical health subscale, there were no significant Group × Time interactions detected ($SF\text{-}12_{PH}$: $F_{1,96} = 3.16$, $p = 0.08$).

3.4. Diagnostic Status Pre- and Post-Treatment

In total, 51 participants filled out the post-treatment questionnaire (Active, $n = 16$ (33%), CAU, $n = 35$ (70%)). According to the self-report at post-treatment, 15 out of 48 participants in the intervention group (31%) did not meet the criteria for AjD. In contrast, 14 participants in the control group (28%) could be considered remitted after four weeks.

3.5. Program Usage and Usability

The intensity in which the intervention was used shows a high degree of heterogeneity within the user group. The average time spent in the intervention (total) was 43 min (SD = 106.6), while the average duration of a session was 8 min (SD = 11). The average number of sessions (total) was 2.7 (SD = 5.2). The usability of the intervention was rated as above average by the users. The average SUS score was 73 (SD = 18), which translates to an adjective rating of "good" [51].

3.6. Predictors of Outcome

To investigate potential predictors of outcome, we used regression analyses, predicting 4-week primary and secondary outcomes, controlled for baseline scores. For these analyses, we only used data of participants that logged in at least once and completed the post-treatment questionnaires. None of the pre-treatment variables such as age, sex, marital status, occupational situation, education or psychotherapeutic treatment had any significant relation to the primary outcome (all *ps* > 0.24). At the same time, none of the indicators of program usage such as number of sessions or time spent in the intervention were significantly associated with the treatment outcomes for both groups of participants (all *ps* > 0.27).

4. Discussion

The present research aimed to develop a self-guided intervention for adjustment problems and to test its efficacy compared to a control group. Contrary to our hypothesis, there were no significant differences between the intervention group and the control group regarding the primary outcome measure ADNM-20 and its subscales. Both groups showed significantly lower AjD symptom burden from baseline to post-treatment. This result and the within-group effect size of d = 1.04 in the treatment group are in line with the results obtained with the original manual by Bachem and Maercker, what indicates its adequate online implementation [32,33]. The between-group effect size of d = 0.31 was not significant, whereas, the study was underpowered to detect small effects like this.

Although both groups showed similar improvements for the primary outcome, the intervention group showed a significant between-group effect on the reduction of depressive symptoms (d = 0.89). Effects within the intervention group could also be maintained over the three-month follow-up period. This is an encouraging result, which could not yet be shown in previous studies on internet interventions for AjD [22].

Likewise, there was a significant between-group effect regarding the improvement of mental health-related quality of life at post (d = 0.74). Within-group comparisons in the intervention group showed significant improvements over all three points of measurement, respectively ($SF\text{-}12_{MH\_post}$: d = 0.31, $SF\text{-}12_{MH\_fu}$: d = 0.68). For the physically related quality of life, there were no significant effects detected ($SF\text{-}12_{PH}$: d = 0.33, p = 0.08), which again could be related to the lack of power to detect small effect sizes in the present study.

The overall results are further consistent with those of the BADI self-guided approach to AjD treatment by Eimontas et al. [22]. It showed medium effect sizes regarding the AjD symptom reduction, starting from a comparable severity of symptom burden in the pre-treatment evaluation. In contrast to the present study, however, the control group showed no comparable improvements.

In a wider context, the results of the present study stand in accordance with previous research that supports the viability of self-guided approaches in different contexts [52,53]. We were able to show that highly scalable self-guided interventions have a positive effect on users. However, the effects are still small and many dropouts can be expected.

4.1. Limitations

Several limitations to this study need to be acknowledged. First, the sample consisted of self-selected participants. It can be assumed that already a positive opinion regarding internet interventions prevailed. This restricts generalizability, but on the flipside, also reflects a realistic health care scenario. Second, the study suffers from a high dropout rate of 48% (pre-post). Third, the results of the study are solely based on self-report measures, which however allows for scalability of the approach. Fourth, we had a relatively heterogeneous sample of participants regarding symptom burden. Fifth, unexpectedly, the organizational- and time-restrictions of the project did not allow the recruitment efforts to be extended in such a way as to achieve the number of participants required for the assumed effects. This calls for changes in future studies and restricts the generalizability of the current results, demanding their appropriately cautious interpretation. Lastly, from an ethical perspective, we deemed it important to not extend the delay for the waiting list further than needed in the potential period of onset of AjD as a transient disorder. However, this not only made a comparison between experimental and control group at three months impossible, but also clearly limits the informative value on account of the temporal stability of effect beyond this period.

4.2. Implications and Learnings

Even though it is an empirically common phenomenon, especially for self-guided interventions, the low adherence to the intervention, respectively high dropout of the participants, should not be overlooked. Several studies have already demonstrated meaningful relation to treatment outcome [22,54]. Thus, it is a positive sign, that significant effects have been found for ZIEL, despite the relatively small "adherence-dosage". However, a solution-oriented approach to the problem is mandatory and represents an important aspect of the further development of the intervention. We have to assume that we were not able to match the needs of users, e.g., in terms of technical or content-related aspects [55].

To improve adherence, we see different steps that could be implemented in the next iteration [56]. First, the integration of automated reminders should be able to increase engagement [57]. Complementary to this, the addition of automatic feedback on tasks and virtual rewards for favorable actions could be a valuable investment that we want to pursue. On a more general level, we see the need to improve the product-market-fit of the intervention in the broadest sense. To better be able to match user needs, we plan to focus and collaborate with specific target groups, based on classes of AjD-relevant life events like e.g., divorce. This would make it possible to generate greater personal relevance for the user on the one hand. On the other hand, we could target specific needs more directly and learn faster from focused user feedback. An example of such an approach in a guided format is the internet-based intervention for adaption problems after separation or divorce, called LIVIA, which showed significant improvements and moderate effect sizes for participants [58].

A positive and fruitful experience which we gained during the work on the present study, was with the closed loop between the development of both the content and the software. While there is currently a trend in our field towards outsourcing the technical implementation, it has proven very efficient for us to understand the content and IT as two sides of the same coin. Based on an agile strategy, one can make early decisive decisions for later developments. In other words, the hope is that initial investment in interdisciplinary teams will pay off several times over, in the lifecycle of fruitful projects. The approach becomes even more relevant in an academic context, with a multitude of parallel projects, changing financing situations and continuously changing teams.

In conclusion, the present study supports the current positive findings of efficient internet-based treatment of AjD. It expands the current state of knowledge with an extension of possible approaches to treatment and conceptual considerations regarding the process of realization. Given the potential reach and impact of a low threshold, high scalability intervention for AjD, sustainable research efforts are required.

Author Contributions: R.B. and A.M. developed the original intervention manual and its theoretical framework. C.M. developed the intervention platform and revised the content. A.M. and T.B. were involved in planning and supervised the work. C.M. wrote the manuscript with input from all authors.

Appendix A

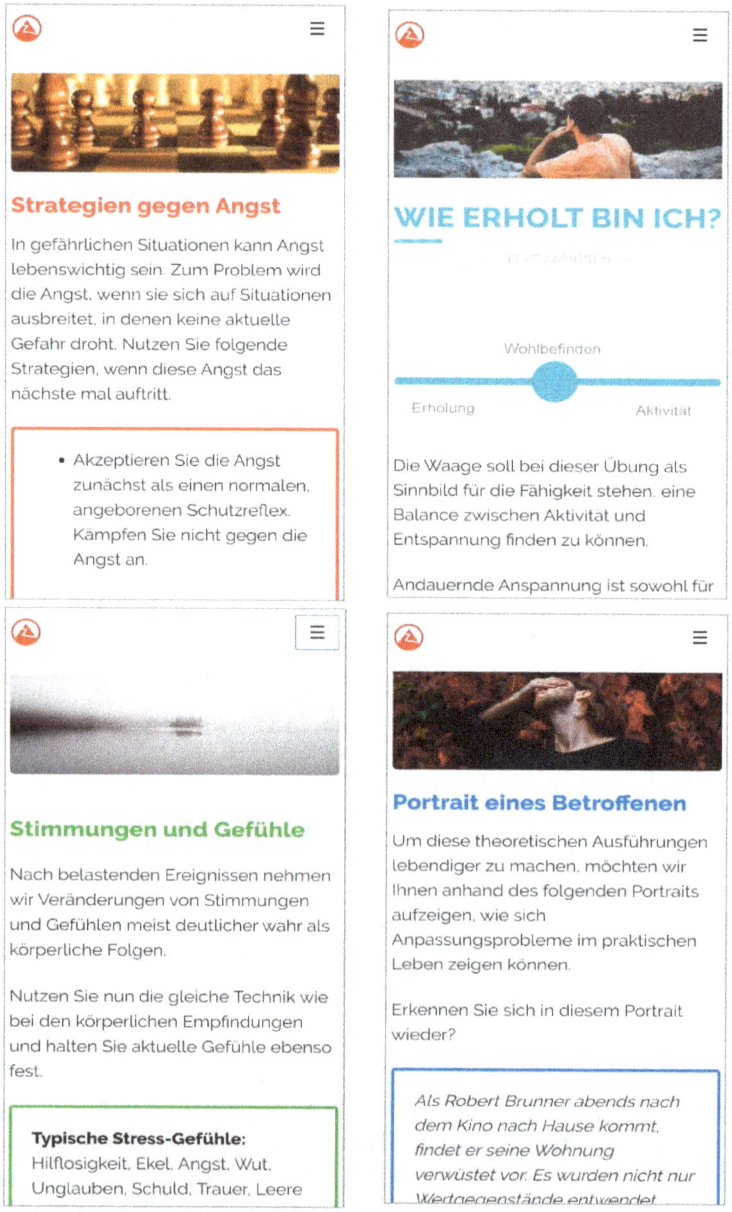

Figure A1. Illustrative Screenshots of the ZIEL Intervention.

References

1. Stoker, A. *Dracula*; Archibald Constable & Company: Dublin, OH, USA, 1897.
2. Casey, P.; Bailey, S. Adjustment disorders: The state of the art. *World Psychiatry* **2011**, *10*, 11–18. [CrossRef]
3. Keeley, J.W.; Reed, G.M.; Roberts, M.C.; Evans, S.C.; Robles, R.; Matsumoto, C.; Brewin, C.R.; Cloitre, M.; Perkonigg, A.; Rousseau, C.; et al. Disorders specifically associated with stress: A case-controlled field study for ICD-11 mental and behavioural disorders. *Int. J. Clin. Health Psychol.* **2016**, *16*, 109–127. [CrossRef] [PubMed]
4. Bachem, R.; Casey, P. Adjustment disorder: A diagnosis whose time has come. *J. Affect. Disord.* **2018**, *227*, 243–253. [CrossRef] [PubMed]
5. Evans, S.C.; Reed, G.M.; Roberts, M.C.; Esparza, P.; Watts, A.D.; Correia, J.M.; Ritchie, P.; May, M.; Saxena, S. Psychologists' perspectives on the diagnostic classification of mental disorders: Results from the WHO-IUPsyS Global Survey. *Int. J. Psychol.* **2013**, *48*, 177–193. [CrossRef] [PubMed]

6. Casey, P. *Adjustment Disorders: From Controversy to Clinical Practice*; Oxford University Press: Oxford, UK, 2018.
7. Strain, J.J.; Diefenbacher, A. The adjustment disorders: The conundrums of the diagnoses. *Compr. Psychiatry* **2008**, *49*, 121–130. [CrossRef] [PubMed]
8. World Health Organization. *The ICD-10 Classification of Mental and Behavioural Disorders: Clinical Descriptions and Diagnostic Guidelines*; World Health Organization: Geneva, Switzerland, 1992.
9. Association, A.P. *Diagnostic and Statistical Manual of Mental Disorders (DSM-5®)*; American Psychiatric Pub: Washington, DC, USA, 2013.
10. Casey, P.; Maracy, M.; Kelly, B.D.; Lehtinen, V.; Ayuso-Mateos, J.L.; Dalgard, O.S.; Dowrick, C. Can adjustment disorder and depressive episode be distinguished? Results from ODIN. *J. Affect. Disord.* **2006**, *92*, 291–297. [CrossRef] [PubMed]
11. Polyakova, I.; Knobler, H.Y.; Ambrumova, A.; Lerner, V. Characteristics of suicidal attempts in major depression versus adjustment reactions. *J. Affect. Disord.* **1998**, *47*, 159–167. [CrossRef]
12. O'Donnell, M.L.; Alkemade, N.; Creamer, M.; McFarlane, A.C.; Silove, D.; Bryant, R.A.; Felmingham, K.; Steel, Z.; Forbes, D. A longitudinal study of adjustment disorder after trauma exposure. *Am. J. Psychiatry* **2016**, *173*, 1231–1238. [CrossRef] [PubMed]
13. Runeson, B.S.; Beskow, J.; Waern, M. The suicidal process in suicides among young people. *Acta Psychiatr. Scand.* **1996**, *93*, 35–42. [CrossRef]
14. World Health Organization. *International Statistical Classification of Diseases and Related Health Problems*; World Health Organization: Geneva, Switzerland, 2018.
15. Carta, M.G.; Balestrieri, M.; Murru, A.; Hardoy, M.C. Adjustment Disorder: Epidemiology, diagnosis and treatment. *Clin. Pract. Epidemiol. Ment. Health* **2009**, *5*, 15. [CrossRef]
16. Strain, J.J.; Smith, G.C.; Hammer, J.S.; McKenzie, D.P.; Blumenfield, M.; Muskin, P.; Newstadt, G.; Wallack, J.; Wilner, A.; Schleifer, S.S. Adjustment disorder: A multisite study of its utilization and interventions in the consultation-liaison psychiatry setting. *Gen. Hosp. Psychiatry* **1998**, *20*, 139–149. [CrossRef]
17. Dalgaard, L.; Eskildsen, A.; Carstensen, O.; Willert, M.V.; Andersen, J.H.; Glasscock, D.J. Changes in self-reported sleep and cognitive failures: A randomized controlled trial of a stress management intervention. *Scand. J. Work Environ. Health* **2014**, *40*, 569–581. [CrossRef] [PubMed]
18. Cvetek, R. EMDR treatment of distressful experiences that fail to meet the criteria for PTSD. *J. EMDR Pract. Res.* **2008**, *2*, 2. [CrossRef]
19. Altenhöfer, A.; Schulz, W.; Schwab, R.; Eckert, J. Psychotherapie von Anpassungsstörungen. *Psychotherapeut* **2007**, *52*, 24–34. [CrossRef]
20. Gabbard, G.O. *Gabbard's Treatments of Psychiatric Disorders*; American Psychiatric Pub: Washington, DC, USA, 2007.
21. Baños, R.M.; Guillen, V.; Quero, S.; Garcia-Palacios, A.; Alcaniz, M.; Botella, C. A virtual reality system for the treatment of stress-related disorders: A preliminary analysis of efficacy compared to a standard cognitive behavioral program. *Int. J. Hum. Comput. Stud.* **2011**, *69*, 602–613. [CrossRef]
22. Eimontas, J.; Rimsaite, Z.; Gegieckaite, G.; Zelviene, P.; Kazlauskas, E. Internet-based self-help intervention for ICD-11 adjustment disorder: Preliminary findings. *Psychiatr. Q.* **2018**, *89*, 451–460. [CrossRef] [PubMed]
23. Rachyla, I.; Quero Castellano, S.; Pérez Ara, M.Á.; Molés Amposta, M.; Campos, D.; Mira Pastor, A. *Web-Based, Self-Help Intervention for Adjustment Disorders: Acceptance and Usability*; Interactive Media Institute (IMI): San Diego, CA, USA, 2017.
24. Lindsäter, E.; Axelsson, E.; Salomonsson, S.; Santoft, F.; Ejeby, K.; Ljótsson, B.; Akerstedt, T.; Lekander, M.; Hedman-Lagerlöf, E. Internet-Based Cognitive Behavioral Therapy for Chronic Stress: A Randomized Controlled Trial. *Psychother. Psychosom.* **2018**, *87*, 296–305. [CrossRef] [PubMed]
25. Berger, T. *Internetbasierte Interventionen bei Psychischen Störungen*; Hogrefe Verlag: Göttingen, Germany, 2015.
26. Maercker, A.; Bachem, R.C.; Lorenz, L.; Moser, C.T.; Berger, T. Adjustment disorders are uniquely suited for ehealth interventions: Concept and case study. *JMIR Ment. Health* **2015**, *2*, e15. [CrossRef]
27. Gega, L.; Marks, I.; Mataix-Cols, D. Computer-aided CBT self-help for anxiety and depressive disorders: Experience of a London clinic and future directions. *J. Clin. Psychol.* **2004**, *60*, 147–157. [CrossRef]
28. Petersen, K.; Wohlin, C. The effect of moving from a plan-driven to an incremental software development approach with agile practices. *Empir. Softw. Eng.* **2010**, *15*, 654–693. [CrossRef]
29. Christensen, H.; Griffiths, K. The Internet and mental health literacy. *Aust. N. Z. J. Psychiatry* **2000**, *34*, 975–979. [CrossRef] [PubMed]

30. Christensen, H.; Petrie, K. Information technology as the key to accelerating advances in mental health care. *Aust. N. Z. J. Psychiatry* **2013**, *47*, 114–116. [CrossRef] [PubMed]
31. ClinicalTrials.gov. Identifier NCT03379155. Available online: https://clinicaltrials (accessed on 28 August 2019).
32. SealedEnvelope.com. Available online: www.sealedenvelope (accessed on 28 August 2019).
33. Bootstrap. Open Source Toolkit for Developing with HTML, CSS, and JS. 2019. Available online: www.getbootstrap (accessed on 28 August 2019).
34. Bachem, R.; Maercker, A. *Ist das Noch Mein Zuhause*; Mobiliar Versicherung: Bern, Switzerland, 2013.
35. Bachem, R.; Maercker, A. Self-help interventions for adjustment disorder problems: A randomized waiting-list controlled study in a sample of burglary victims. *Cogn. Behav. Ther.* **2016**, *45*, 397–413. [CrossRef] [PubMed]
36. Glaesmer, H.; Romppel, M.; Brähler, E.; Hinz, A.; Maercker, A. Adjustment disorder as proposed for ICD-11: Dimensionality and symptom differentiation. *Psychiatry Res.* **2015**, *229*, 940–948. [CrossRef] [PubMed]
37. Einsle, F.; Köllner, V.; Dannemann, S.; Maercker, A. Development and validation of a self-report for the assessment of adjustment disorders. *Psychol. Health Med.* **2010**, *15*, 584–595. [CrossRef] [PubMed]
38. Lorenz, L.; Bachem, R.C.; Maercker, A. The adjustment disorder–new module 20 as a screening instrument: Cluster analysis and cut-off values. *Int. J. Occup. Environ. Med. (IJOEM)* **2016**, *7*, 215–220. [CrossRef] [PubMed]
39. Spitzer, C.; Hammer, S.; Löwe, B.; Grabe, H.J.; Barnow, S.; Rose, M.; Wingenfeld, K.; Freyberger, H.J.; Franke, G.H. The short version of the Brief Symptom Inventory (BSI-18): Preliminary psychometric properties of the German translation. *Fortschr. Neurol. Psychiatr.* **2011**, *79*, 517–523. [CrossRef] [PubMed]
40. Beck, A.T.; Ward, C.H.; Mendelson, M.; Mock, J.; Erbaugh, J. An inventory for measuring depression. *Arch. Gen. Psychiatry* **1961**, *4*, 561–571. [CrossRef]
41. Beck, A.T.; Steer, R.A.; Carbin, M.G. Psychometric properties of the Beck Depression Inventory: Twenty-five years of evaluation. *Clin. Psychol. Rev.* **1988**, *8*, 77–100. [CrossRef]
42. Ware, J.E.; Kosinski, M.; Keller, S.D. A 12-Item Short-Form Health Survey: Construction of Scales and Preliminary Tests of Reliability and Validity. *Med Care* **1996**, *34*, 220–233. [CrossRef]
43. Gandek, B.; Ware, J.E.; Aaronson, N.K.; Apolone, G.; Bjorner, J.B.; Brazier, J.E.; Bullinger, M.; Kaasa, S.; Leplege, A.; Prieto, L.; et al. Cross-validation of item selection and scoring for the SF-12 Health Survey in nine countries: Results from the IQOLA Project. *J. Clin. Epidemiol.* **1998**, *51*, 1171–1178. [CrossRef]
44. Devilly, G.J.; Borkovec, T.D. Psychometric properties of the credibility/expectancy questionnaire. *J. Behav. Ther. Exp. Psychiatry* **2000**, *31*, 73–86. [CrossRef]
45. Jordan, P.W.; Thomas, B.; McClelland, I.L.; Weerdmeester, B. *Usability Evaluation in Industry*; CRC Press: Boca Raton, FL, USA, 1996.
46. Brooke, J. SUS-A quick and dirty usability scale. *Usability Eval. Ind.* **1996**, *189*, 4–7.
47. Faul, F.; Erdfelder, E.; Buchner, A.; Lang, A.G. Statistical power analyses using G* Power 3.1: Tests for correlation and regression analyses. *Behav. Res. Methods* **2009**, *41*, 1149–1160. [CrossRef]
48. Gueorguieva, R.; Krystal, J.H. Move over anova: Progress in analyzing repeated-measures data andits reflection in papers published in the archives of general psychiatry. *Arch. Gen. Psychiatry* **2004**, *61*, 310–317. [CrossRef] [PubMed]
49. Team, R.C. *R: A Language and Environment for Statistical Computing*; R Foundation for Statistical Computing: Vienna, Austria, 2016.
50. Bates, D.; Mächler, M.; Bolker, B.; Walker, S. Fitting linear mixed-effects models using lme4. *arXiv* **2014**, arXiv:1406.5823.
51. Bangor, A.; Kortum, P.; Miller, J. Determining what individual SUS scores mean: Adding an adjective rating scale. *J. Usability Stud.* **2009**, *4*, 114–123.
52. Karyotaki, E.; Riper, H.; Twisk, J.; Hoogendoorn, A.; Kleiboer, A.; Mira, A.; Mackinnon, A.; Meyer, B.; Botella, C.; Littlewood, E.; et al. Efficacy of self-guided internet-based cognitive behavioral therapy in the treatment of depressive symptoms: A meta-analysis of individual participant data. *JAMA Psychiatry* **2017**, *74*, 351–359. [CrossRef]
53. Berger, T.; Hämmerli, K.; Gubser, N.; Andersson, G.; Caspar, F. Internet-based treatment of depression: A randomized controlled trial comparing guided with unguided self-help. *Cogn. Behav. Ther.* **2011**, *40*, 251–266. [CrossRef]

54. Rachyla, I.; Pérez-Ara, M.; Molés, M.; Campos, D.; Mira, A.; Botella, C.; Quero, S. An internet-based intervention for adjustment disorder (TAO): Study protocol for a randomized controlled trial. *BMC Psychiatry* **2018**, *18*, 161. [CrossRef]
55. Christensen, H.; Griffiths, K.M.; Farrer, L. Adherence in internet interventions for anxiety and depression: Systematic review. *J. Med. Internet Res.* **2009**, *11*, e13. [CrossRef] [PubMed]
56. Baumel, A.; Birnbaum, M.L.; Sucala, M. A systematic review and taxonomy of published quality criteria related to the evaluation of user-facing eHealth programs. *J. Med. Syst.* **2017**, *41*, 128. [CrossRef] [PubMed]
57. Fogg, B.J. A behavior model for persuasive design. In Proceedings of the 4th international Conference on Persuasive Technology, Claremont, CA, USA, 26–29 April 2009; p. 40.
58. Brodbeck, J.; Berger, T.; Biesold, N.; Rockstroh, F.; Znoj, H.J. Evaluation of a guided internet-based self-help intervention for older adults after spousal bereavement or separation/divorce: A randomised controlled trial. *J. Affect. Disord.* **2019**, *252*, 440–449. [CrossRef] [PubMed]

11

A Low-Intensity Internet-Based Intervention Focused on the Promotion of Positive Affect for the Treatment of Depression in Spanish Primary Care: Secondary Analysis of a Randomized Controlled Trial

Mª Dolores Vara [1,2,*], Adriana Mira [3], Marta Miragall [2,3], Azucena García-Palacios [2,4], Cristina Botella [2,4], Margalida Gili [5,6,7], Pau Riera-Serra [5,6], Javier García-Campayo [7,8], Fermín Mayoral-Cleries [9] and Rosa Mª Baños [1,2,3]

1 Polibienestar Research Institute, University of Valencia, 46022 Valencia, Spain; banos@uv.es
2 CIBERObn Physiopathology of Obesity and Nutrition, Instituto de Salud Carlos III, 28029 Madrid, Spain; marta.miragall@uv.es (M.M.); azucena@uji.es (A.G.-P.); botella@uji.es (C.B.)
3 Department of Personality, Evaluation and Psychological Treatment, Faculty of Psychology, University of Valencia, 46010 Valencia, Spain; adriana.mira@uv.es
4 Department of Basic and Clinical Psychology and Psychobiology, Faculty of Health Sciences, Jaume I University, 12071 Castellon de la Plana, Spain
5 Institut Universitari d'Investigació en Ciències de la Salut, University of Balearic Islands, E-07122 Palma de Mallorca, Spain; mgili@uib.es (M.G.); pau.riera@uib.es (P.R.-S.)
6 Institut d'Investigació Sanitaria Illes Balears, 07120 Palma de Mallorca, Spain
7 Primary Care Prevention and Health Promotion Research Network, RedIAPP, 28029 Madrid, Spain; jgarcamp@unizar.es
8 Aragon Institute for Health Research (IIS Aragón), Miguel Servet Hospital, University of Zaragoza, 50009 Zaragoza, Spain
9 Mental Health Unit, Hospital Regional of Malaga, Biomedicine Research Institute (IBIMA), 29010 Málaga, Spain; fermin.mayoral.sspa@juntadeandalucia.es
* Correspondence: m.dolores.vara@uv.es

Abstract: *Background*: A large number of low-intensity Internet-based interventions (IBIs) for the treatment of depression have emerged in Primary Care; most of them focused on decreasing negative emotions. However, recent studies have highlighted the importance of addressing positive affect (PA) as well. This study is a secondary analysis of a randomized control trial. We examine the role of an IBI focused on promoting PA in patients with depression in Primary Care (PC). The specific objectives were to explore the profile of the patients who benefit the most and to analyze the change mechanisms that predict a significantly greater improvement in positive functioning measures. *Methods*: 56 patients were included. Measures of depression, affect, well-being, health-related quality of life, and health status were administered. *Results*: Participants who benefited the most were those who had lower incomes and education levels and worse mental health scores and well-being at baseline (7.9%–39.5% of explained variance). Improvements in depression severity and PA were significant predictors of long-term change in well-being, $F\ (3,55) = 17.78$, $p < 0.001$, $R^2 = 47.8\%$. *Conclusions*: This study highlights the importance of implementing IBIs in PC and the relevance of PA as a key target in Major Depressive Disorder treatment.

Keywords: depression; primary care; internet-based intervention; positive affect

1. Introduction

Major depressive disorder (MDD) is one of the most prevalent mental disorders worldwide, and it is associated with significant personal and social costs [1,2]. Specifically, the prevalence of depression in Spanish Primary Care (PC) is between 13.9 and 29% [3]. Even though there are effective treatments for this disorder (pharmacotherapy, psychotherapy, or both) [4,5], only half the people with depression receive adequate care [6], only two-thirds of patients respond to treatment, and only about one-third experience remission of their depressive symptoms [7,8]. Therefore, it is important to continue to explore different ways to improve these treatment outcomes.

Currently, there are evidence-based psychological treatments (e.g., cognitive-behavioral therapy, interpersonal therapy, problem-solving therapy) for depressive disorders in PC [9]. However, their therapeutic approaches have focused mainly on improving negative affect (NA) (e.g., depression, anxiety), paying less attention to the role of promoting positive affect (PA) and building positive resources (e.g., well-being, strengths) [10,11]. The literature indicates that MDD is related to low levels of positive emotions and that depression is more associated with low levels of PA than other emotional disorders [12]. Several studies point out the importance of promoting PA—as well as gratitude, resilience, and positive functioning—as core elements of interventions to facilitate recovery from depression [13,14].

A possible alternative in understanding MDD is to consider it a heterogeneous diagnostic construct with different underlying functional domains that may require different therapeutic strategies, as proposed in the Research Domain Criteria (RDoC) and transdiagnostic approaches [15]. Within this framework, MDD is proposed as resulting from alterations in two partly dissociable neurobiological dimensions: the upregulation of a negative valence system that promotes NA and leads to a pervasive depressed mood; and the downregulation of a positive valence system that guides the focus toward rewarding stimuli or PA, leading to loss of interest or pleasure (anhedonia) [16,17]. In the same vein, to effectively treat depression, research needs to propose psychotherapeutic interventions that include elements to downregulate NA and upregulate PA.

Several therapeutic approaches from the positive psychology (PP) field [18] are emerging with the aim of enhancing positive emotional human functioning (e.g., well-being, resilience, satisfaction with life), especially PA. Some reviews and meta-analyses show that PP interventions are effective in reducing depressive symptoms and increasing well-being [19–22], emphasizing their role alongside standard treatments for clinical depression [23].

One of the most important obstacles to integrating these treatments in PC settings is the lack of time and resources [24]. Many of the empirically validated treatments for MDD consist of 15–20 sessions requiring one hour per week [25,26]. Although this treatment length is considered quite brief compared to previous approaches, it has been argued that it is still too intense to be implemented in PC. One way to reduce the high costs of MDD treatment and overcome the limitations of traditional treatments in PC (e.g., logistical, geographical, and access difficulties) is to propose the use of brief or low-intensity psychological interventions for the treatment of MDD. Internet-based interventions (IBIs) are an example of low-intensity interventions that have been shown to be appropriate and cost-effective options within the stepped care model for the treatment of MDD [27]. Given the potential of IBIs as low-intensity interventions in PC, we conducted a randomized control trial (RCT) in a sample of patients diagnosed with MDD in different PC settings in Spain [28]. In this study, we examined the effectiveness of three low-intensity IBIs (PA promotion vs. healthy lifestyle vs. mindfulness) along with improved treatment as usual (iTAU), compared to iTAU alone, and the results were promising [29]. Specifically, healthy lifestyle and mindfulness interventions were effective in reducing depression severity, compared to iTAU, at post-treatment. Moreover, all the interventions were also effective in improving medium- and long-term quality of life. Finally, the PA promotion intervention was found to be effective in improving well-being at the six-month follow-up and NA at the 12-month follow-up, compared to iTAU.

The present study is a secondary analysis of the RCT carried out by Gili et al. [29]. More specifically, this study carries out an in-depth examination of the role of a specific IBI to promote PA as an adjunct therapy to iTAU in PC settings, given PA's potential as a strategy to improve well-being in MDD patients. Hence, the specific objectives are to determine: (1) which patient profile (i.e., sociodemographic and clinical baseline variables) predicts the improvement in depression severity and positive functioning in the post-treatment and follow-up sessions (Objective 1); and (2) which change mechanism predicts the greatest change in measures related to positive functioning in the post-treatment and follow-up sessions (Objective 2). The results on the efficacy of the PA intervention (vs. iTAU condition) can be found in Gili et al. [29]. Nevertheless, we will also analyze the changes in the primary and secondary outcomes from pre-treatment to post-treatment and at the 6- and 12-month follow-ups to provide a better understanding of the results of Objective 1 and 2. No specific hypotheses are proposed due to the exploratory nature of the analyses.

2. Materials and Methods

2.1. Study Design

This is a secondary analysis study of an RCT with repeated measures (baseline, post-treatment, 6-month and 12-month follow-ups) with four independent conditions: (a) PA promotion IBI + iTAU; (b) healthy lifestyle psychoeducational IBI + iTAU; (c) mindfulness IBI + iTAU; and (d) only iTAU group, in PC ([29]; Current Controlled Trials ISRCTN82388279). In the present study, we will only focus on the condition of the PA promotion IBI + iTAU.

2.2. Participants

In the original study, a total of 221 participants were recruited in PC settings from the Spanish regions of Aragon, Andalusia, and the Balearic Islands. The present study included 56 participants (78.6% women) who completed the PA intervention. Ages ranged between 19 and 68 years, with a mean of 44.14 years (SD = 10.38). In addition, 55.4% of the participants were married, 80.4% lived with family or a partner, 28.6% had higher education, 44.6% were employed, and 23.2% had an income below the national minimum wage. Regarding depression severity at baseline, the average on the Spanish Patient Health Questionnaire-9 (PHQ-9) was 15.79 (SD = 6.21).

Inclusion criteria were: (a) having mild or moderately severe depressive symptoms according to the Spanish Patient Health Questionnaire-9 (PHQ-9; [30]) (5–9 = Mild depression; 10–14 = moderate depression); (b) age between 18–65 years; (c) ability to use a computer; (d) having Internet and an email account; and (e) being able to read and understand Spanish. The Mini International Neuropsychiatric Interview (MINI) 5.0 [31,32] was used to assess different mental disorders and establish the diagnosis. Patients were excluded from the study if they had (a) severe depression (score ≥14 on the PHQ-9); (b) a severe Axis I psychiatric disorder (e.g., psychotic disorders, presence of suicidal ideation or plan, alcohol/substance abuse or dependence); (c) any disease that can affect the central nervous system (e.g., brain pathology, traumatic brain injury, dementia); or (d) if they were currently receiving psychological treatment.

Full information on the participant flow of the PA intervention is shown in Figure 1.

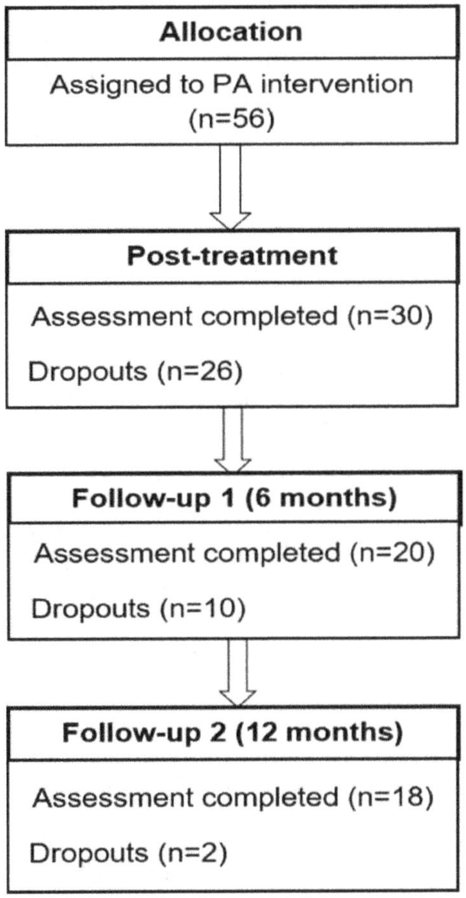

Figure 1. Patient flow diagram. PA: positive affect

2.3. Interventions

All the participants in the PA condition completed the low-intensity IBI and received iTAU from their general practitioner (GP).

2.3.1. Low-Intensity Internet-Based Computerized Intervention (IBI) Focused on the Promotion of PA

Before starting the online treatment, participants received a 90-min (3–5 patients) group face-to-face session conducted by a clinical psychologist. The objective of this session was to explain the program structure and the main components of the treatment, clarify the instructions for the use of the online platform, and motivate participants to change.

The online self-guided program consisted of four therapeutic modules (60 min per module approximately). The program duration could vary among the users, but it was usually completed in 4 to 8 weeks (maximum of 2 weeks per module). These modules contained multimedia elements (videos, images, texts) that provided information about MDD and coping strategies. These modules were sequential so that users could move step by step through the program. Moreover, users could review the module's contents after they had finished.

To enhance adherence, participants received two weekly automated mobile phone messages encouraging them to proceed with the program and reminding them of the importance of doing the homework tasks. In addition, the participants received automated emails encouraging them to continue with the modules if they had not accessed the program for a week.

Specifically, this intervention was based on PP techniques, and it was mainly designed to decrease depression severity and prevent relapse by promoting PA and subjective well-being. Table 1 shows each module, its objectives, and its specific content. For more information about the protocol for promoting PA, see García-Palacios, Mira, Mayoral, Baños, and Botella [33].

Table 1. Modules, objectives, and therapeutic content of Internet-Based Computerized Intervention (IBI).

Module	Objectives	Therapeutic Content
1. Learning to live	- Understanding the role of activity in mood regulation and our well-being. - Establishing and maintaining an adequate activity level and the relevance of choosing activities that are significant, with a personal meaning for the individual. - Learning the procedure to follow to schedule meaningful activities in daily life.	1. The role of activity in our well-being. 2. Things we should do and things we can do: meaningful activities. 3. The importance of daring, of getting involved with life. 4. Seeking social support. 5. Overcoming obstacles.
2. Learning to enjoy	- Learning about the effect of positive emotions in our lives. - Learning procedures to increase the likelihood of experiencing positive emotions, promoting the occurrence of pleasant activities to learn to enjoy the present moment.	1. Positive emotions, such as seeds or life anchors. 2. Satisfaction with the present. 3. Learning to generate good moments. 4. The importance of smiling. 5. Learn to identify, capture, and save good times.
3. Accepting to live	- Focusing on positive emotions related to the past (e.g., gratitude) or the future (such as optimism). - Identification and management of beliefs and behaviors that disturb the good moments.	1. Satisfaction with the past. 2. Satisfaction with the future. 3. Psychological well-being as a result of being active and practicing learned strategies.
4. Living and learning	- Understanding life as a continuous process of learning and personal growth. - Emphasizing the training in strategies to promote psychological strengths, resilience, and meaningful goals linked to important values.	1. Finding psychological well-being. 2. Potential, talents, and life goals. 3. Living with others, finding support in others. 4. What do I want my future to be like?

2.3.2. iTAU

The Treatment as Usual (TAU) in PC settings was improved. The participating GP received a training program on how to diagnose and treat depression in PC, based on the Spanish Guide for the Treatment of Depression in Primary Care [34]. Participants could receive medication for at least two months, and they had at least four visits with the GP that lasted an average of 30 min each. In cases with suicide risk, severe social dysfunction, or worsening of symptoms, the GP had to refer the patient to mental health facilities.

2.4. *Measures*

2.4.1. Primary Outcome Measure

Depression severity: The Patient Health Questionnaire-9 (PHQ-9; [35]) is a 9-item self-administered test for screening, diagnosing, monitoring, and measuring depression severity. Patients describe their state, taking into account the two weeks before the evaluation. Items are rated from 0 to 3, denoting "not at all", "several days", "more than half the days", and "nearly every day", respectively. Cut-off points of 5, 10, 15, and 20 represent mild, moderate, moderately severe, and severe depression

(DSM-IV-TR; [36]). The Spanish version has been shown to have good psychometric properties (for the diagnosis of any disorder, k = 0.74; overall accuracy, 88%; sensitivity, 87%; specificity, 88%) [30]. In the current study, the alpha coefficient was very satisfactory (α = 0.86).

2.4.2. Secondary Outcomes Measures

Affect: The Positive and Negative Affect Scale (PANAS; [37]) consists of 20 items that evaluate two independent dimensions: PA (10 items) and NA (10 items). The total score for each subscale ranges from 5 to 50, using a 5-point Likert-type scale (1 = very slightly or not at all, 5 = very much). The Spanish version by Sandín et al. [38] showed adequate internal consistency. In the current study, alpha coefficients were very satisfactory for both scales (αs = 0.87 and 0.86 for positive and negative subscales, respectively).

Well-being: The Pemberton Happiness Index (PHI; [39]) consists of 11 items related to different domains of remembered well-being (general, hedonic, eudaimonic, and social well-being), each with an 11-point Likert-type scale (0 = strongly disagree, 10 = strongly agree), and 10 items related to experienced well-being (positive and negative emotional events that may have happened the day before), with dichotomous response options (yes/no). The sum of the remembered and experienced well-being scores yields a combined well-being index (total well-being) ranging from 0 to 10. The validated Spanish version showed adequate psychometric properties [39]. In the current study, the alpha coefficient was very satisfactory (α = 0.86). In the current study, the alpha coefficient was very satisfactory (αs = 0.80).

Health-related quality of life: The Short Form 12 Health Survey (SF-12; [40]) is a 12-item questionnaire that measures aspects of health-related quality of life from the patient's perspective in two dimensions: physical health (general health, bodily pain, role-physical, physical functioning) and mental health (mental health, role-emotional, social-functioning, vitality). Scores > 50 represent better physical or mental health than the mean, and scores <50 represent worse physical or mental health than the mean. The Spanish version has been found to be a valid and reliable measure, showing good internal consistency [41]. In the current study, alpha coefficients were acceptable for both scales (αs = 0.80 for the physical health dimension and 0.66 for the mental health dimension, respectively).

Health status: The EuroQoL (EQ-5D; [42]) is a 5-item instrument to assess general health status (mobility, self-care, pain, usual activities, and psychological status) with three possible answers for each item (1 = no problem, 2 = moderate problem, 3 = severe problem). A summary index with a maximum score of 1 can be derived from these five dimensions using a conversion table [42]. The maximum score of 1 indicates the best health state, in contrast to the scores on individual questions, where higher scores indicate more severe or frequent problems. In addition to the descriptive system, the EQ-5D includes a visual analog scale (EQ VAS). The EQ VAS is a rating scale ranging from 0 (worst imaginable health state) to 100 (best imaginable health state), and it represents the evaluation of the patient's health state from his/her point of view. The validated Spanish version of the EQ-5D was used [42]. In this study, only the EQ VAS was taken into account.

2.4.3. Screening Related Measures

Sociodemographic data: Personal data that includes information such as age, sex, marital status, living alone or with others, educational level, employment, and income level.

Diagnostic interview: The MINI International Neuropsychiatric Interview version 5.0 (M.I.N.I. 5.0; [31]) is used in the screening to assess current depression and comorbid disorders. This measure is a structured diagnostic interview based on the DSM-IV and ICD-10 criteria. The Spanish version [32] was used for this study.

2.5. Procedure

Patients were recruited in Spanish PC settings from three different regions between March 2015 and March 2016. GPs detected possible participants with MDD using the PHQ-9. After a few days, an independent researcher used the MINI to assess the participants, taking into account the inclusion and exclusion criteria. Participants gave their signed written informed consent to be part of the study. Then, randomization was carried out by another independent researcher. All participants completed the pre-treatment assessment integrated into a web system (https://psicologiaytecnologia.labpsitec.es/). At the end of the treatment, they also completed the post-treatment and follow-up assessments through the website. The PHQ-9, PANAS, and SF-12 were administered at baseline, post-treatment, and 6-month and 12-month follow-ups. The PHI and EQ-5D were administered only at baseline and in the follow-up sessions. The Ethical Review Board of the regional health authority approved the study (Ref: IB 2144/13PI). More details about the study design, recruitment, and randomization methods are included in the protocol study by Castro et al. [28].

2.6. Data Analyses

All statistical analyses were performed using the SPSS v.26 (IBM Corp, Armonk, NY, USA). First, we implemented Multiple Imputation with Chained Equations (MICE) to replace the outcomes' missing values, performing 100 imputation models with 100 iterations per model [43].

Second, preliminary analyses were conducted to ensure that relevant assumptions of repeated-measures ANOVAs and multiple regression were met (i.e., normality, sphericity, and absence of multicollinearity). We tested normality, carrying out a visual inspection of the Q-Q (quantile-quantile) plots, verifying that the observed data was approximately closed to the expected data (i.e., the distance between the observed and expected data was not extreme). Hence, we assured that we met the normality assumption to carry out a repeated-measures ANOVA and multiple regression. Moreover, we tested the assumption of sphericity using Mauchly's test. If Mauchly's test statistic was significant (i.e., sphericity was not met), the degrees of freedom were adjusted using the Greenhouse–Geisser correction. Finally, we tested the absence of multicollinearity using the Variance Inflation Factor (VIF).

Third, seven repeated-measures ANOVA with time as within-factor—pre-treatment (Pre), post-treatment (Post), 6-month follow-up (FW6), and 12-month follow up (FW12)—were conducted to analyze the changes in each primary (i.e., PHQ-9) and secondary (i.e., PANAS-PA, PANAS-NA, PHI, SF-12 mental and physical health, EQ-5D) outcomes. Post-hoc analyses using Bonferroni corrections were carried out when significant effects were found. Within-group Cohen's d effect sizes with a 95% Confidence Interval were calculated.

Fourth, seven hierarchical multiple regression analyses with a stepwise selection of predictors within each block were conducted to explore which sociodemographic variables (i.e., sex, age, marital status, living alone or with others, educational level, employment, and income level) and pre-treatment scores on each primary and secondary outcome predicted the pre-post treatment, pre-FW6, and pre-FW12 change. The seven sociodemographic variables were entered in the first block, and six pre-treatment scores were entered in the second block to test the relevance of the extra explained variance of these variables in the dependent variables once the effects of the sociodemographic variables were controlled for. Given the small sample size to the number of predictors, a consideration of all predictors simultaneously in each regression was not tenable. Therefore, within each block, a statistical inclusion criterion for relevant predictors (stepwise method) was used. Creating two blocks in the regression analyses allowed us to test a lower number of predictors in each regression (i.e., seven instead of thirteen predictors).

To carry out correlation and regression analyses, categorical sociodemographic variables were transformed into recoded binary variables; that is, the correlation and regression analyses included: dichotomous variables (i.e., sex), continuous variables (i.e., age and scores in PHQ-9, PANAS-PA, PANAS-NA, PHI, SF-12 mental and physical health, EQ-5D) and recoded binary variables (i.e., ordinal or categorical variables were recoded into dichotomous variables with 0 and 1). Regarding the recoded binary variables, the categories were recategorized as follows: (a) marital status: 0 = not married (i.e., single, divorced, widowed); 1 = married or in a relationship; (b) *living alone or with others:* 0 = living alone; 1 = living with others (i.e., partner, sons, relatives, friends); (c) *educational level:* 0 = lower level (i.e., no education or primary school); 1 = higher level (i.e., secondary school or university studies); (d) *work status:* 0 = "not-working" (i.e., unemployed, retired, housekeeper, disability, student); 1 = employed; (e) *income level*: 0 = "lower than the minimum income (i.e., <641.40€); 1 = higher than the minimum income. We recoded into binary variables (instead of doing dummy variables) because the pair comparisons we constructed were theoretically appropriate, and a smaller number of predictors should be tested in the regression analyses. That is, if binary variables are used, only one predictor should be tested (e.g., 0 = "lower than the minimum income (i.e., <641.40€) vs. 1 = higher than the minimum income); however, if dummy variables are used, more than one predictor should be included in the regression equation (e.g., *dummy 1*: 0 = "lower than the minimum income < 641.40€ vs. 1 = between 1–2 minimum incomes; *dummy 2*: 0 = "lower than the minimum income < 641.40€ vs. 1 = between 2–4 minimum incomes). Moreover, the change in each primary and secondary outcome was calculated as follows: pre-post (post-treatment scores—pre-treatment scores), pre-FW6 (6-month follow up—pre-treatment scores), and pre-FW12 (12-month follow-up—pre-treatment scores). Negative values for the changes in PHQ and PANAS-NA meant improvements in these measures, whereas negative values for the changes in PANAS-PA, PHI, SF-12, and 5Q-5D meant a deterioration in these measures. The pairwise deletion method was used (i.e., whenever the variables of interest are present, they are analyzed) to deal with missing values and preserve all the data available in the regression analyses. The pre-treatment score on the corresponding dependent variable was not introduced in the equation regression model (e.g., the PHQ-9 pre score was not introduced as a predictor when the change in PHQ-9 was tested as a dependent variable).

Finally, four stepwise multiple regression analyses were conducted to analyze whether the changes in PHQ, PANAS-PA, or PANAS-NA were predictors of the change in PHI, SF-12 (mental and physical health), and EQ-5D. Changes in pre-post predictors were introduced for changes in pre-post dependent variables; changes in pre-post and pre-FW6 predictors were introduced for changes in pre-FW6 dependent variables; and changes in pre-post, pre-FW6, and pre-FW-12 predictors were introduced for changes in pre-FW12 dependent variables. All predictor variables were entered in the same block using the stepwise method.

It should be noted that the stepwise approach was used because we did not have an a priori hypotheses of which specific independent variables would predict the dependent variables, and consequently, we decided to identify the predictor variables relying on a statistical criterion.

3. Results

3.1. Sociodemographic Characteristics of the Sample

Table 2 shows a detailed description of the sociodemographic variables.

Table 2. Sociodemographic characteristics of the sample.

Sociodemographic Variables	%	n = 56
Sex		
Women	78.6%	44
Men	21.4%	12
Age (years)	44.14 (10.38) [a]	
Marital status		
Single	16.1% [b]	31
In a relationship/Married	55.4%	9
Divorced/Separated	16.1%	9
Widowed	1.8%	1
Income level		
Lower than the minimum income (<641,40€)	23.2%	13
Between 1–2 minimum incomes [c]	25.0%	14
Between 2–4 minimum incomes	21.4%	12

Table 2. *Cont.*

Sociodemographic Variables	%	n = 56
Work status		
Student	3.6%	2
Housekeeper	3.6%	2
Subsidized unemployed	5.4%	3
Unemployed with no subsidy	12.5%	7
Employee	44.6%	25
Sick leave	8.9%	5
Retired	3.6%	2
Disability	3.6%	2
Others	3.6%	2
Educational Level		
No education	5.4%	3
Primary school	16.1%	9
Secondary school	33.9%	19
University studies	28.6%	16
Living alone or with others		
Alone	8.9%	5
Living with partner	16.1%	9
Living with partner and children	53.6%	30
Living with relatives	8.9%	5
Living with friends or neighbors	1.8%	1

Note. [a] These values are the mean and standard deviation of age, which is a continuous variable. [b] Due to missing values, the sum of the percentages of the categories of the "marital status", "income level", "work status", "educational level", or "living alone or with others" are not 100%. That is, we do not have the 30.4% of the information regarding "income level" ($n = 17$); the 10.7% of the information regarding "marital status", "work status", and "living alone or with others" ($n = 6$); and the 16.1% of the information regarding the "educational level ($n = 9$). [c] Between "1–2 or "2–4" minimum incomes means that the minimum income level is equivalent to "641,40€ (641,40€x 1)–1282,80€ (641,40€x 2)" or "1282,80€ (641,40€x 2)–2.565,60€ (641,40€x 4)", respectively.

3.2. Primary and Secondary Outcome Scores at Pre-Treatment, Post-Treatment, and 6- and 12-Month Follow-Ups

Descriptive statistics, repeated-measures ANOVA results, and within-group effect sizes with 95% CI are shown in Table 3 for primary and secondary outcomes. The main effects of time were found for all the primary and secondary outcomes, with increases in the PANAS-PA, PHI, SF-12, and EQ-5D scores and decreases in the PHQ-9 and PANAS-NA scores.

Post-hoc analyses using the Bonferroni correction showed that there were significant differences from pre-treatment to post-treatment, FW6, and FW12 in depression severity (PHQ-9), PA (PANAS-PA), NA (PANAS-NA), and Mental Health (SF-12) ($p < 0.05$). Significant differences from pre-treatment to FW12 were found for Physical Health (SF-12), but not from pre-treatment to post-treatment or FW6. Finally, significant differences from baseline to the 6- and 12-month follow-ups were found for well-being (PHI) and health status (EQ-5D).

Table 3. Descriptive statistics and repeated-measures ANOVA results of the primary and secondary outcomes.

	Pre*M (SD)*	Post*M (SD)*	FW6*M (SD)*	FW12*M (SD)*	*F*	Within-Group Effect Size, d [95% CI] Pre–Post	Within-Group Effect Size, d [95% CI] Pre-FW6	Within-Group Effect Size, d [95% CI] Pre-FW12
1. Depression Severity (PHQ-9)	15.79 (6.21)	10.57 (6.68)	8.63 (6.11)	9.75 (5.65)	$F(2.51, 137.89) = 33.15$, MSE = 20.32, $p < 0.001$	0.83 [0.55, 1.11]	1.14 [0.78, 1.49]	0.96 [0.61, 1.31]
2. Positive Affect (PANAS-PA)	17.63 (6.11)	20.75 (7.92)	22.27 (8.23)	22.95 (9.66)	$F(2.37, 130.09) = 9.61$, MSE = 41.42, $p < 0.001$	−0.50 [−0.78, −0.22]	−0.75 [−1.06, −0.43]	−0.86 [−1.15, −0.57]
3. Negative Affect (PANAS-NA)	26.82 (8.56)	22.23 (8.07)	21.21 (7.30)	22.02 (8.56)	$F(2.54, 139.72) = 11.37$, MSE = 37.47, $p < 0.001$	0.53 [0.28, 0.78]	0.65 [0.34, 0.96]	0.55 [0.25, 0.85]
4. Well-being (PHI)	4.21 (1.72)	-	5.70 (1.89)	5.59 (1.78)	$F(2110) = 33.48$, MSE = 1.15, $p < 0.001$	-	−0.85 [−1.12, −0.59]	−0.79 [−1.09, −0.49]
5. Mental Health (SF-12)	26.22 (8.08)	30.50 (10.43)	38.61 (10.83)	35.26 (13.42)	$F(2.53, 139.31) = 20.65$, MSE = 94.52, $p < 0.001$	−0.52 [−0.79, −0.26]	−1.51 [−1.98, −1.04]	−1.10 [−1.47, −0.74]
6. Physical Health (SF-12)	42.45 (9.83)	45.11 (11.32)	45.58 (10.15)	47.04 (10.66)	$F(3, 165) = 4.66$, MSE = 44.02, $p = 0.004$	−0.27 [−0.50, −0.03]	−0.31 [−0.59, −0.04]	−0.46 [−0.70, −0.22]
7. Health Status (EQ-5D)	47.86 (20.34)	-	62.68 (15.24)	66.57 (19.04)	$F(1.65, 90.64) = 24.68$, MSE = 268.55, $p <$ 0.001	-	−0.72 [−1.00, −0.44]	−0.91 [−1.29, −0.53]

Notes. PHQ-9 = Patient Health Questionnaire-9; PANAS = The Positive and Negative Affect Scale; PHI = Pemberton Happiness Index; SF-12 = Short Form 12 Health Survey; EQ-5D = EuroQoL; PA = Positive affect; NA = Negative affect; Pre = Pre-treatment; Post = Post-treatment; FW6 = 6-month follow-up; FW12 = 12-month follow-up. MSE: Mean Squared Error.

3.3. *Sociodemographic Variables and Pre-Treatment Scores as Predictors of the Changes in Primary and Secondary Outcomes in the PA Intervention*

Point-Biserial and Pearson's correlations between potential predictors (sociodemographic and pre-treatment scores) are shown in Table 4. Positive significant relationships were found between age and educational level and income level; being married or in a relationship correlated positively with well-being (PHI) and with living with someone, and income level correlated positively with health status (5Q-5D). A negative significant relationship was found between age and physical health (SF-12). Negative significant relationships were found between depression severity (PHQ-9) and positive affect (PANAS), well-being (PHI), mental health and physical health (SF-12), and health status (5Q-5D). Finally, a positive significant relationship was found between depression severity (PHQ-9) and NA (PANAS).

Regarding hierarchical multiple regression analysis, coefficients of determination, unstandardized coefficients, standard errors, standard coefficients, and *t*-statistics are shown in Table 5. The statistical models for predicting the change in each primary and secondary outcome are described in the following paragraphs. Variance Inflation Factor ranged from 0.95 to 1.06 for all the regression analyses, indicating no problems with multicollinearity [44,45].

Models for predicting change in depression severity (PHQ). Level of income positively predicted the change from Pre-Post, $F(1,38) = 10.35$, $p = 0.003$, R^2 Adjusted = 19.7%; Level of income positively predicted the change from Pre-FW6, $F(1,38) = 5.50$, $p = 0.024$, R^2 Adjusted = 10.6%, and level of income positively predicted the change from Pre-FW12, $F(1,38) = 16.00$, $p < 001$, R^2 Adjusted = 28.3%. Once the sociodemographic variables were controlled, only well-being (PHI) positively predicted the change in PHQ from Pre-FW12, $F(2,38) = 13.39$, $p < 0.001$, R^2 Adjusted = 39.5%, which significantly increased the explained variance in 12.5% ($p = 0.008$). Lower level incomes predicted greater improvements in depression severity at post-treatment, and the 6- and 12-month follow-ups; and lower well-being predicted greater improvements in depression severity at the 12-month follow-up.

Models for predicting change in PA (PANAS). None of the variables entered predicted the Pre-Post, Pre-FW6, or Pre-FW12 change.

Models for predicting change in NA (PANAS). None of the variables entered predicted the Pre-Post, Pre-FW6, or Pre-FW12 change.

Models for predicting change in well-being (PHI). Mental health (SF-12) negatively predicted the change Pre-FW6 change, $F(1,38) = 4.27$, $p = 0.046$, R^2 Adjusted = 7.9%. None of the variables entered predicted the Pre-FW12 change. Lower mental health predicted greater improvements in well-being at the 6-month follow-up.

Models for predicting change in mental health (SF-12). Level of income negatively predicted the Pre-FW6 change, $F(1,38) = 5.71$, $p = 0.022$, R^2 Adjusted = 11.0%. None of the variables entered predicted the Pre-FW12 change. Lower income levels predicted greater improvements in mental health at the 6-month follow-up.

Models for predicting change in physical health (SF-12). Educational level predicted negatively the change from Pre-Post, $F(1,38) = 4.33$, $p = 0.044$, R^2 Adjusted = 8.1%; Pre-FW6, $F(1,38) = 8.23$, $p = 0.007$, R^2 Adjusted = 16.0%, and Pre-FW12, $F(1,38) = 9.04$, $p = 0.005$, R^2 Adjusted = 17.5%. Lower levels of education predicted greater improvements in physical health at post-treatment and 6- and 12-month follow-ups.

Models for predicting change in health status (EQ-5D). Level of income negatively predicted the Pre-FW6 change, $F(1,38) = 10.20$, $p = 0.003$, R^2 Adjusted = 19.5%. None of the variables entered predicted the Pre-FW12 change. Lower income levels predicted greater improvements in health status at the 6-month follow-up.

Table 4. Point-Biserial and Pearson's correlations between proposed predictor variables.

Sociodemographic Variables and Pre-Treatment Scores	1	2	3	4	5	6	7	8	9	10	11	12	13	14
1. Sex	—													
2. Age	−0.13	—												
3. Marital status (binary variable)	−0.05	0.03	—											
4. Living alone or not (binary variable)	0.13	−0.04	0.29 *	—										
5. Educational level (binary variable)	−0.19	0.33 *	0.04	−0.04	—									
6. Work status (binary variable)	−0.17	0.03	0.02	−0.14	0.02	—								
7. Income level (binary variable)	−0.13	0.50 **	0.26	0.05	0.21	0.22	—							
8. Depression Severity (PHQ-9)	0.02	−0.09	-0.23	0.05	−0.20	−0.12	−0.24	—						
9. Positive Affect (PANAS-PA)	−0.03	0.04	0.07	0.08	0.08	0.15	0.25	−0.33 *	—					
10. Negative Affect (PANAS-NA)	−0.05	−0.20	0.04	0.26	−0.16	0.04	−0.14	0.55 ***	−0.33 *	—				
11. Well-being (PHI)	0.04	0.10	0.33 *	−0.15	0.13	0.15	0.23	−0.51 ***	0.50 ***	−0.40 **	—			
12. Mental Health (SF-12)	0.13	0.08	0.26	0.11	0.09	0.05	0.28	−0.43 **	0.50 ***	−0.21	0.53 ***	—		
13. Physical Health (SF-12)	−0.05	−0.30 *	0.15	0.15	0.23	0.22	0.08	−0.36 **	0.15	−0.25	0.09	−0.09	—	
14. Health Status (EQ-5D)	−0.03	−0.12	0.20	0.07	0.15	0.26	0.44 **	−0.43 **	0.36 **	−0.16	0.42 **	0.26	0.40 **	—

Notes. PHQ-9 = Patient Health Questionnaire-9; PANAS = The Positive and Negative Affect Scale; PHI = Pemberton Happiness Index; SF-12 = Short Form 12 Health Survey; EQ-5D = EuroQoL; PA = Positive affect; NA = Negative affect. Point-Biserial's correlations were carried out among dichotomous and recoded binary variables and between dichotomous/recoded binary variables and continuous variables. Pearson's correlations were carried out among continuous variables. * $p < 0.05$, ** $p < 0.01$, *** $p < 0.001$.

Table 5. Models for sociodemographic variables and pre-treatment scores as predictors of change in primary and secondary outcomes.

Outcomes	Predictors	R	Adjusted R^2	R^2 Change	B	SE	β	t
Change in PHQ								
Pre-Post	Constant				−8.93	1.41		6.32 ***
	Level of incomes (binary variable)	0.47	0.20	0.22	5.57	1.73	0.47	3.22 **
Pre-FW6	Constant				−10.49	1.74		6.04 ***
	Level of incomes (binary variable)	0.36	0.11	0.13	4.99	2.13	0.36	2.35 *
Pre-FW12	Constant				−16.40	2.36		6.95 ***
	Level of incomes (binary variable)	0.55	0.28	0.30	6.57	1.83	0.47	3.60 **
	PHI	0.65	0.40	0.13	1.42	0.51	0.36	2.80 **
Change in PANAS positive								
Pre-Post	-	-	-	-	-	-	-	-
Pre-FW6	-	-	-	-	-	-	-	-

Table 5. *Cont.*

Outcomes	Predictors	R	Adjusted R^2	R^2 Change	B	SE	β	t
Pre-FW12	-	-	-	-	-	-	-	-
Change in PANAS negative								
Pre-Post	-	-	-	-	-	-	-	-
Pre-FW6	-	-	-	-	-	-	-	-
Pre-FW12	-	-	-	-	-	-	-	-
Change in PHI								
Pre-FW6	Constant				2.97	0.75		3.97 ***
	SF-12 (Mental Health)	0.32	0.08	0.10	−0.06	0.03	−0.32	2.07 *
Pre-FW12	-	-	-	-	-	-	-	-
Change in SF-12 (Mental Health)								
Pre-Post	-	-	-	-	-	-	-	-
Pre-FW6	Constant				19.23	3.51		5.48 ***
	Level of incomes (binary variable)	0.37	0.11	0.13	−10.26	4.29	−0.37	2.39 *
Pre-FW12	-	-	-	-	-	-	-	-
Change in SF-12 (Physical Health)								
Pre-Post	Constant				7.77	2.85		2.73 *
	Education level (binary variable)	0.32	0.08	0.11	−6.87	3.30	−0.32	2.08 *
Pre-FW6	Constant				10.58	3.010		3.52 **
	Education level (binary variable)	0.43	0.16	0.18	−10.01	3.490	−0.43	2.87 **
Pre-FW12	Constant				11.11	2.51		4.42 ***
	Education level (binary variable)	0.44	0.18	0.20	−8.76	2.91	−0.44	3.01 **
Change in EQ-5D								
Pre-FW6	Constant				26.30	4.40		5.98 ***
	Level of incomes (binary variable)	0.47	0.20	0.22	−17.21	5.39	−0.47	3.19 **
Pre-FW12	-	-	-	-	-	-	-	-

Notes. * $p < 0.05$; ** $p < 0.01$; *** $p < 0.001$. PHQ-9 = Patient Health Questionnaire-9; PANAS = The Positive and Negative Affect Scale; PHI = Pemberton Happiness Index; SF-12 = Short Form 12 Health Survey; EQ-5D = EuroQoL; PA = Positive affect; NA = Negative affect; Pre = Pre-treatment; Post = Post-treatment; FW6 = 6-month follow-up; FW12 = 12-month follow-up.

3.4. Change in Depression Severity and PA and NA as Predictors of Change in Well-Being, Mental and Physical Health, and Health Status

Coefficients of determination, unstandardized coefficients, standard errors, standard coefficients, and *t*-statistics for each stepwise multiple regression analysis are shown in Table 6. The statistical models to explain the changes in well-being, mental and physical health and health status are described in the following paragraphs. Variance Inflation Factor ranged from 1.01 to 2.37 for all the regression analyses, indicating no problems with multicollinearity.

Models for predicting change in well-being (PHI). The Pre–Post change in depression severity (PHQ-9) negatively predicted the Pre-FW6 change in well-being, $F(1,55) = 6.60$, $p = 0.013$, R^2 Adjusted = 9.2%. The Pre-12FW change in depression severity (PHQ-9) and PA (PANAS-PA), and the Pre-6FW change in depression severity (PHQ-9) (negatively, positively and negatively -respectively-) predicted the Pre-FW12 change in well-being, $F(3,55) = 17.78$, $p < 0.001$, R^2 Adjusted = 47.8%. Greater improvements in depression severity at post-treatment predicted greater improvements in well-being at the 6-month follow-up and greater improvements in depression severity and PA at the 12-month follow-up, and greater improvements in depression severity at the 6-month follow-up predicted greater improvements in well-being at the 12-month follow-up.

Models for predicting change in mental health (SF-12). The Pre-FW6 change in depression severity (PHQ-9) negatively predicted the Pre-FW6 change in mental health, $F(1,55) = 7.37$, $p = 0.009$, R^2 Adjusted = 10.4%. Greater improvements in depression severity at the 6-month follow-up predicted greater improvements in mental health at the 6-month follow-up.

Models for predicting change in physical health (SF-12). Changes in Pre-Post treatment scores for depression severity (PHQ-9) and NA (PANAS-NA) negatively predicted the Pre-Post change in physical health, $F(1,55) = 5.19$, $p = 0.009$, R^2 Adjusted = 13.2%. Greater improvements in depression severity and NA at post-treatment predicted greater improvements in physical health at post-treatment.

Models for predicting change in health status (EQ-5D). The Pre-FW12 change in depression severity (PHQ-9) negatively predicted the Pre-FW12 change in health status, $F(1,55) = 5.91$ $p = 0.018$, R^2 Adjusted = 8.2%. Greater improvements in depression severity at the 12-month follow-up predicted greater improvements in health status at the 12-month follow-up.

Table 6. Models for changes in depression severity (PHQ-9) and affect (PANAS) as predictors of change in well-being (PHI), health-related quality of life (SF-12), and health status (EQ-5D).

Outcomes	Predictors	R	Adjusted R^2	R^2 Change	B	SE	β	t
Change in PHI								
Pre-FW6	Constant				1.06	0.25		4.33 ***
	Change in PHQ-9 *Pre-Post*	0.33	0.09	0.11	−0.08	0.03	−0.33	2.57 *
Pre-FW12	Constant				0.57	0.27		2.14 *
	Change in PHQ-9 *Pre-FW12*	0.50	0.24	0.25	−0.22	0.04	−0.88	5.84 ***
	Change in PANAS-PA *Pre-FW12*	0.63	0.37	0.14	0.08	0.02	0.37	3.73 ***
	Change in PHQ *Pre-FW6*	0.71	0.48	0.12	0.14	0.04	0.52	3.50 **
Change in SF-12 (Mental Health)								
Pre-Post	-	-	-	-	-	-	-	-
Pre-FW6	Constant				7.37	2.51		2.94 **
	Change in PHQ-9 *Pre-FW6*	0.35	0.10	0.12	−0.70	0.26	−0.35	2.72 **
Pre-FW12	-	-	-	-	-	-	-	-
Change in SF-12 (Physical Health)								
Pre-Post	Constant				−1.18	1.68		0.70
	Change in PHQ-9 *Pre-Post*	0.31	0.08	0.10	−0.44	0.21	−0.27	2.10 *
	Change in PANAS-NA *Pre-Post*	0.41	0.13	0.07	−0.34	0.17	−0.26	2.04 *
Pre-FW6	-							
Pre-FW12	-							
Change in EQ-5D								
Pre-FW6	-	-	-	-	-	-	-	-
Pre-FW12	Constant				11.56	4.39		2.64 *
	Change in PHQ-9 *Pre-FW12*	0.31	0.08	0.10	−1.19	0.49	−0.31	2.43 *

Notes. * $p < 0.05$; ** $p < 0.01$; *** $p < 0.001$. PHQ-9 = Patient Health Questionnaire-9; PANAS = The Positive and Negative Affect Scale; PHI = Pemberton Happiness Index; SF-12 = Short Form 12 Health Survey; EQ-5D = EuroQoL; PA = Positive affect; NA = Negative affect; Pre = Pre-treatment; Post = Post-treatment; FW6 = 6-month follow-up; FW12 = 12-month follow-up.

4. Discussion

The purpose of this study was to shed light on the *patient profiles* (Objective 1) and *change mechanisms* (e.g., PA or NA) (Objective 2) that predicted a significantly greater improvement in depressive severity and positive functioning variables in an IBI focused on promoting PA, along with iTAU, in patients with MDD.

The efficacy of this intervention was tested in Gili et al. [29], where the PA intervention is compared to other interventions and a control group. However, in this study, we analyzed the change in the primary and secondary treatment outcomes to contextualize the secondary analyses of the present study. The results showed that participants improved on all the variables evaluated from pre- to post-treatment (depression, NA, PA, and mental health) significantly, except physical health, and the improvements were maintained until the follow-ups. The same thing occurred with the variables evaluated at pre-treatment and the 6- and 12-month follow-ups (well-being and general health status) because both variables improved significantly from pre to follow-ups. Hence, it is important to highlight that the PA intervention was not only able to decrease negative functioning measures significantly (PHQ-9 and PANAS-NA) but also to increase the positive functioning variables (PANAS-PA, quality of life, and well-being).

Our results showed that PP-based strategies focusing especially on the promotion of PA might have an impact on the decline in clinical symptomatology and the increase in positive functioning variables, which is consistent with other studies [46,47]. These results emphasize the benefits of including PP exercises and techniques in conventional treatments to promote positive emotions and positive functioning measures [19,20]. Recent studies suggest the importance of directly working on the promotion of positive emotions to improve depressive symptoms and achieve greater changes in positive emotion outcomes [48–50]. Nevertheless, the role of PP in interventions for depression has been poorly studied. The majority of the interventions for depression focus on reducing distress and negative emotions; however, it is has been recognized that well-being and the increase in positive emotions and behaviors contribute to mitigating negative emotions in life [51] and help to reduce stress reactivity [52,53]. Depression is characterized by high levels of NA. However, patients suffering from depression also have low PA, which, if not addressed, increases the consequences of the problem [11,54,55]. Moreover, PA has been found to contribute to better physical and psychological health and well-being [56], and so its improvement should be considered a core element of depression treatment. Our results show that depression can be addressed effectively not only by managing negative symptoms but also by increasing positive emotions [57,58].

Regarding the profile of patients who benefited more from this kind of intervention, sociodemographic variables and baseline scores on specific psychological measures were predictors of the changes in the primary and secondary outcomes. Overall, patients with lower income levels (i.e., under the minimum income level), lower educational levels (i.e., no education or only primary school), and worse scores on mental health and well-being before starting the intervention benefited more from the intervention. More specifically, *lower income levels* predicted greater improvements in depression severity at post-treatment (19.7% of variance), 6-month follow-up (10.6% of variance), and 12-month follow-up (28.3% of variance), as well as greater improvements in mental health and health status at the 6-month follow-up (11.0% and 21.6% of variance, respectively); *worse mental health* predicted greater improvements in well-being at the 6-month follow-up (7.9% of variance); *lower well-being* predicted greater improvements in depression severity at the 12-month follow-up (11.2% of variance); and finally, *lower education levels* predicted greater improvements in physical health at post-treatment (8.1% of variance), 6-month follow-up (16.0% of variance), and 12-month follow-up (19.6% of variance).

Regarding the education and income levels, our results pointed out that these variables were associated with intervention efficacy. In addition, we should highlight that this PA intervention was implemented in public PC contexts, where health status, education level, and income level are usually lower than in other psychological treatment settings. Thus, this study suggests that a brief self-guided

IBI could help people in more disadvantaged situations. None of the other sociodemographic variables examined predicted treatment outcomes. This means that the PA intervention is equally useful for people of different ages, marital status, work status, and sexes, which supports its dissemination. This result is in line with previous studies that found no sociodemographic variables that moderated the results of IBIs for depression [59].

Regarding mental health and well-being status, our findings are congruent with the results obtained by an Individual Patient Data (IPD) meta-analysis of low-intensity interventions for depression [60]. This study found that higher severity of depressive symptoms at baseline was associated with a greater decrease after the completion of the treatment. Nevertheless, because the effect was relatively small, the authors remarked that it is more cautious to conclude that low-intensity interventions work similarly across all the ranges of depression severity. By contrast, another recent IPD meta-analysis found that baseline depressive symptom scores did not moderate treatment outcomes [59]. This finding does not agree with our results because it suggests that characteristics of the intervention (e.g., focused only on PA) or the participants (e.g., patients from public PC settings) could explain these differences. More research with larger samples and different IBIs is needed to draw firm conclusions.

Regarding the mechanism of change, the improvement in depression severity was the most common predictor of the change in quality of life (mental and physical), well-being, and health status. More specifically, greater improvements in *depression severity and NA at post-treatment* predicted greater improvements in physical health at post-treatment (8.2% and 5% of variance, respectively); greater improvements in *depression severity at the 6-month follow-up* predicted greater improvements in mental health and well-being at the 6-month follow-up (10.4% and 9.2% of variance, respectively) and well-being at the 12-month follow-up (11.1% of variance); greater improvements in *depression severity at the 12-month follow-up* predicted greater improvements in well-being and health status at the 12-month follow-up (23.9% and 8.2% of variance, respectively). Furthermore, the increase in PA was also a relevant variable in increasing well-being in the long term. Specifically, greater improvements in *PA at the 12-month follow-up* predicted greater improvements in well-being at the 12-month follow-up (12.8% of variance). Hence, our results point out two important mechanisms of change in well-being in the long term (12-month follow-up): the improvement in depressive symptoms (PHQ-9) and the improvement in PA. These findings suggest that even though our intervention is focused on PA, changes in well-being are explained by changes in both depressive symptoms and PA.

This study has some limitations. First, the sample was small, and so the results should be interpreted with caution. Future PP research needs to focus on increasing sample sizes [61]. Second, the predictions of the multiple regression analyses were based on the stepwise method, so the conclusion should be taken as preliminary (i.e., the stepwise method is based on a mathematical criterion and not a theoretical criterion). Third, in our sample, participants had mild or moderate depressive symptoms; thus, it would be important to investigate the effect of PP strategies on patients with more severe depression [22]. Finally, it was not possible to record the number of face-to-face sessions focused on treating depression with the GP (although the available information indicated that they were very scarce and brief) or the medication dose administered to each patient in the iTAU condition. Future studies should consider these variables and analyze whether participants in IBIs receive less medical attention, which could be a cost-effectiveness variable of this treatment. Future research could explore the efficacy of this PP intervention, but in a completely self-guided way, without the support of the GP [59].

Despite the exploratory nature of this work, we consider that this study has several strengths. It may be relevant to the field of PP interventions, as it provides preliminary data on the profile of patients who benefit most of them. It also identifies the mechanisms of change of the intervention showing the improvement in PA, and not only in depression, as a significant predictor of long-term change in well-being. Finally, the study was carried out in a real context in a naturalistic way, which informs us regarding the utility of low-intensity IBIs in PC settings. The findings of the present study suggest that PA promotion can be an effective approach to treat depression by helping to improve both negative symptoms and positive emotions [62]. Furthermore, the PP intervention can be delivered using the Internet and self-guided formats, thus responding to an essential challenge in the field of depression treatments: reaching everyone in need by using new and alternative ways to apply psychological interventions. Therefore, the use of digital interventions helps to fulfill this proposal by contributing to the accessibility and dissemination of evidence-based treatments in the PC context.

5. Conclusions

In conclusion, this was the first study to explore a low-intensity IBI based on PA promotion in the PC setting in Spain. The results suggest that PP strategies might have an impact on clinical symptomatology, but they also contribute to improvements in positive functioning measures. Moreover, income level, education level, mental health, and well-being were significant predictors of the changes in depression severity and positive functioning measures at the end of the treatment and in the follow-up period. In addition, two mechanisms were identified as being responsible for the change in long-term well-being: the improvement in depression severity and the improvement in PA. Nevertheless, these findings should be interpreted with caution given the exploratory nature of the analyses and the small sample size used. Finally, this study highlights the importance of implementing IBIs in PC to produce changes in both negative and positive dimensions of human psychological functioning and promote more comprehensive psychotherapy for depression [63]. Overall, this study provides further support for the application of PP techniques using an IBI [62–64]. Future research should take into account the profile and unique characteristics of each patient to provide reliable tools to guide the choice of effective treatments.

Author Contributions: Conceptualization, A.G.-P., C.B., M.G., J.G.-C., F.M.-C., and R.M.B.; methodology, M.G. and A.G.-P.; software, C.B. and R.M.B.; formal analysis, M.D.V., A.M., M.M., and P.R.-S.; resources, A.G.-P., C.B., and R.M.B.; data curation, M.D.V., A.M., M.M., and P.R.-S.; writing—original draft preparation, M.D.V., A.M., and M.M.; writing—review and editing, all authors; supervision, A.G.-P., C.B., M.G., J.G.-C., F.M.-C., and R.M.B.; funding acquisition, A.G.-P., C.B., M.G., and R.M.B. All authors have read and agreed to the published version of the manuscript.

Acknowledgments: We would like to thank CIBERObn, an initiative of the ISCIII (ISC III CB06 03/0052), and "INTERSABIAS" Project (PROMETEO/2018/110).

References

1. Kessler, R.C. The Costs of Depression. *Psychiatr. Clin. N. Am.* **2012**, *35*, 1–14. [CrossRef]
2. Mrazek, D.A.; Hornberger, J.C.; Altar, C.A.; Degtiar, I. A Review of the Clinical, Economic, and Societal Burden of Treatment-Resistant Depression: 1996–2013. *Psychiatr. Serv.* **2014**, *65*, 977–987. [CrossRef] [PubMed]
3. Roca, M.; Gili, M.; García-García, M.; Salva, J.; Vives, M.; Campayo, J.G.; Comas, A. Prevalence and comorbidity of common mental disorders in primary care. *J. Affect. Disord.* **2009**, *119*, 52–58. [CrossRef] [PubMed]
4. Cuijpers, P.; Van Straten, A.; Andersson, G.; Van Oppen, P. Psychotherapy for depression in adults: A meta-analysis of comparative outcome studies. *J. Consult. Clin. Psychol.* **2008**, *76*, 909–922. [CrossRef] [PubMed]
5. Cuijpers, P.; Beekman, A.T.F.; Reynolds, C.F. Preventing Depression. *JAMA* **2012**, *307*, 1033–1034. [CrossRef] [PubMed]
6. Craven, M.; Bland, R. Depression in Primary Care: Current and Future Challenges. *Can. J. Psychiatry* **2013**, *58*, 442–448. [CrossRef]
7. Al-Harbi, K.S. Treatment-resistant depression: Therapeutic trends, challenges, and future directions. *Patient Prefer Adher* **2012**, *6*, 369–388. [CrossRef] [PubMed]

8. Cuijpers, P.; Karyotaki, E.; Weitz, E.; Andersson, G.; Hollon, S.D.; Van Straten, A. The effects of psychotherapies for major depression in adults on remission, recovery and improvement: A meta-analysis. *J. Affect. Disord.* **2014**, *159*, 118–126. [CrossRef] [PubMed]
9. Linde, K.; Sigterman, K.; Kriston, L.; Rücker, G.; Jamil, S.; Meissner, K.; Schneider, A. Effectiveness of Psychological Treatments for Depressive Disorders in Primary Care: Systematic Review and Meta-Analysis. *Ann. Fam. Med.* **2015**, *13*, 56–68. [CrossRef]
10. Carl, J.R.; Soskin, D.P.; Kerns, C.; Barlow, D.H. Positive emotion regulation in emotional disorders: A theoretical review. *Clin. Psychol. Rev.* **2013**, *33*, 343–360. [CrossRef]
11. Ruini, C. *Positive Psychology in the Clinical Domains*; Springer Science and Business Media LLC: Berlin/Heidelberg, Germany, 2017.
12. Watson, D.; Naragon-Gainey, K. On the specificity of positive emotional dysfunction in psychopathology: Evidence from the mood and anxiety disorders and schizophrenia/schizotypy. *Clin. Psychol. Rev.* **2010**, *30*, 839–848. [CrossRef]
13. Werner-Seidler, A.; Banks, R.; Dunn, B.D.; Moulds, M.L. An investigation of the relationship between positive affect regulation and depression. *Behav. Res. Ther.* **2013**, *51*, 46–56. [CrossRef]
14. Pressman, S.D.; Jenkins, B.N.; Moskowitz, J.T. Positive Affect and Health: What Do We Know and Where Next Should We Go? *Annu. Rev. Psychol.* **2019**, *70*, 627–650. [CrossRef]
15. Dalgleish, T.; Black, M.; Johnston, D.; Bevan, A. Transdiagnostic approaches to mental health problems: Current status and future directions. *J. Consult. Clin. Psychol.* **2020**, *88*, 179–195. [CrossRef]
16. Gray, J.A. Précis ofThe neuropsychology of anxiety: An enquiry into the functions of the septo-hippocampal system. *Behav. Brain Sci.* **1982**, *5*, 469–484. [CrossRef]
17. Watson, D.; Wiese, D.; Vaidya, J.; Tellegen, A. The two general activation systems of affect: Structural findings, evolutionary considerations, and psychobiological evidence. *J. Pers. Soc. Psychol.* **1999**, *76*, 820–838. [CrossRef]
18. Seligman, M.E.; Csikszentmihalyi, M. Special issue on happiness, excellence, and optimal human functioning. *Am. Psychol.* **2000**, *55*, 5–183. [CrossRef] [PubMed]
19. Sin, N.L.; Lyubomirsky, S. Enhancing well-being and alleviating depressive symptoms with positive psychology interventions: A practice-friendly meta-analysis. *J. Clin. Psychol.* **2009**, *65*, 467–487. [CrossRef]
20. Bolier, L.; Haverman, M.; Westerhof, G.J.; Riper, H.; Smit, F.; Bohlmeijer, E. Positive psychology interventions: A meta-analysis of randomized controlled studies. *BMC Public Health* **2013**, *13*, 119. [CrossRef]
21. Weiss, L.A.; Westerhof, G.J.; Bohlmeijer, E.T. Can We Increase Psychological Well-Being? The Effects of Interventions on Psychological Well-Being: A Meta-Analysis of Randomized Controlled Trials. *PLoS ONE* **2016**, *11*, e0158092. [CrossRef]
22. Chakhssi, F.; Kraiss, J.T.; Sommers-Spijkerman, M.; Bohlmeijer, E.T. The effect of positive psychology interventions on well-being and distress in clinical samples with psychiatric or somatic disorders: A systematic review and meta-analysis. *BMC Psychiatry* **2018**, *18*, 1–17. [CrossRef]
23. Johnson, J.; Wood, A.M. Integrating Positive and Clinical Psychology: Viewing Human Functioning as Continua from Positive to Negative Can Benefit Clinical Assessment, Interventions and Understandings of Resilience. *Cogn. Ther. Res.* **2015**, *41*, 335–349. [CrossRef]
24. Wakida, E.K.; Talib, Z.; Akena, D.; Okello, E.S.; Kinengyere, A.; Mindra, A.; Obua, C. Barriers and facilitators to the integration of mental health services into primary health care: A systematic review. *Syst. Rev.* **2018**, *7*, 211. [CrossRef]
25. Beck, J.S. *Cognitive Therapy: Basics and Beyond*; Guilford Press: New York, NY, USA, 1995.
26. Weissman, M.M.; Markowitz, J.C.; Klerman, G.L. *Comprehensive Guide to Interpersonal Psychotherapy*; Basic Books: New York, NY, USA, 2000.
27. Andrews, G.; Williams, A.D. Up-scaling clinician assisted internet cognitive behavioural therapy (iCBT) for depression: A model for dissemination into primary care. *Clin. Psychol. Rev.* **2015**, *41*, 40–48. [CrossRef]
28. Castro, A.; Garcia-Palacios, A.; Campayo, J.G.; Mayoral, F.; Botella, C.; Garcia-Herrera, J.M.; Pérez-Yus, M.-C.; Vives, M.; Baños, R.; Roca, M.; et al. Efficacy of low-intensity psychological intervention applied by ICTs for the treatment of depression in primary care: A controlled trial. *BMC Psychiatry* **2015**, *15*, 1–10. [CrossRef]
29. Gili, M.; Castro, A.; García-Palacios, A.; García-Campayo, J.; Mayoral-Cleries, F.; Botella, C.; Roca, M.; Barceló-Soler, A.; Hurtado, M.M.; Navarro, M.T.; et al. In primary care: Randomized Controlled Trial. *J. Med. Internet Res.* **2020**, *22*, e15845. [CrossRef]

30. Diez-Quevedo, C.; Rangil, T.; Sanchez-Planell, L.; Kroenke, K.; Spitzer, R.L. Validation and Utility of the Patient Health Questionnaire in Diagnosing Mental Disorders in 1003 General Hospital Spanish Inpatients. *Psychosom. Med.* **2001**, *63*, 679–686. [CrossRef]
31. Sheehan, D.V.; Lecrubier, Y.; Sheehan, K.H.; Amorim, P.; Janavs, J.; Weiller, E.; Hergueta, T.; Baker, R.; Dunbar, G.C. The Mini-International Neuropsychiatric Interview (M.I.N.I.): The development and validation of a structured diagnostic psychiatric interview for DSM-IV and ICD-10. *J. Clin. Psychiatry* **1998**, *59*, 22–33.
32. Bobes, J. A Spanish validation study of the mini international neuropsychiatric interview. *Eur. Psychiatry* **1998**, *13*, 198S–199S. [CrossRef]
33. García-Palacios, A.; Mira, A.; Mayoral, F.; Baños, R.M.; Botella, C. *Psychological Intervention in Primary Care for Mild-Moderate Depression. Protocol for the Promotion of Positive Affect. Therapist's Manual*; Publications of the University Jaume I: Castellón de la Plana, Spain, 2017. (In Spanish)
34. Fernández, A.; Haro, J.M.; Codony, M.; Vilagut, G.; Martinez-Alonso, M.; Autonell, J.; Salvador-Carulla, L.; Ayuso-Mateos, J.L.; Fullana, M.A.; Alonso, J. Treatment adequacy of anxiety and depressive disorders: Primary versus specialised care in Spain. *J. Affect. Disord.* **2006**, *96*, 9–20. [CrossRef]
35. Kroenke, K.; Spitzer, R.L.; Williams, J.B. The PHQ-9: Validity of a brief depression severity measure. *J. Gen. Intern. Med.* **2001**, *16*, 606–613. [CrossRef] [PubMed]
36. American Psychiatric Association. *Diagnostic and Statistical Manual of Mental Disorders, Fourth Edition, Text Revision (DSM-IV-TR)*; Masson: Barcelona, Spain, 1995.
37. Watson, D.; Clark, L.A.; Tellegen, A. Development and Validation of Brief Measures of Positive and Negative Affect: The PANAS Scales. *J. Pers. Soc. Psychol.* **1988**, *54*, 1063–1070. [CrossRef]
38. Sandín, B.; Chorot, P.; Lostao, L.; Joiner, T.E.; Santed, M.A.; Valiente, R.M. Escalas PANAS de afecto positivo y negativo: Validación factorial y convergencia transcultural. *Psicothema* **1999**, *11*, 37–51.
39. Hervás, G.; Vázquez, C. Construction and validation of a measure of integrative well-being in seven languages: The Pemberton Happiness Index. *Heal. Qual. Life Outcomes* **2013**, *11*, 66. [CrossRef]
40. Ware, J.E.; Kosinski, M.; Keller, S.D. A 12-Item Short-Form Health Survey. *Med Care* **1996**, *34*, 220–233. [CrossRef] [PubMed]
41. Vilagut, G.; Valderas, J.M.; Ferrer, M.; Garin, O.; López-García, E.; Alonso, J. Interpretación de los cuestionarios de salud SF-36 y SF-12 en España: Componentes físico y mental. *Medicina Clínica* **2008**, *130*, 726–735. [CrossRef]
42. Badia, X.; Roset, M.; Montserrat, S.; Herdman, M.; Segura, A. [The Spanish version of EuroQol: A description and its applications. European Quality of Life scale]. *Medicina Clínica* **1999**, *112*, 79–85.
43. Azur, M.J.; Stuart, E.A.; Frangakis, C.; Leaf, P.J. Multiple imputation by chained equations: What is it and how does it work? *Int. J. Methods Psychiatr. Res.* **2011**, *20*, 40–49. [CrossRef]
44. Bowerman, B.L.; O'Connell, R.T. *Linear Statistical Models: An. Applied Approach*; Duxbury: Belmont, CA, USA, 1990.
45. Myers, R. *Classical and Modern Regression with Applications*; Duxbury: Boston, MS, USA, 2000.
46. Santos, V.; Paes, F.; Pereira, V.; Arias-Carrión, O.; Silva, A.C.; Carta, M.G.; Nardi, A.E.; Machado, S. The Role of Positive Emotion and Contributions of Positive Psychology in Depression Treatment: Systematic Review. *Clin. Pr. Epidemiology Ment. Heal.* **2013**, *9*, 221–237. [CrossRef]
47. Chaves, C.; Lopez-Gomez, I.; Hervas, G.; Vazquez, C. A Comparative Study on the Efficacy of a Positive Psychology Intervention and a Cognitive Behavioral Therapy for Clinical Depression. *Cogn. Ther. Res.* **2016**, *41*, 417–433. [CrossRef]
48. Geschwind, N.; Arntz, A.; Bannink, F.; Peeters, F. Positive cognitive behavior therapy in the treatment of depression: A randomized order within-subject comparison with traditional cognitive behavior therapy. *Behav. Res. Ther.* **2019**, *116*, 119–130. [CrossRef]
49. Mira, A.; Bretón-López, J.; Enrique, Á.; Castilla, D.; Garcia-Palacios, A.; Baños, R.; Botella, C. Exploring the Incorporation of a Positive Psychology Component in a Cognitive Behavioral Internet-Based Program for Depressive Symptoms. Results Throughout the Intervention Process. *Front. Psychol.* **2018**, *9*, 2360. [CrossRef]
50. Proyer, R.T.; Wellenzohn, S.; Gander, F.; Ruch, W. Toward a better understanding of what makes positive psychology interventions work: Predicting happiness and depression from the person × intervention fit in a follow-up after 3.5 years. *Appl. Psychol. Health Well Being.* **2015**, *7*, 108–128. [CrossRef]
51. Bower, J.E.; Moskowitz, J.T.; Epel, E. Is benefit finding good for your health? Pathways linking positive life changes after stress and physical health outcomes. *Curr. Dir. Psychol. Sci.* **2009**, *18*, 337–341. [CrossRef]

52. Craske, M.G.; Meuret, A.E.; Ritz, T.; Treanor, M.; Dour, H.; Rosenfield, D. Positive affect treatment for depression and anxiety: A randomized clinical trial for a core feature of anhedonia. *J. Consult. Clin. Psychol.* **2019**, *87*, 457–471. [CrossRef] [PubMed]
53. Craske, M.G.; Meuret, A.E.; Ritz, T.; Treanor, M.; Dour, H.J. Treatment for Anhedonia: A Neuroscience Driven Approach. *Depress. Anxiety* **2016**, *33*, 927–938. [CrossRef] [PubMed]
54. Gilbert, K.; Nolen-Hoeksema, S.; Gruber, J. Positive emotion dysregulation across mood disorders: How amplifying versus dampening predicts emotional reactivity and illness course. *Behav. Res. Ther.* **2013**, *51*, 736–741. [CrossRef]
55. Fredrickson, B.L. The role of positive emotions in positive psychology: The broaden-and-build theory of positive emotions. *Am. Psychol.* **2001**, *56*, 218–226. [CrossRef]
56. Seligman, M.E.P.; Rashid, T.; Parks, A.C. Positive psychotherapy. *Am. Psychol.* **2006**, *61*, 774–788. [CrossRef]
57. Ryff, C.D. Psychological Well-Being Revisited: Advances in the Science and Practice of Eudaimonia. *Psychother. Psychosom.* **2014**, *83*, 10–28. [CrossRef]
58. Taylor, C.T.; Lyubomirsky, S.; Stein, M.B. Upregulating the positive affect system in anxiety and depression: Outcomes of a positive activity intervention. *Depress. Anxiety* **2017**, *34*, 267–280. [CrossRef]
59. Karyotaki, E.; Riper, H.; Twisk, J.; Hoogendoorn, A.; Kleiboer, A.; Mira, A.; MacKinnon, A.; Meyer, B.; Botella, C.; Littlewood, E.; et al. Efficacy of Self-guided Internet-Based Cognitive Behavioral Therapy in the Treatment of Depressive Symptoms. *JAMA Psychiatry* **2017**, *74*, 351–359. [CrossRef]
60. Bower, P.; Kontopantelis, E.; Sutton, A.; Kendrick, T.; Richards, D.A.; Gilbody, S.; Knowles, S.; Cuijpers, P.; Andersson, G.; Christensen, H.; et al. Influence of initial severity of depression on effectiveness of low intensity interventions: Meta-analysis of individual patient data. *BMJ* **2013**, *346*, f540. [CrossRef]
61. White, C.A.; Uttl, B.; Holder, M.D. Meta-analyses of positive psychology interventions: The effects are much smaller than previously reported. *PLoS ONE* **2019**, *14*, e0216588. [CrossRef]
62. Wood, A.M.; Tarrier, N. Positive Clinical Psychology: A new vision and strategy for integrated research and practice. *Clin. Psychol. Rev.* **2010**, *30*, 819–829. [CrossRef] [PubMed]
63. Rashid, T. Positive interventions in clinical practice. *J. Clin. Psychol.* **2009**, *65*, 461–466. [CrossRef]
64. Fava, G.A.; Ruini, C. Development and characteristics of a well-being enhancing psychotherapeutic strategy: Well-being therapy. *J. Behav. Ther. Exp. Psychiatry* **2003**, *34*, 45–63. [CrossRef]

12

From Research to Practice: Ten Lessons in Delivering Digital Mental Health Services

Nickolai Titov [1,*], Heather D. Hadjistavropoulos [2], Olav Nielssen [1], David C. Mohr [3], Gerhard Andersson [4,5] and Blake F. Dear [1]

1 MindSpot Clinic and Department of Psychology, Macquarie University, Sydney, NSW 2109, Australia
2 Online Therapy Unit, Department of Psychology, University of Regina, Regina, Saskatchewan, SK S4S 0A2, Canada
3 Center for Behavioral Intervention Technologies, Department of Preventive Medicine, Northwestern University, Chicago, IL 60611, USA
4 Department of Behavioural Sciences and Learning, Linköping University, Linköping SE-581 83, Sweden
5 Department of Clinical Neuroscience, Karolinska Institute, Stockholm 171 77, Sweden
* Correspondence: nick.titov@mq.edu.au

Abstract: There is a large body of research showing that psychological treatment can be effectively delivered via the internet, and Digital Mental Health Services (DMHS) are now delivering those interventions in routine care. However, not all attempts to translate these research outcomes into routine care have been successful. This paper draws on the experience of successful DMHS in Australia and Canada to describe ten lessons learned while establishing and delivering internet-delivered cognitive behavioural therapy (ICBT) and other mental health services as part of routine care. These lessons include learnings at four levels of analysis, including lessons learned working with (1) consumers, (2) therapists, (3) when operating DMHS, and (4) working within healthcare systems. Key themes include recognising that DMHS should provide not only treatment but also information and assessment services, that DMHS require robust systems for training and supervising therapists, that specialist skills are required to operate DMHS, and that the outcome data from DMHS can inform future mental health policy. We also confirm that operating such clinics is particularly challenging in the evolving funding, policy, and regulatory context, as well as increasing expectations from consumers about DMHS. Notwithstanding the difficulties of delivering DMHS, we conclude that the benefits of such services for the broader community significantly outweigh the challenges.

Keywords: delivery; implementation; internet-delivered cognitive behaviour therapy; psychological treatment; routine care; depression; anxiety disorders

---

1. Introduction

Globally, mood and anxiety disorders affect more than 700 million people each year and are associated with considerable burden and disability [1,2]. However, in a 12-month period, fewer than half of those affected seek or receive evidence-based treatments [3–5] for reasons that include cost, limited availability of services in many areas, limited awareness of both illness and the potential benefit of treatment, stigma and preference to self-manage [6].

Delivering psychological services via the internet is one way of increasing access to care. A large number of randomised controlled trials have demonstrated that internet-delivered cognitive behavioural therapy (ICBT) is effective at treating anxiety and depression [7–10]. However, attempts to extend ICBT to routine care have produced mixed results. Several attempts at implementation have either been unsuccessful [11] or were not found to have added value to existing face to face services [12], which has raised doubt as to whether internet-delivered psychological services can be implemented successfully in typical health care settings [13]. Notwithstanding the challenges, the successful use of ICBT as part of routine clinical care has been reported in Sweden [14–17], the Netherlands [18,19], Norway, Denmark [20,21], Canada [22–25], and Australia [26–30]. In addition to reports of outcomes from individual clinics, and reflecting the maturing state of the field, there is now an increasing number of studies describing barriers [20,23,31,32], guidelines for implementation [33,34], and comparisons of clinics across different countries [35]. The successful clinics typically deliver ICBT interventions via so-called virtual or digital mental health services (DMHS). Common features of the successful clinics include high standards of both clinical and organisational governance, and robust systems for staff training and supervision [35].

This paper describes key lessons learned during our own efforts to develop and deliver DMHS. The MindSpot Clinic, Australia, and the Online Therapy Unit (OTU) in the province of Saskatchewan, Canada accept referrals directly from consumers as well as via general practitioners. Together, these DMHS have provided assessments to more than 100,000 people and treatment to more than 30,000 people. The authors have worked closely together for several years and have served on advisory bodies to each other's services. The lessons we describe draw on our shared experiences in service development, delivery and collaboration.

We narrowed down our experience to ten key lessons that were not fully described in other papers. These lessons were not immediately apparent to us when we set about translating our research findings to routine care but have been of fundamental importance in how we developed and now operate our DMHS. Hence, we anticipate that these lessons may help those launching similar clinics.

We intentionally avoided specific frameworks of reporting [36,37], because an aim of this paper was to describe the experiences of operating mature services, rather than just the implementation phase. We also acknowledge that some of these lessons overlap, may not apply in other jurisdictions or even to other DMHS within our own countries.

2. Lessons

We chose to organise our lessons according to the model shown in Table 1, which represents the lessons learned from working with (1) consumers, (2) therapists, (3) operating DMHS, and (4) when operating in the broader health systems, including when engaging with funders and policy makers.

Table 1. Lessons learned at four levels of analysis of digital mental health services (DMHS).

Level	Lesson
1. Consumers	1. DMHS can improve access to care for those who really need care 2. DMHS deliver more than treatment services 3. DMHS are used by a broad cross-section of the population
2. Therapists	1. DMHS require specialised therapist skills 2. DMHS require specialised clinical processes
3. Operating DMHS	1. The operation of DMHS require specialised systems and skills 2. DMHS evolve
4. Health Systems, Funders, and Policy Makers	1. Integrating DMHS within health systems is challenging 2. DMHS may change the mental health system 3. DMHS are not a panacea

Before further describing the lessons learned, key aspects of the MindSpot Clinic and OTU are summarised below.

2.1. *The MindSpot Clinic, Sydney, Australia*

MindSpot was launched in 2013 and operates from Macquarie University, Sydney. MindSpot is funded by the Australian Government Department of Health, with funding initially provided for a 3-year period as a result of the competitive tender process. MindSpot aims to improve access to evidence-based education, triage, assessment, referral, and treatment services throughout Australia to adults with symptoms of depression and anxiety [28,29]. Clinic services are provided free of charge.

Patients can either self-refer after learning about MindSpot via the website (mindspot.org.au), online advertising, links from other mental health websites, recommendations by previous users or can take up referrals from health professionals. Patients first register online or via telephone and complete a detailed assessment questionnaire followed by telephone or secure email contact with a therapist to discuss symptoms and treatment options. Patients then choose between information to assist with self-management, referral to another service or ICBT. The clinic offers seven ICBT programs that have been validated in clinical trials, including transdiagnostic treatments designed to treat symptoms of anxiety and depression in several age groups [24,38–47] and disorder-specific treatments for obsessive compulsive disorder [48,49], post-traumatic stress disorder [50], and chronic pain [51]. All the treatment programs comprise of five lessons which provide the core information, delivered over eight-weeks. Additional resources targeting specific symptoms or difficulties are made available during treatment to assist patients tailor treatment to their own needs. Outcomes are measured using validated symptom scales that are administered weekly during treatment, on completion, and at a three-month follow-up. The therapists are all registered or provisionally registered mental health professionals who contact and monitor participants weekly during treatment via a secure email system or by telephone. The treatment patients are enrolled in cohorts every two weeks, with therapists each responsible for 50 or so patients. To date, more than 100,000 people have registered to use the clinic, and 25,000 have opted to receive ICBT.

2.2. *Online Therapy Unit, Canada*

The OTU has operated from the University of Regina in Saskatchewan since October 2010. Initial funding was provided by a federal research grant, but since 2015, the OTU has received stable funding from the Saskatchewan Ministry of Health. The OTU aims to provide therapist-guided ICBT for depression and anxiety and to educate providers of mental health care and conduct research on ICBT in routine practice [25]. Clinic services are also provided to patients free of charge.

The OTU promotes services to patients via word of mouth primarily from health care providers, media reports, and both digital and print communication. Patients are encouraged to visit the clinic online (onlinetherapyuser.ca) and can either self-refer or are referred by a health professional. Patients first complete an online screening followed by telephone assessment.

The OTU delivers several ICBT programs including an adaptation of the Wellbeing course developed at Macquarie University and used at the MindSpot Clinic [44,47,52]. Clinically validated patient reported outcome measures (PROMS) of anxiety and depression are administered regularly during treatment, at post-treatment, and at three-month follow-up. Therapists are registered mental health professionals or graduate students under supervision employed by the clinic or by publicly funded community clinics located in other parts of Saskatchewan. During treatment, patients receive weekly therapist contact primarily via secure email or by telephone to assist in applying the skills taught during treatment. Since October 2010, the clinic had assessed more than 5400 patients, 4200 of whom have received ICBT [23,24,35].

3. The Ten Lessons

3.1. *Level 1: Lessons Working with Consumers*

The first three lessons refer to the way DMHS can improve access to care and serve a broad section of the community, and how they deliver services other than treatment.

3.1.1. Lesson 1: DMHS Can Improve Access to Care for Those Who Really Need Care

One of the most profound lessons we learned is that DMHS improve access to mental health services for many people who would not otherwise seek care. For example, at least a third of the users of both MindSpot and OTU report that they have not previously spoken to a health professional about symptoms and 80% of MindSpot and 55% of OTU users are not using other mental health services at the time of assessment [28,53].

The users of these services often have chronic and disabling symptoms. A third of MindSpot users have been troubled by their symptoms for between one and five years with a further third reporting symptoms for more than six years. Among users of the OTU, 45% report symptoms for two or more years and those in paid employment report an average of 7 days off work in the last 30 days due to symptoms. Moreover, the mean symptom scores reported by users of MindSpot are in the moderate–severe range, a quarter report suicidal thoughts and 2.4% disclose suicidal plans.

We were also surprised at how people use our DMHS. While most users access content online, many others download information and refer to it when they do not have internet access [54]. In addition, for those who prefer or require printed materials, we send all the treatment course content in printed form [28]. For these reasons, we sometimes think of our services as delivering *virtual* rather than *digital* care, however, we are reluctant to introduce new terms to describe this already definitionally challenged field.

3.1.2. Lesson 2: DMHS Deliver More than Treatment

Contrary to our expectations, not all consumers using our DMHS seek treatment, especially in Australia, where most users report they are primarily seeking a confidential assessment and recommendations about treatment options. This should not have come as a complete surprise, given the high proportion who had not previously sought treatment. However, we learned that for many people, the assessment itself serves as a brief but helpful clinical intervention, particularly when the consumer and therapist create a shared clinical formulation, discuss treatment options that include self-help strategies, and explore barriers and facilitators to recovery. This assessment process is highly regarded by the patients of both clinics.

Consumers also frequently report enormous difficulty understanding and navigating the existing mental health service eco-system and some report using our services to seek advice about other health services, a theme which we return to below. Consequently, our second lesson is that DMHS need to offer a range of services in addition to online treatment, including information, assessment, triage and referral to other services. It should be noted that there are differences between our two clinics, with more people using the OTU reporting they are seeking treatment compared with users of MindSpot [55]. Thus, the specific services offered by DMHS may vary between jurisdictions, possibly reflecting differences in how the clinics are perceived and promoted, and differences in the needs of the local community.

3.1.3. Lesson 3: DMHS are used by a Broad Cross Section of the Population

Our third lesson is that a diverse cross section of our communities access our services, including indigenous Australians and Canadians [56], people on low incomes, people living in rural and remote regions, and other groups who often under-utilise traditional health services. We stress that our DMHS are not a panacea in this regard. Instead, we note that the widespread use of internet-enabled devices to access a range of services, including education, banking, entertainment and other domains, has extended to healthcare. In a similar way, DMHS have considerable potential to reduce, to some degree, the inequality of access to mental health.

A striking example is the ability of DMHS to reach people living in rural areas. Almost 40% of MindSpot users report living outside major metropolitan areas, with many living in rural or remote parts of Australia, including islands off the mainland. Similarly, 28% of OTU users are from rural locations and 32% from small cities. Collectively, these people live in locations where access to health services is limited or sometimes non-existent [55]. A further example relates to engagement by older adults. Across both clinics, approximately 6% of users are over the age of 60, which is a group that often experience difficulty accessing mental health services, including for reasons related to physical impairments. The experience at both clinics is that older adults strongly engage in treatments and often obtain large improvements in symptoms [42].

A final example relates to socio-economic disadvantage. A recent analysis of MindSpot data found that users come from all socio-economic backgrounds, including 33% from the lower four deciles of socio-economic status, a group who are more prone to experience a disadvantage and difficulties accessing mental health services.

3.2. *Level 2: Lessons Working with Therapists*

Both clinics have now trained large numbers of therapists, previously experienced in delivering face-to-face care, to deliver DMHS. Key lessons have been that therapists working in DMHS require specialised skills and therefore, require specialised training and supervision to acquire and maintain those skills.

3.2.1. Lesson 4: DMHS Require Specialised Therapist Skills

An important lesson is that the skills and knowledge required for effective delivery of DMHS are sufficiently different to those associated with traditional models of care to warrant specialised training and supervision [57]. Obvious examples include the need for DMHS therapists to become competent in the use of clinical software platforms and in engaging with patients via telephone or text-based communication, including responding appropriately to very long messages or technical questions, skills that are not taught in most clinical training programs [23,40,58].

However, there are less obvious reasons for providing specialised training and supervision. First, therapists new to DMHS often intellectually understand that DMHS treatments can result in similar outcomes to face-to-face treatment [10,59] but may initially expect DMHS treatments to produce poorer outcomes, a sentiment they may communicate to consumers [23]. New therapists also often find that their assumptions about mechanisms or facilitators of recovery are challenged, particularly when they learn that DMHS patients can develop very strong therapeutic alliances [60] and may obtain large clinical improvements, even after choosing not to have regular therapist contact [55]. Related to this, therapists are often surprised to learn that the structured educational aspects and resources associated with DMHS offer significant advantages over traditional clinical care where such resources may not be used.

A second reason for providing specialised training and supervision is to support DMHS therapists to successfully process the transference and other dynamics that occur when delivering DMHS to large groups of patients at once. An example of this is the temporary increase in symptoms experienced by many consumers at mid-treatment when they begin to apply skills learned in treatment in their everyday lives. These lapses usually resolve and most continue to recover. This process is familiar to experienced therapists, who can help patients understand this trajectory and can manage their own reactions. However, the effect can be magnified by the large numbers of patients in each treatment cohort, leading to feelings of intense elation or sometimes disillusionment, particularly when some patients choose not to engage with the therapist but have not made this clear at the outset. A strong framework of training and supervision can assist therapists to understand and adapt to these patterns and maintain confidence in both their own performance and the effectiveness of the treatment programs.

3.2.2. Lesson 5: DMHS Require Specialised Clinical Processes

This lesson reflects important differences in the clinical procedures and processes used in DMHS compared to traditional mental health clinics. An obvious example is the use of structured ICBT interventions, questionnaires and outcome measures used in DMHS, the delivery of which are governed by procedures which regulate therapists' actions more than they would in typical in face-to-face services.

This level of structure reflects how DMHS attempt to manage both quality assurance and treatment to large numbers of consumers. Therapists experienced in working at DMHS can efficiently deliver individualised care within these structured frameworks, but this is more difficult for less experienced therapists. Another lesson has been the importance of robust systems for not only training and supervision [58,61], but also the recruitment and retention of clinicians who are comfortable with relatively high levels of structure and process [23].

Another example of how DMHS differ from traditional face-to-face mental health services, at least in our jurisdictions, relates to the use of PROMS and patient-reported experience measures (PREMS) [62–64]. Despite the documented utility of PROMS and PREMS in clinical care, they are infrequently used in traditional services, and rarely as a therapeutic tool for guiding discussions or decisions about treatment or as a method for improving the quality of care. Since our clinics routinely administer PROMS and PREMS during and after treatment, we provide specific training for new therapists to increase their comfort and competence in using measures of outcome and experience [61].

3.3. Level 3: Lessons Operating Services

3.3.1. Lesson 6: The Operation of DMHS Require Specialised Systems and Skills

This lesson is obvious, but we include it here because we underestimated the complexity of developing and delivering safe and effective DMHS. We expected that our DMHS would be similar to traditional face-to-face clinical mental health services or an extension of the operations used in our large-scale clinical research trials. However, we quickly learned that safely and effectively operating DMHS required attention in at least four areas.

First, DMHS require robust procedures to define and effectively manage safety risks for people presenting with more severe and complex needs than seen in our clinical trials [30] and who often live in remote locations. This requires developing expertise in evaluation of risk via telephone or online communication, the ability to contact emergency services that are available near where the patient is located, how to refer to such services, and how to stay abreast of changes in their referral and contact details.

Second, although operating DMHS involve similar skills as those required for operating traditional mental health services, including management, human resources, marketing and IT [25], we found that DMHS were sufficiently different to warrant employing people with additional expertise, including skills relevant to telehealth, social media and online marketing.

Third, and in addition to the urgent requirement for establishing robust systems of organizational and clinical governance we recognised that in order to effectively lead our services, we personally needed to develop commercial and management skills, domains in which we, as clinical researchers, had little or no experience. We also needed to address challenges relating to regulation; for example at MindSpot, we needed to determine which of the myriad of possible regulatory frameworks applied to our activities [65] given that most [66] had been developed for traditional face-to-face services. Within the OTU, a similar issue requiring attention was how to meet the different regulatory requirements for services provided by therapists from psychology and social work.

Establishing, maintaining, and subsequently improving our operational systems has required a considerable work effort. Whilst we have recruited specialist staff to assist with such efforts, due to the novelty of DMHS, we often also sometimes found it necessary to train and develop our own staff in these operational and managerial roles.

3.3.2. Lesson 7: Digital Mental Health Clinics Evolve

This lesson represents another difference between DMHS and traditional clinical services. Traditional services may change frequently, but the change is usually limited to organisational structure or branding, with less frequent changes to the service or delivery models. By contrast, our DMHS regularly undergo significant changes in procedures, systems, and even service delivery models due to developments in research, technology, the changing expectations of consumers, and changes in the policy priorities of the funding bodies. However, the most frequent changes stem from reviewing our outcomes and procedures.

For example, within the OTU, changes within recent years include (1) replacing disorder-specific ICBT programs with a transdiagnostic treatment program in light of the extensive comorbidity found among patients seeking services and the efficiency of delivery compared to disorder-specific programs [24], (2) ongoing trials to determine the best level of support and specialisation by therapists [40,67], and (3) the expansion of services to address other needs in the community, such as ICBT for pain [22].

Regular change has significant implications for the operation of our clinics. For example, management needs systems for reliably collecting and analysing data, the ability to develop and test alternative models, and the skills and authority to make decisions. The individuals given the task of implementing change need project leadership and change management skills and procedures to plan and deploy changes. Furthermore, therapists and other staff need to be prepared for and willing to implement changes. This means that all staff members need to be adaptable and change needs to become part of the culture of the DMHS.

3.4. Level 4: Lessons Working with Health Systems, Funders, and Policy Makers

This final group of lessons summarises key learnings derived from working with and influencing health systems, in particular, the future role and value of DMHS within health systems.

3.4.1. Lesson 8: Integrating DMHS within Health Systems Is Challenging

Our DMHS reside within enormously complex health systems which might be more accurately described as interconnected nodes of care rather than true *systems*. For example, mental health services, while all purporting to share the aim of improving mental wellbeing, often target different groups and may be accountable to different policy and regulatory frameworks. Health services also differ with respect to funding, and in both Canada and Australia, funding for different types of mental health services can be provided by the federal government, state/provincial government, state mental health commissions, non-governmental organisations and individual consumers. As a result, mental health services are often fragmented, poorly connected, and difficult for consumers to navigate.

The complexity of health systems and their resistance to change created a number of threats to the sustainability and stability of our DMHS, particularly in our early years of service delivery. We were able to overcome such challenges by building strong relationships with key stakeholders and in particular, by publishing outcome data that documented the value of the services. This data has also assisted in defining the role of DMHS in the broader mental healthcare system, including as services which improve access to patients who would otherwise not access mental health services.

These so-called external-facing activities have required considerable time and effort. Participation in such activities has required us to learn the sometimes-subtle rules of engaging with other organisations, to commit to regular participation in networking activities, and to make frequent efforts to build and maintain collaborations. Such activities can be enormously time consuming but we have found that they are an essential component of successfully delivering our DMHS.

3.4.2. Lesson 9: DMHS May Change the Mental Health System

By providing services to large numbers of consumers and because of our routine collection of outcome data, our clinics are having a growing influence on the health system and are increasingly seen as agents or examples of change. In Canada, the experiences and activities of the OTU have influenced the development of e-mental health in several ways [68]. In Australia, data from MindSpot has helped inform long-term government planning and funding strategies for mental health services [69], not only DMHS. The data and outcome driven reports prepared by our services are often in marked contrast to submissions by other groups, which may be based more on opinion rather than on evidence. Hence, an important role of DMHS is to inform policy makers and funders to help improve the broader mental health system by presenting data drawn from a broad cross section of the community and also to nudge traditional services to adopt systems of measurement and reporting of outcomes.

3.4.3. Lesson 10: DMHS Are Not a Panacea

We are struck by how often mental health funders and policy makers, when presented with the evidence from our DMHS, become enthusiastic about their potential without an appreciation of their limits. These limits include the so-called digital divide, that is, the group in society who does not use digital devices, those with very low levels of literacy, and those in crisis, who can benefit from contact with DMHS, but may be better off with a mental health service that includes direct human interaction, as well as those who prefer to see someone face-to-face.

In all our communication, we emphasise that DMHS should complement and not replace existing services. We also emphasise that attention must be paid to systematically evaluating delivery methods that combine the best elements of DMHS with traditional services, including blended care [70–74]. We also stress that consumer knowledge of DMHS is still limited and that even brief education about DMHS can improve consumer perceptions and uptake of services [75]. These observations lead to our final lesson that whilst acknowledging that DMHS can significantly improve access to safe, clinical and cost-effective care, our DMHS are not a panacea.

4. General Discussion

This paper aimed to assist other emerging DMHS by sharing ten lessons we learned from successfully delivering DMHS to very large numbers of consumers. Some of these lessons might seem obvious, but their importance was not always apparent when we started our services. Several key themes are discussed below, followed by recommendations.

One theme is that we expect that demand for this service model will grow. The number of patients treated using ICBT in the OTU has more than doubled in the past four years. The threshold for accessing this model of care is significantly lower than traditional face-to-face services and consumers are becoming increasingly comfortable with using technology to access a broad range of services, including health services. Along with a growth in numbers, we expect that existing DMHS will become more tailored to different populations, for example, people in certain occupations, different cultures, or who have been referred from different pathways, although our experience is that the extent to which the treatment course materials need to be customised is considerably less than expected [56,76–78].

A second theme is that the workforce requires specialised training, clinical supervision and support. This raises broader issues about workforce planning and training programs. We note that many professional bodies have recognised the importance of education and training of mental health professionals and standards in this model of care [79–82] but that few training programs in any mental health discipline offer courses or training opportunities specifically for digital mental health. The absence of such training opportunities poses significant risks for the future sustainability and quality of the field.

A third theme is that the delivery of DMHS requires specialist skills in both clinical and operational domains. We also note that although the costs to entry of developing a DMHS, especially a low volume service, might be relatively low, the costs of maintaining quality services can be high. Inadequate funding and inadequate organisational governance can affect the reputation, credibility, and therefore, the potential of the emerging field of DMHS [83]. Hence, we strongly encourage anyone seeking to launch a DMHS to carefully consider the governance frameworks that will ensure the safe and sustainable delivery of services, or to consider licensing their interventions to groups who have proven success in implementing similar services.

Another theme is that the field of DMHS is rapidly evolving. We encourage those seeking to start a DMHS to consider trialing different models of care to those currently used by existing DMHS, including testing different levels of therapist support [24,40,55] and testing care which combines both face-to-face and online delivery. We note the important work conducted by our European colleagues on blended care [70–74] and by others on mobile services [13] and encourage collaboration in order to collectively develop the most effective models of care.

Our final theme relates to recognising the true value proposition of DMHS. We maintain that they are not a panacea but instead serve several valuable functions, including as a useful complement to existing services, as a way of improving equity of access to mental health care for common psychological disorders, and as a stepping stone to other services. Over-promising may increase the likelihood of short-term funding, but poorly designed and delivered services might harm consumers, disappoint stakeholders and risk the future of DMHS.

4.1. Recommendations

These observations lead to several recommendations which we encourage those contemplating developing DMHS to consider. First, we recommend that new DMHS recruit not only appropriately skilled therapists, but also people with commercial and professional skills, ideally with experience in digital service delivery. Second, given the unique challenges of DMHS, we recommend the development of both thorough initial training of therapists, as well as of systems for ongoing training and supervision. Third, given the likelihood that demand for DMHS will grow, we strongly encourage that organisations involved in training and certification of mental health professionals add content and training opportunities relevant to the competencies required in DMHS.

Fourth, we recommend that emerging DMHS measure and publish their outcomes, including disappointing and negative effects outcomes [84]. We also encourage DMHS to engage with policy makers and funders to develop mental health policy grounded in evidence rather than in opinion. Finally, we strongly encourage DMHS to engage with their consumers in appropriate co-design and evaluation activities to ensure services are not only effective but acceptable to consumers.

4.2. Strengths and Limitations

We believe that the main strength of this paper stems from the authors' shared experience in launching and steadily improving successful high volume DMHS. However, we acknowledge several weaknesses, including that the list of lessons is non-exhaustive and did not include some of the significant challenges associated with managing funding insecurity or bureaucratic and professional challenges within the field of mental health, topics we will return to in a subsequent publication. We also acknowledge that our experiences may not reflect those of other DMHS.

4.3. Conclusions

This paper described ten key lessons learned by the authors when developing, delivering, and evaluating DMHS. Despite the challenges, provided they are delivered safely, effectively and with strong clinical, operational and organisational governance, we remain highly optimistic about the potential of DMHS to reduce the global burden of the high prevalence of mental disorders.

Author Contributions: Conceptualisation, N.T. and B.F.D.; Writing—Original Draft Preparation, N.T., H.D.H., O.N., and B.F.D.; Writing—Review & Editing, N.T., H.D.H., O.N., D.C.M., G.A. and B.F.D.

Acknowledgments: The Online Therapy Unit is funded by Saskatchewan Ministry of Health. Research conducted by the Unit is currently funded by the Canadian Institutes of Health Research (152917), the Saskatchewan Health Research Foundation, and the Saskatchewan Centre for Patient-Oriented Research. The MindSpot Clinic is funded by the Australian Department of Health and supported by MQ Health, Macquarie University. The authors gratefully acknowledge their funders, supporting institutions, the patients for allowing the use of their data, and their clinical, management, and technical teams for their efforts in launching and operating the Clinics. We also acknowledge the achievements and leadership shown by early and current researchers in the field of psychological internet interventions. Their work has strongly influenced the models and outcomes reported here and continue to inspire our attempts at reducing barriers to evidence-based psychological services.

References

1. Kessler, R.C.; Aguilar-Gaxiola, S.; Alonso, J.; Chatterji, S.; Lee, S.; Ormel, J.; Üstün, T.B.; Wang, P.S. The global burden of mental disorders: An update from the WHO World Mental Health (WMH) surveys. *Epidemiol. E Psichiatr. Soc.* **2009**, *18*, 23–33. [CrossRef]
2. Whiteford, H.A.; Degenhardt, L.; Rehm, J.; Baxter, A.J.; Ferrari, A.J.; Erskine, H.E.; Charlson, F.J.; Norman, R.E.; Flaxman, A.D.; Johns, N.; et al. Global burden of disease attributable to mental and substance use disorders: Findings from the Global Burden of Disease Study 2010. *Lancet* **2013**, *382*, 1575–1586. [CrossRef]
3. Urbanoski, K.; Inglis, D.; Veldhuizen, S. Service Use and Unmet Needs for Substance Use and Mental Disorders in Canada. *Can J. Psychiat.* **2017**, *62*, 551–559. [CrossRef] [PubMed]
4. Wang, P.S.; Matthias, A.; Borges, G.; Bruffaerts, R.; Chiu, T.; De Girolamo, W.; Fayyad, G.; John, G.; Ronald, C.; Kovess, V.; et al. Steven Delay and failure in treatment seeking after first onset of mental disorders in the World Health Organization's World Mental Health Survey Initiative. *World Psychiatry.* **2007**, *6*, 177–185. [PubMed]
5. Whiteford, H.A.; Buckingham, W.J.; Harris, M.G.; Burgess, P.M.; Pirkis, J.E.; Barendregt, J.J.; Hall, W.D. Estimating treatment rates for mental disorders in Australia. *Aust. Health Rev.* **2014**, *38*, 80–85. [CrossRef] [PubMed]
6. Mojtabai, R.; Olfson, M.; Sampson, N.A.; Jin, R.; Druss, B.; Wang, P.S.; Wells, K.B.; Pincus, H.A.; Kessler, R.C. Barriers to mental health treatment: Results from the National Comorbidity Survey Replication. *Psychol. Med.* **2011**, *41*, 1751–1761. [CrossRef] [PubMed]
7. Andrews, G.; Cuijpers, P.; Craske, M.G.; McEvoy, P.; Titov, N. Computer therapy for the anxiety and depressive disorders is effective, acceptable and practical health care: A meta-analysis. *PLoS ONE* **2010**, *5*, e13196. [CrossRef]
8. Andersson, G.; Titov, N. Advantages and limitations of Internet-based interventions for common mental disorders. *World Psychiatry Off. J. World Psychiatr. Assoc.* **2014**, *13*, 4–11. [CrossRef]
9. Andersson, G.; Carlbring, P.; Titov, N.; Lindefors, N. Internet Interventions for Adults with Anxiety and Mood Disorders: A Narrative Umbrella Review of Recent Meta-Analyses. *Can. J. Psychiatry* **2019**, *64*, 465–470. [CrossRef]
10. Carlbring, P.; Andersson, G.; Cuijpers, P.; Riper, H.; Hedman-Lagerlöf, E. Internet-based vs. face-to-face cognitive behavior therapy for psychiatric and somatic disorders: An updated systematic review and meta-analysis. *Cogn. Behav. Ther.* **2018**, *47*, 1–18. [CrossRef]
11. Gilbody, S.; Littlewood, E.; Hewitt, C.; Brierley, G.; Tharmanathan, P.; Araya, R.; Barkham, M.; Bower, P.; Cooper, C.; Gask, L.; et al. Computerised cognitive behaviour therapy (cCBT) as treatment for depression in primary care (REEACT trial): Large scale pragmatic randomised controlled trial. *BMJ* **2015**. [CrossRef]
12. Kenter, R.M.F.; Van De Ven, P.M.; Cuijpers, P.; Koole, G.; Niamat, S.; Gerrits, R.S.; Willems, M.; Van Straten, A. Costs and effects of Internet cognitive behavioral treatment blended with face-to-face treatment: Results from a naturalistic study. *Internet Interv.* **2015**, *2*, 77–83. [CrossRef]

13. Mohr, D.C.; Weingardt, K.R.; Reddy, M.; Schueller, S.M. Three Problems with Current Digital Mental Health Research and Three Things We Can Do About Them. *Psychiatr. Serv.* **2017**, *68*, 427–429. [CrossRef]
14. El Alaoui, S.; Hedman, E.; Kaldo, V.; Hesser, H.; Kraepelien, M.; Andersson, E.; Rück, C.; Andersson, G.; Ljótsson, B.; Lindefors, N. Effectiveness of Internet-based cognitive–behavior therapy for social anxiety disorder in clinical psychiatry. *J. Consult. Clin. Psychol.* **2015**, *83*, 902. [CrossRef]
15. Hedman, E.; Ljótsson, B.; Kaldo, V.; Hesser, H.; El Alaoui, S.; Kraepelien, M.; Andersson, E.; Rück, C.; Svanborg, C.; Andersson, G.; et al. Effectiveness of Internet-based cognitive behaviour therapy for depression in routine psychiatric care. *J. Affect. Disord.* **2014**, *155*, 49–58. [CrossRef]
16. Hedman, E.; Ljótsson, B.; Rück, C.; Bergström, J.; Andersson, G.; Kaldo, V.; Jansson, L.; Andersson, E.; Andersson, E.; Blom, K.; et al. Effectiveness of Internet-based cognitive behaviour therapy for panic disorder in routine psychiatric care. *Acta Psychiatri. Scand.* **2013**, *128*, 457–467. [CrossRef]
17. Hedman, E.; Ljótsson, B.; Andersson, E.; Rück, C.; Andersson, G.; Lindefors, N. Effectiveness and cost offset analysis of group CBT for hypochondriasis delivered in a psychiatric setting: An open trial. *Cogn. Behav. Ther.* **2010**, *39*, 239–250. [CrossRef]
18. Ruwaard, J.; Lange, A.; Schrieken, B.; Dolan, C.V.; Emmelkamp, P. The Effectiveness of Online Cognitive Behavioral Treatment in Routine Clinical Practice. *Plos One* **2012**, *7*, e40089. [CrossRef]
19. Ruwaard, J.; Lange, A.; Schrieken, B.; Emmelkamp, P.M. Efficacy and effectiveness of online cognitive behavioral treatment: A decade of interapy research. *Stud. Health Technol. Inform.* **2011**, *167*, 9–14.
20. Folker, A.P.; Mathiasen, K.; Lauridsen, S.M.; Stenderup, E.; Dozeman, E.; Folker, M.P. Implementing internet-delivered cognitive behavior therapy for common mental health disorders: A comparative case study of implementation challenges perceived by therapists and managers in five European internet services. *Internet Interv.* **2018**, *11*, 60–70. [CrossRef]
21. Mathiasen, K.; Riper, H.; Ehlers, L.H.; Valentin, J.B.; Rosenberg, N.K. Internet-based CBT for social phobia and panic disorder in a specialised anxiety clinic in routine care: Results of a pilot randomised controlled trial. *Internet Interv.* **2016**, *4*, 92–98. [CrossRef]
22. Hadjistavropoulos, H.D.; Schneider, L.H.; Hadjistavropoulos, T.; Titov, N.; Dear, B.F. Effectiveness, acceptability and feasibility of an Internet-delivered cognitive behavioral pain management program in a routine online therapy clinic in Canada. *Can. J. Pain* **2018**, *2*, 62–73. [CrossRef]
23. Hadjistavropoulos, H.; Nugent, M.; Dirkse, D.; Pugh, N. Implementation of internet-delivered cognitive behavior therapy within community mental health clinics: A process evaluation using the consolidated framework for implementation research. *BMC Psychiatry* **2017**, *17*, 331. [CrossRef]
24. Hadjistavropoulos, H.; Nugent, M.; Alberts, N.; Staples, L.; Dear, B.; Titov, N. Transdiagnostic Internet-delivered cognitive behaviour therapy in Canada: An open trial comparing results of a specialized online clinic and nonspecialized community clinics. *J. Anxiety Disord.* **2016**, *42*, 19–29. [CrossRef]
25. Hadjistavropoulos, H.D.; Thompson, M.; Ivanov, M.; Drost, C.; Butz, C.J.; Klein, B.; Austin, D.W. Considerations in the Development of a Therapist-Assisted Internet Cognitive Behavior Therapy Service. *Prof. Psycol. Res. Pr.* **2011**, *42*, 463–471. [CrossRef]
26. Newby, J.M.; Mackenzie, A.; Williams, A.D.; McIntyre, K.; Watts, S.; Wong, N.; Andrews, G. Internet cognitive behavioural therapy for mixed anxiety and depression: A randomized controlled trial and evidence of effectiveness in primary care. *Psychol. Med.* **2013**, *43*, 2635–2648. [CrossRef]
27. Williams, A.D.; Andrews, G. The Effectiveness of Internet Cognitive Behavioural Therapy (iCBT) for Depression in Primary Care: A Quality Assurance Study. *PloS One* **2013**, *8*, e57447. [CrossRef]
28. Titov, N.; Dear, B.F.; Staples, L.G.; Bennett-Levy, J.; Klein, B.; Rapee, R.M.; Andersson, G.; Purtell, C.; Bezuidenhout, G.; Nielssen, O.B. The first 30 months of the MindSpot Clinic: Evaluation of a national e-mental health service against project objectives. *Aust. New Zealand J. Psychiatry* **2017**, *51*, 1227–1239. [CrossRef]
29. Titov, N.; Dear, B.F.; Staples, L.G.; Bennett-Levy, J.; Klein, B.; Rapee, R.M.; Shann, C.; Richards, D.; Andersson, G.; Ritterband, L.; et al. MindSpot Clinic: An Accessible, Efficient, and Effective Online Treatment Service for Anxiety and Depression. *Psychiatr. Serv.* **2015**, *66*, 1043–1050. [CrossRef]
30. Nielssen, O.; Dear, B.F.; Staples, L.G.; Dear, R.; Ryan, K.; Purtell, C.; Titov, N. Procedures for risk management and a review of crisis referrals from the MindSpot Clinic, a national service for the remote assessment and treatment of anxiety and depression. *BMC Psychiatry* **2015**, *15*, 304. [CrossRef]

31. Mathiasen, K.; Riper, H.; Andersen, T.E.; Roessler, K.K. Evaluation of Clinical Effect in Routine Secondary Care of Guided Internet Based CBT for Adult Depression and Anxiety: An Observational Study. *JMIR Preprints.* **2018**. [CrossRef]
32. Vis, C.; Mol, M.; Kleiboer, A.; Bührmann, L.; Finch, T.; Smit, J.; Riper, H. Improving Implementation of eMental Health for Mood Disorders in Routine Practice: Systematic Review of Barriers and Facilitating Factors. *JMIR Ment. Health* **2018**, *5*, e20. [CrossRef]
33. Vis, C.; Ruwaard, J.; Finch, T.; Rapley, T.; de Beurs, D.; van Stel, H.; van Lettow, B.; Mol, M.; Kleiboer, A.; Riper, H.; et al. Toward an Objective Assessment of Implementation Processes for Innovations in Health Care: Psychometric Evaluation of the Normalization Measure Development (NoMAD) Questionnaire Among Mental Health Care Professionals. *J. Med. Int. Res.* **2019**, *21*, e12376. [CrossRef]
34. ImpleMentAll: Getting eHealth implementation right. Available online: https://www.implementall.eu/ (accessed on 25 June 2019).
35. Titov, N.; Dear, B.; Nielssen, O.; Staples, L.; Hadjistavropoulos, H.; Nugent, M.; Adlam, K.; Nordgreen, T.; Bruvik, K.H.; Hovland, A.; et al. ICBT in routine care: A descriptive analysis of successful clinics in five countries. *Internet Interv.* **2018**, *13*, 108–115. [CrossRef]
36. Damschroder, L.J.; Aron, D.C.; Keith, R.E.; Kirsh, S.R.; Alexander, J.A.; Lowery, J.C. Fostering implementation of health services research findings into practice: A consolidated framework for advancing implementation science. *Implement. Sci.* **2009**, *4*, 50. [CrossRef]
37. Gaglio, B.; Shoup, J.A.; Glasgow, R.E. The RE-AIM framework: A systematic review of use over time. *Am. J. Public Health* **2013**, *103*, e38–e46. [CrossRef]
38. Staples, L.G.; Dear, B.F.; Johnson, B.; Fogliati, V.; Gandy, M.; Fogliati, R.; Nielssen, O.; Titov, N. Internet-delivered treatment for young adults with anxiety and depression: Evaluation in routine clinical care and comparison with research trial outcomes. *J. Affect. Disord.* **2019**, *256*, 103–109. [CrossRef]
39. Dear, B.F.; Fogliati, V.J.; Fogliati, R.; Johnson, B.; Boyle, O.; Karin, E.; Gandy, M.; Kayrouz, R.; Staples, L.G.; Titov, N. Treating anxiety and depression in young adults: A randomised controlled trial comparing clinician-guided versus self-guided Internet-delivered cognitive behavioural therapy. *Aust. New Zealand J. Psychiatry* **2018**, *52*, 668–679. [CrossRef]
40. Hadjistavropoulos, H.D.; Schneider, L.H.; Edmonds, M.; Karin, E.; Nugent, M.N.; Dirkse, D.; Dear, B.F.; Titov, N. Randomized controlled trial of internet-delivered cognitive behaviour therapy comparing standard weekly versus optional weekly therapist support. *J. Anxiety Disord.* **2017**, *52*, 15–24. [CrossRef]
41. Fogliati, V.J.; Dear, B.F.; Staples, L.G.; Terides, M.D.; Sheehan, J.; Johnston, L.; Kayrouz, R.; Dear, R.; McEvoy, P.M.; Titov, N. Disorder-specific versus transdiagnostic and clinician-guided versus self-guided internet-delivered treatment for panic disorder and comorbid disorders: A randomized controlled trial. *J. Anxiety Disord.* **2016**, *39*, 88–102. [CrossRef]
42. Staples, L.G.; Fogliati, V.J.; Dear, B.F.; Nielssen, O.; Titov, N. Internet-delivered treatment for older adults with anxiety and depression: Implementation of the Wellbeing Plus Course in routine clinical care and comparison with research trial outcomes. *Brit. J. Psychiat. Open* **2016**, *2*, 307–313. [CrossRef]
43. Dear, B.; Staples, L.; Terides, M.; Fogliati, V.; Sheehan, J.; Johnston, L.; Kayrouz, R.; Dear, R.; McEvoy, P.; Titov, N. Transdiagnostic versus disorder-specific and clinician-guided versus self-guided internet-delivered treatment for social anxiety disorder and comorbid disorders: A randomized controlled trial. *J. Anxiety Disord.* **2016**, *42*, 30–44. [CrossRef]
44. Titov, N.; Dear, B.F.; Staples, L.G.; Terides, M.D.; Karin, E.; Sheehan, J.; Johnston, L.; Gandy, M.; Fogliati, V.J.; Wootton, B.M.; et al. Disorder-specific versus transdiagnostic and clinician-guided versus self-guided treatment for major depressive disorder and comorbid anxiety disorders: A randomized controlled trial. *J. Anxiety Disord.* **2015**, *35*, 88–102. [CrossRef]
45. Titov, N.; Fogliati, V.J.; Staples, L.G.; Gandy, M.; Johnston, L.; Wootton, B.; Nielssen, O.; Dear, B.F. Treating anxiety and depression in older adults: randomised controlled trial comparing guided v. self-guided internet-delivered cognitive–behavioural therapy. *Brit. J. Psychiat. Open* **2016**, *2*, 50–58. [CrossRef]
46. Titov, N.; Dear, B.F.; Johnston, L.; McEvoy, P.M.; Wootton, B.; Terides, M.D.; Gandy, M.; Fogliati, V.; Kayrouz, R.; Rapee, R.M. Improving adherence and clinical outcomes in self-guided internet treatment for anxiety and depression: A 12-month follow-up of a randomised controlled trial. *PLoS ONE* **2014**, *9*, e89591. [CrossRef]

47. Titov, N.; Dear, B.F.; Johnston, L.; Lorian, C.; Zou, J.; Wootton, B.; Spence, J.; McEvoy, P.M.; Rapee, R.M. Improving adherence and clinical outcomes in self-guided internet treatment for anxiety and depression: Randomised controlled trial. *PloS One* **2013**, *8*, e62873. [CrossRef]
48. Wootton, B.M.; Dear, B.F.; Johnston, L.; Terides, M.D.; Titov, N. Self-guided internet-delivered cognitive behavior therapy (iCBT) for obsessive–compulsive disorder: 12 month follow-up. *Internet Interv.* **2015**, *2*, 243–247. [CrossRef]
49. Wootton, B.M.; Dear, B.F.; Johnston, L.; Terides, M.D.; Titov, N. Remote treatment of obsessive-compulsive disorder: A randomized controlled trial. *J. Obs. Compuls. Relat. Disord.* **2013**, *2*, 375–384. [CrossRef]
50. Spence, J.; Titov, N.; Johnston, L.; Jones, M.P.; Dear, B.F.; Solley, K. Internet-based trauma-focused cognitive behavioural therapy for PTSD with and without exposure components: A randomised controlled trial. *J. Affect. Disord.* **2014**, *162*, 73–80. [CrossRef]
51. Dear, B.F.; Titov, N.; Perry, K.N.; Johnston, L.; Wootton, B.M.; Terides, M.D.; Rapee, R.M.; Hudson, J.L. The Pain Course: A randomised controlled trial of a clinician-guided Internet-delivered cognitive behaviour therapy program for managing chronic pain and emotional well-being. *Pain* **2013**, *154*, 942–950. [CrossRef]
52. Dear, B.; Staples, L.; Terides, M.; Karin, E.; Zou, J.; Johnston, L.; Gandy, M.; Fogliati, V.; Wootton, B.; McEvoy, P. Transdiagnostic versus disorder-specific and clinician-guided versus self-guided internet-delivered treatment for generalized anxiety disorder and comorbid disorders: A randomized controlled trial. *J. Anxiety Disord.* **2015**, *36*, 63–77. [CrossRef]
53. Hadjistavropoulos, H.D. *Online Therapy Unit Outcome Report 2013-2017*; University of Regina: Regina, SK, Canada, 2018.
54. Hadjistavropoulos, H.D.; Faller, Y.N.; Klatt, A.; Nugent, M.N.; Dear, B.F.; Titov, N. Patient Perspectives on Strengths and Challenges of Therapist-Assisted Internet-Delivered Cognitive Behaviour Therapy: Using the Patient Voice to Improve Care. *Community Ment. Health J.* **2018**, *54*, 944–950. [CrossRef]
55. Hadjistavropoulos, H.D.; Schneider, L.H.; Mehta, S.; Karin, E.; Dear, B.F.; Titov, N. Preference trial of internet-delivered cognitive behaviour therapy comparing standard weekly versus optional weekly therapist support. *J. Anxiety Disord.* **2019**, *63*, 51–60. [CrossRef]
56. Titov, N.; Schofield, C.; Staples, L.; Dear, B.F.; Nielssen, O. A comparison of Indigenous and non-Indigenous users of MindSpot: An Australian digital mental health service. *Australas. Psychiatry* **2018**, *27*, 352–357. [CrossRef]
57. Hadjistavropoulos, H.D.; Thompson, M.J.; Klein, B.; Austin, D.W. Dissemination of Therapist-Assisted Internet Cognitive Behaviour Therapy: Development and Open Pilot Study of a Workshop. *Cog. Behav. Ther.* **2012**, *41*, 230–240. [CrossRef]
58. Hadjistavropoulos, H.D.; Gullickson, K.M.; Schneider, L.H.; Dear, B.F.; Titov, N. Development of the Internet-Delivered Cognitive Behaviour Therapy Undesirable Therapist Behaviours Scale (ICBT-UTBS). *Internet Interv.* **2019**. [CrossRef]
59. Andersson, G.; Cuijpers, P.; Carlbring, P.; Riper, H.; Hedman, E. Guided Internet-based vs. face-to-face cognitive behavior therapy for psychiatric and somatic disorders: A systematic review and meta-analysis. *World Psychiatry* **2014**, *13*, 288–295. [CrossRef]
60. Hadjistavropoulos, H.D.; Pugh, N.E.; Hesser, H.; Andersson, G. Therapeutic Alliance in Internet-Delivered Cognitive Behaviour Therapy for Depression or Generalized Anxiety. *Clin. Psychol. Psychother.* **2016**, *24*, 451–461. [CrossRef]
61. Hadjistavropoulos, H.D.; Schneider, L.H.; Klassen, K.; Dear, B.F.; Titov, N. Development and evaluation of a scale assessing therapist fidelity to guidelines for delivering therapist-assisted Internet-delivered cognitive behaviour therapy. *Cogn. Behav. Ther.* **2018**, *47*, 447–461. [CrossRef]
62. Hatfield, D.R.; Ogles, B.M. The Use of Outcome Measures by Psychologists in Clinical Practice. *Prof. Psychol. Res. Pract.* **2004**, *35*, 485–491. [CrossRef]
63. Boswell, J.F.; Kraus, D.R.; Miller, S.D.; Lambert, M.J. Implementing routine outcome monitoring in clinical practice: Benefits, challenges, and solutions. *Psychother. Res.* **2015**, *25*, 6–19. [CrossRef]
64. Jensen-Doss, A.; Haimes, E.M.B.; Smith, A.M.; Lyon, A.R.; Lewis, C.C.; Stanick, C.F.; Hawley, K.M. Monitoring Treatment Progress and Providing Feedback is Viewed Favorably but Rarely Used in Practice. *Adm. Policy Ment. Health Ment. Health Serv. Res.* **2018**, *45*, 48–61. [CrossRef]
65. Australian Government. *National Standards for Mental Health Services*; Department of Health, Ed.; Australian Government: Canberra, Australian, 2010.

66. Commonwealth of Australia. *Quality Framework for Telephone Counselling and Internet-based Support Services*; Department of Health and Ageing, Australian Government: Canberra, Australian, 2009.
67. Hadjistavropoulos, H.D.; Pugh, N.E.; Hesser, H.; Andersson, G. Predicting Response to Therapist-Assisted Internet-Delivered Cognitive Behavior Therapy for Depression or Anxiety Within an Open Dissemination Trial. *Behav. Ther.* **2016**, *47*, 155–165. [CrossRef]
68. Mental Health Commission of Canada. *E-Mental Health in Canada: Transforming the Mental Health System Using Technology*; Mental Health Commission of Canada: Ottawa, ON, Canada, 2014.
69. National Mental Health Service Planning Framework. Available online: https://nmhspf.org.au/ (accessed on 27 June 2019).
70. Urech, A.; Krieger, T.; Möseneder, L.; Biaggi, A.; Vincent, A.; Poppe, C.; Meyer, B.; Riper, H.; Berger, T. A patient post hoc perspective on advantages and disadvantages of blended cognitive behaviour therapy for depression: A qualitative content analysis. *Psychother. Res.* **2018**, *31*, 1–13. [CrossRef]
71. Mol, M.; Dozeman, E.; Provoost, S.; van Schaik, A.; Riper, H.; Smit, J.H. Behind the Scenes of Online Therapeutic Feedback in Blended Therapy for Depression: Mixed-Methods Observational Study. *J. Med Internet Res.* **2018**, *20*, e174. [CrossRef]
72. Erbe, D.; Eichert, H.C.; Riper, H.; Ebert, D.D. Blending face-to-face and internet-based interventions for the treatment of mental disorders in adults: Systematic review. *J. Med Internet Res.* **2017**, *19*, e306. [CrossRef]
73. Mathiasen, K.; Andersen, T.E.; Riper, H.; Kleiboer, A.A.M.; Roessler, K.K. Blended CBT versus face-to-face CBT: A randomised non-inferiority trial. *BMC Psychiatry* **2016**, *16*, 432. [CrossRef]
74. Kleiboer, A.; Smit, J.; Bosmans, J.; Ruwaard, J.; Andersson, G.; Topooco, N.; Berger, T.; Krieger, T.; Botella, C.; Baños, R.; et al. European COMPARative Effectiveness research on blended Depression treatment versus treatment-as-usual (E-COMPARED): Study protocol for a randomized controlled, non-inferiority trial in eight European countries. *Trials* **2016**, *17*, 387. [CrossRef]
75. Soucy, J.N.; Owens, V.A.M.; Hadjistavropoulos, H.D.; Dirkse, D.A.; Dear, B.F. Educating patients about Internet-delivered cognitive behaviour therapy: Perceptions among treatment seekers and non-treatment seekers before and after viewing an educational video. *Internet Interv.* **2016**, *6*, 57–63. [CrossRef]
76. Choi, I.; Zou, J.; Titov, N.; Dear, B.F.; Li, S.; Johnston, L.; Andrews, G.; Hunt, C. Culturally attuned Internet treatment for depression amongst Chinese Australians: A randomised controlled trial. *J. Affect. Disord.* **2012**, *136*, 459–68. [CrossRef]
77. Kayrouz, R.; Dear, B.F.; Kayrouz, B.; Karin, E.; Gandy, M.; Titov, N. Meta-analysis of the efficacy and acceptability of cognitive-behavioural therapy for Arab adult populations experiencing anxiety, depression or post-traumatic stress disorder. *Cogn. Behav. Ther.* **2018**, *47*, 412–430. [CrossRef]
78. Kayrouz, R.; Dear, B.F.; Karin, E.; Fogliati, V.J.; Titov, N. A pilot study of a clinician-guided internet-delivered cognitive behavioural therapy for anxiety and depression among Arabs in Australia, presented in both English and Arabic languages. *Internet Interv.* **2016**, *5*, 5–11. [CrossRef]
79. American Psychological Association, Guidelines for the Practice of Telepsychology. *Am. Psychol.* **2013**, *68*, 791–800. [CrossRef]
80. Association of Canadian Psychology Regulatory Organizations. *Model Standards for Telepsychology Service Delivery*; ACPRO: Saskatchewan, Canadian, 2011; pp. 1–3.
81. Royal Australian and New Zealand College of Psychiatrists. *Benefits of E-Mental Health Treatments and Interventions*; RANZCP: Melbourne, Australian, 2019.
82. Available online: http://www.emhprac.org.au/e-MentalHealthinPractice (accessed on 26 June 2019).
83. Ruwaard, J.; Kok, R. Wild West eHealth: Time to hold our horses? *Eur. Health Psychol.* **2015**, *17*, 45–49.
84. Rozental, A.; Andersson, G.; Boettcher, J.; Ebert, D.D.; Cuijpers, P.; Knaevelsrud, C.; Ljótsson, B.; Kaldo, V.; Titov, N.; Carlbring, P. Consensus statement on defining and measuring negative effects of Internet interventions. *Internet Interv.* **2014**, *1*, 12–19. [CrossRef]

13

Use of Virtual Reality for the Management of Anxiety and Pain in Dental Treatments

Nansi López-Valverde [1], Jorge Muriel Fernández [1], Antonio López-Valverde [1,*], Luis F. Valero Juan [2], Juan Manuel Ramírez [3], Javier Flores Fraile [1], Julio Herrero Payo [1], Leticia A. Blanco Antona [1], Bruno Macedo de Sousa [4] and Manuel Bravo [5]

1 Department of Surgery, University of Salamanca, Instituto de Investigación Biomédica de Salamanca (IBSAL), 37007 Salamanca, Spain; nlovalher@usal.es (N.L.-V.); murimuriel@gmail.com (J.M.F.); j.flores@usal.es (J.F.F.); jhpayo@usal.es (J.H.P.); lesablantona@gmail.com (L.A.B.A.)
2 Department of Biomedical and Diagnostic Sciences, University of Salamanca, Avda. Alfonso X El Sabio S/N, 37007 Salamanca, Spain; luva@usal.es
3 Department of Morphological Sciences, University of Cordoba, Avenida Menéndez Pidal s/n, 14071 Cordoba, Spain; jmramirez@uco.es
4 Institute for Occlusion and Orofacial Pain Faculty of Medicine, University of Coimbra, Polo I - Edifício Central Rua Larga, 3004-504 Coimbra, Portugal; brunomsousa@usal.es
5 Department of Preventive and Community Dentistry, Facultad de Odontología, Campus de Cartuja s/n, 18071 Granada, Spain; mbravo@ugr.es
* Correspondence: anlopezvalverde@gmail.com

Abstract: Background: Dental treatments often cause pain and anxiety in patients. Virtual reality (VR) is a novel procedure that can provide distraction during dental procedures or prepare patients to receive such type of treatments. This meta-analysis is the first to gather evidence on the effectiveness of VR on the reduction of pain (P) and dental anxiety (DA) in patients undergoing dental treatment, regardless of age. Methods: MEDLINE, CENTRAL, PubMed, EMBASE, Wiley Library and Web of Science were searched for scientific articles in November 2019. The keywords used were: "virtual reality", "distraction systems", "dental anxiety" and "pain". Studies where VR was used for children and adults as a measure against anxiety and pain during dental treatments were included. VR was defined as a three-dimensional environment that provides patients with a sense of immersion, transporting them to appealing and interactive settings. Anxiety and pain results were assessed during dental treatments where VR was used, and in standard care situations. Results: 31 studies were identified, of which 14 met the inclusion criteria. Pain levels were evaluated in four studies ($n = 4$), anxiety levels in three ($n = 3$) and anxiety and pain together in seven ($n = 7$). Our meta-analysis was based on ten studies ($n = 10$). The effect of VR was studied mainly in the pediatric population (for pain SMD = −0.82). In the adult population, only two studies (not significant) were considered. Conclusions: The findings of the meta-analysis show that VR is an effective distraction method to reduce pain and anxiety in patients undergoing a variety of dental treatments; however, further research on VR as a tool to prepare patients for dental treatment is required because of the scarcity of studies in this area.

Keywords: virtual reality; distraction systems; dental anxiety; pain

---

1. Introduction

Pain suppression during dental interventions has been a major accomplishment for humankind. In 1842, William E. Clarke gave ether to a patient for the removal of a tooth; later, in 1844, a dentist named Horace Wells used nitrous oxide as an anesthetic for dental extractions; and in 1846, another dentist, William T. G. Morton, became a pioneer in the use of inhaled ether as an anaesthetic at the Massachusetts General Hospital [1].

Patient anxiety when facing dental procedures is determined by two circumstances: on the one hand, the prior act of anesthetizing, which in itself frequently causes a state of phobia [2] and, on the other hand, the subsequent dental treatment. The number of studies on this pathology has exponentially increased over the last few years, growing from a very low number in the 1940s to the more than 6000 papers that are currently available, according to the U.S. National Library of Medicine (Figure 1).

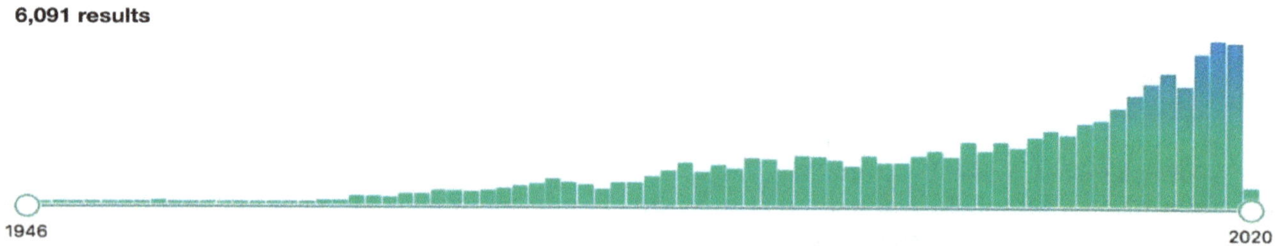

Figure 1. Increasing tendency of publications, according the U.S. National Library of Medicine database, using "dental phobia" as the keyword.

Different therapies have been proposed for the prevention and treatment of P and DA, among them virtual reality (VR) distraction techniques [3].

Although it is a concept that is difficult to define, VR is generally accepted as a three-dimensional environment generated by means of computer technology that creates a sense of immersion in the user, transporting the individual to appealing and interactive settings [4].

The benefits of using VR for the reduction of dental anxiety (DA) and pain (P) levels during dental procedures has been extensively addressed in scientific literature [5–9], and its usefulness as a distraction tool is receiving increasing attention in medical contexts [9]. During aversive experiences, VR can improve pain management [10] and reduce the perceived duration of the procedure [11]. Moreover, a recent systematic review examined the effectiveness of virtual reality distraction in reducing pain [12]. This could be an advantage for many patients who reject DA control using anti-anxiety drugs because of their disadvantages or side effects, which can be, among others, impaired cognitive function and coordination, since they act as depressants on specific areas of the central nervous system [13–15].

The purpose of this study was to conduct a systematic review of literature comparing the effectiveness of the use of VR as a method for reducing anxiety and pain levels during dental treatment. This systematic review constitutes an essential tool to synthesize the scientific information available, increasing the validity of the conclusions and of individual studies, and identifying areas of uncertainty, where research is necessary. Meta-analysis (when possible) provides very useful information, to facilitate understanding of the effect of a treatment or intervention, both in general and in specific groups of patients. In addition, it allows us to increase the precision in the estimation of the effect, detecting effects of moderate magnitude, but of clinical importance, that could go unnoticed in primary studies.

2. Methods

The study selection process was carried out according to the Preferred Reporting Items for Systematic Review and Meta-Analyses (PRISMA) guidelines for systematic reviews and meta-analysis [16].

2.1. Protocol

The search strategy was conducted using the population, intervention, comparison and outcome (PICO) framework, based on the following question:

"Are distraction techniques using VR effective against the anxiety and pain caused by dental procedures?"

To answer this question, a population of patients undergoing dental treatment, with no age limit, were selected. The intervention consisted in using audio–visual or VR distraction methods. Controls were patients who were not subjected to audio–visual or VR distraction methods. The results revised in the literature were the DA or P values obtained using different validated scales:

- For pain: Visual Analogic Scale (VAS), Wong–Baker Faces Scale (W–BFS) and Faces Pain Scale-Revise (FPS-R).
- For anxiety: Consolability Scale (FLACC), Verbal Rating Scale (VRS), Modified Dental Anxiety Scale (MDAS), (Norman Corah's anxiety questionnaire (NCAQ) and Venham's Clinical Anxiety Rating Scale (VCARS).

2.2. *Search Method for the Identification of Studies*

A search of the MEDLINE, CENTRAL, PubMed, EMBASE, Wiley Library and Web of Science electronic databases was conducted in November 2019 to identify relevant scientific articles. The search terms used were: "virtual reality", "distraction systems", "dental anxiety", "pain".

2.3. *Inclusion and Exclusion Criteria*

Inclusion criteria:

(a) Articles published in English.
(b) Randomized controlled clinical trials related to dental anxiety and pain associated with dental procedures in children and adults.
(c) Studies assessing anxiety in said procedures.

Exclusion criteria:

(a) Non-randomized studies or non-controlled clinical trials.
(b) Comparative studies.
(c) Narrative reviews and systematic reviews.
(d) Case studies.
(e) Irrelevant and duplicate studies and those that did not meet the established inclusion criteria.

2.4. *Data Extraction and Analysis*

Studies that made no reference to the research question were removed, and the titles and abstracts of the articles selected were obtained and entered in an Excel spreadsheet. Two reviewers (NL-V and JMF) selected the titles and abstracts independently. Discrepancies in terms of study inclusion were discussed between the two mentioned reviewers until consensus was reached. Subsequently, the full texts of the selected studies were obtained for their review and inclusion.

2.5. *Risk of Bias (RoB) of Included Articles*

The Cochrane Collaboration, London, UK, tool was used to assess the methodology of the scientific evidence in all the selected studies [17].

2.6. *Quality of the Reports of the Included Studies*

This was assessed according to the modified Strengthening the Reporting of Observational studies in Epidemiology (STROBE) statement [18], which includes a total of 22 items. Each item was assessed by reviewers NL-V and JMF, who attributed scores of 0 (not reported) or 1 (reported), carrying out a complete count of all the studies included (Table 1).

Table 1. Checklist of Reporting of Observational studies in Epidemiology (STROBE) criteria reported by the included studies. Each item was judged as "0" (not reported) or "1" (reported). The total score of each of included studies was also recorded.

Authors	Asl Aminabadi et al. [22]	Tanja-Dijkstra et al. [9]	Nunna et al. [23]	Gujjar et al. [6]	Niharika et al. [24]	Al-Halabi et al. [20]	Raghav et al. [7]	Tanja-Dijkstra et al. [19]	Shetty et al. [25]	Al-Khotani et al. [26]	Mitrakul et al. [27]	Asvanund et al. [28]	Bentsen et al. [21]	Sweta et al. [2]
Section and item														
1. Title and Abstract	1	1	1	1	1	1	1	1	1	1	1	1	1	1
Introduction														
2. Background	1	1	1	1	1	1	1	1	1	1	1	1	1	1
3. Objectives	1	1	1	1	1	1	1	1	1	1	1	1	1	1
Methods														
4. Study design	1	1	1	1	1	1	1	1	1	1	1	1	1	1
5. Setting	1	1	1	1	1	1	1	0	1	1	1	1	1	1
6. Participants	1	1	1	1	1	1	1	1	1	1	1	1	1	1
7. Variables	1	1	1	1	1	1	1	1	1	1	1	1	1	1
8. Data sources/ Measurement	1	1	1	1	1	1	1	1	1	1	1	1	1	1
9. Bias	1	0	0	0	0	1	0	0	0	1	1	0	1	0
10. Study Size	1	1	1	1	1	1	1	1	1	1	1	1	1	1
11.Quantitative variables	1	1	1	1	1	1	1	1	1	1	1	1	1	1
12. Statistical Methods	1	1	1	1	1	1	1	1	1	1	1	1	1	1
Results														
13. Participants	1	1	1	1	1	1	1	1	1	1	1	1	1	1
14. Descriptive data	1	1	1	1	1	1	1	1	1	1	1	1	1	1
15. Outcome data	1	1	1	1	1	1	1	1	1	1	1	1	1	1
16. Main results	1	1	1	1	1	1	1	1	1	1	1	1	1	1
17. Other analyses	0	0	1	1	1	1	1	0	1	0	1	1	0	1
Discussion														
18. Key results	1	1	1	1	1	1	1	1	1	1	1	1	1	1
19. Limitations	1	0	0	0	0	1	0	0	0	1	1	0	1	0
20. Interpretation	1	1	1	1	1	1	1	1	1	1	1	1	1	1
21. Generalisability	1	1	1	1	1	1	1	1	1	1	1	1	1	1
Other information														
22. Funding	1	1	1	1	1	1	1	1	1	1	1	1	1	1
Total score	21	19	20	20	20	22	20	18	20	21	22	20	21	20

Mode Value: 27.4 (± 0.85).

2.7. Statistical Analysis

In the meta-analysis, four studies were excluded on the grounds that two of them [7,19] did not present results and the other two [20,21] presented confusing results at the time of their assessment. Physiological data, such as pulse rate, degree of oxygen saturation, blood pressure and more were not included, incorporating data related to pain and anxiety only, during dental treatments. Pain and anxiety were analyzed separately in children and adults. The mean scores and SDs (standard deviations) for pain and anxiety, during the procedure with VR and control, were extracted from the selected articles, using mean scores and interquartile ranges, or reported, directly, by the authors of the studies. Other information not related to VR was not taken into consideration in our meta-analysis. The different measurement scales and VR devices used were not considered. The meta-analysis was performed using Stata v.14.2 (StataCorp LP, College Station, TX, USA) and closely followed the methods proposed by the Cochrane collaboration [17]. The methods can be observed in the different tables and figures. The standardized difference of means (SMD) was used as a measure of effect to account for different measurement scales both for anxiety and pain. Statistical heterogeneity among studies was assessed using the Q test according to Dersimonian and Laird and the I2 index (heterogeneity: I2 > 30% being moderate, >50% substantial and >75% considerable [17]). We decided to pool the study-specific estimates with the random effects model to protect our composite estimates (for anxiety and pain) from heterogeneity in the context of a relatively limited number of studies. We also decided a priori to present the results not only for all the studies together, but also as a subgroup analysis according to age group (children and adults) derived from the different clinical usefulness and interpretation. Finally, funnel graphs (not shown) and p-value calculation (Egger test) were used to assess the publication bias.

3. Results

3.1. Characteristics of the Studies

Until November 2019, a total of 31 studies were gathered and subsequently assessed by the reviewers. Three duplicate studies were removed after an initial detection. A second detection led to the removal of 14 studies, which left a total of 14 full-text studies for the final selection [2,6,7,9,19–28] (Figure 2). Pain levels were assessed in four studies, two in children [20,28] and two in adults [2,21]; anxiety levels in three, two in adults [9,19] and one in children [26]; and anxiety and pain together in seven studies, five in children [22–25,27] and two in adults [6,7].

Table 2 provides a general description of the details of each study. The risk of bias (RoB Cochrane Collaboration Tool) in the studies considered is shown in Figure 3. All the studies complied with random sequence. Two of the studies included [25,28] did not comply with allocation concealment and only 35% complied with blinding of participants and personnel. It should be noted that none of the studies included complied with blinding of outcome assessment.

Table 2. Details of each study.

Study (Year)	Journal	Children Values (Ma, n, Ar)	Adult Values (Ma, n, Ar)	Dental Procedure	VR Device Equipment	Measuring Scales		Outcomes
						DA	P	
Asl Aminabadi et al. 2012 [22]	J Dent Res Dent Clin Dent Prospect	Ma = 5.4 n = 120 Ar = 4–6		Restorative treatment in primary molars.	I-glasses 920HR Ilixco, Inc. Menlo Park, CA, USA.	MDAS	W-BFS	There was a significant decrease in pain perception and anxiety scores with the use of VR eyeglasses during dental treatment.
Tanja-Dijkstra et al 2014 [9]	Plos One J		Ma = 33.1 n = 69 Ar = Nr	A simulated dental treatment.	Eyeglasses EVuzix iWear VR920 headset. Dual-core, 1.3GHz Intel processor with Nvidia GT 540 M graphics card.	MDAS		Participants with higher dental anxiety showed more interested in using VR during real dental treatment than those with lower levels of dental anxiety. Dental patients who have a positive dental treatment experience thanks to VR, might have fewer unpleasant memories and thus be less likely to postpone a future dental visit.
Nunna et al 2019 [23]	J Dent Anesth Pain Med	Ma = Nr n = 70 Ar = 7–11		- Counter-stimulation. - Local anaesthesia administration with virtual reality distraction.	Lenovo smartphone, Sennheiser earphones, and ANTVR glasses.	VCARS	W-BFS	Assessment of mean anxiety scores showed a significant difference in girls belonging to the VR group.
Gujjar et al. 2019 [6]	Journal of Anxiety Disorders		Ma = group 1, 25.3 group 2, 23 n = 30 Ar = Nr	Routine dental treatment.	Eyeglasses. Dell XPS-8700 desktop with 4th Generation Intel Core i7-4790 processor (8M Cache, up to 4.0 GHz) and ASUS NVIDIA GEFORCE GTX 750 TI OC 2GB GDDR5 graphic card.	MDAS	VAS	The results of this study provide evidence to support the efficacy of VR in the treatment of dental phobia. Study limitations: - No blinding of patients or therapist in the interventions. - VR compared with pamphlet information.
Niharika et al. 2018 [24]	J Indian Soc Pedod Prev Dent	Ma = Group A (7.17 ± 0.316) Group B (7.28 ± 0.300) n = 40 Ar = 4–8		Routine dental care (pulp therapy in mandibular primary molars). Local anaesthetic.	Google VR Box and Anti-Tank Virtual Reality 3D Glasses	MDAS	W-BFS	Two groups. Childhood Anxiety-Related Disorders scores did not differ significantly between the two groups. In both groups, a statistically significant difference was detected between the two treatment sessions (with and without VR).
Al-Halabi et al. 2018 [20]	Anaesth Pain & Intensive Care	Ma = 7.4 n = 102 Ar = 7–10		Local anaesthesia in mandibular arch (inferior alveolar nerve block).	Eyeglasses (BlackBug™ Virtual Reality Glasses 3D VR Box Headsets, China)		W-BFS	Three groups. There was no significant difference in the anxiety of groups. There was a statistically significant difference in the anxiety and pain level in pulse rate. Limitations: - No blinding of the external investigator. - The size of the VR Box was a little too big.
Raghav et al. 2016 [7]	BMC Oral Health J		Ma = Nr n = 30 Ar = 19–45	1. Restorative dental procedure which may or may not be requiring local anaesthesia. 2. Extraction procedure requiring local anaesthesia.	Oculus development kit 2HMD, with a resolution of 960 × 1080 per eye and with a 100 degree field of view.	MDAS	VAS	Two groups, VR (Idle, Mirror, Syringe, Soundless Drill, Drill with Sound, 35- second exposures) and informational pamphlet control groups. Efficacy of VR in the treatment of dental phobia in the setting of the dental procedure. A limitation of the present study is the absence of in vivo exposure therapy as gold standard control group.

Table 2. *Cont.*

Study (Year)	Journal	Children Values (Ma, *n*, Ar)	Adult Values (Ma, *n*, Ar)	Dental Procedure	VR Device Equipment	Measuring Scales DA	P	Outcomes
Tanja-Dijkstra et al. 2014 [19]	Trials J		Ma = Nr *n* = 90 Ar = Nr	Dental treatment	Eyeglasses. A Sony personal 3D viewer, connected to an Alienware gaming laptop. Participants can walk around in the virtual environment by using a Zeemote JS1 thumb stick controller.	MDAS		This study compared two types of VR, natural environment and urban environment. It included both referred patients and inhouse patients from a dental clinic and two separate procedures are described, one for each type of patient.
Shetty et al. 2019 [25]	The Journal of Clinical Paediatric Dentistry	Ma = Nr *n* = 120 Ar = 5–8		Dental treatment (vital pulp therapy)	Eyeglasses. VR device (i-glasses 920HR, Ilixco Inc., Menlo Park, CA, USA)	MDAS	W-BFS	Two groups. The group with VR distraction, reported a decrease in the severity of anxiety. Lower pain scores were observed in the VR group.
Al-Khotani et al. 2016 [26]	Acta Odontologica Scandinavica	Ma = 8.2 *n* = 56 Ar = 7–9		Dental examination, oral hygiene information, prophylaxis, restorative treatment.	Eyeglasses. DVD Players, gaming systems like Sony Play Station Pro, Microsoft X-BOX, Nintendo WII	MDAS		Two groups. VR and control group. Significant reduction in anxiety throughout the restorative procedure (including injection with local anaesthesia) in VR group.
Mitrakul et al. 2015 [27]	European Journal of Paediatric Dentistry	Ma = 6.9 ± 0.9 *n* = 42 Ar = 5–8		Restorative dental treatment in maxilla or mandible under local anaesthetic Injection.	Eyeglasses. (Shenzhen Longway Vision Technology Co. Ltd, Shenzhen, China).	FPS-R	FLACC	Two groups. Group 1 received treatment without wearing VR in the first visit and wearing VR in a second visit. In Group 2, VR was used vice versa.
Asvanund et al. 2015 [28]	Quintessence International	Ma= 7 ± 0.8 *n* = 49 Ar = 5–8		Restorative dental treatment (local anaesthetic injection in the maxillary arch or mandibular block).	Eyeglasses (Shenzhen Longway Vision Technology Co. Ltd, Shenzhen, China).	FPS-R	FLACC	Two groups. The study assesses pain and anxiety without making a distinction. The limitation of this study is that the FLACC score was assessed by playing back the video recording of each visit, which was done by two paediatric dentists who could not be blinded to the child's use of VR.
Bentsen et al. 2001 [21]	Eur J of Pain-London		Ma = Nr *n* = 23 Ar = 20–49	Dental treatment	Video glasses (NV-HD 660 PanasonicTM)		VAS	The study was a split-mouth, randomized design (2 dental filling). Dental treatments were performed without anaesthesia. 74% of patients would prefer VR if they were to receive a second dental filling.
Sweta et al. 2019 [2]	Ann Maxillofac Surgery		Ma = 39.72 ± 15.93. *n* = 50 Ar = Nr	Local anaesthesia in patients undergoing a dental procedure.	Nr	NCAQ		Local anaesthesia and extractions reported the highest anxiety levels among the patients. Limitations of this study: - Small sample size. - Patients were not in control of their VR environment.

n (Participant number); Ma (Mean age years); Ar (Age range years); Nr (Not reported); VAS (Visual Analogic Scale); W–BFS (Wong–Baker Faces Scale); FPS-R (Faces Pain Scale-Revised); FLACC (Consolability Scale); VRS (Verbal Rating Scale); MDAS (Modified Dental Anxiety Scale); NCAQ (Norman Corah's anxiety questionnaire); VCARS (Venham's Clinical Anxiety Rating Scale). DA (Dental Anxiety); P (Pain).

FLOWCHART

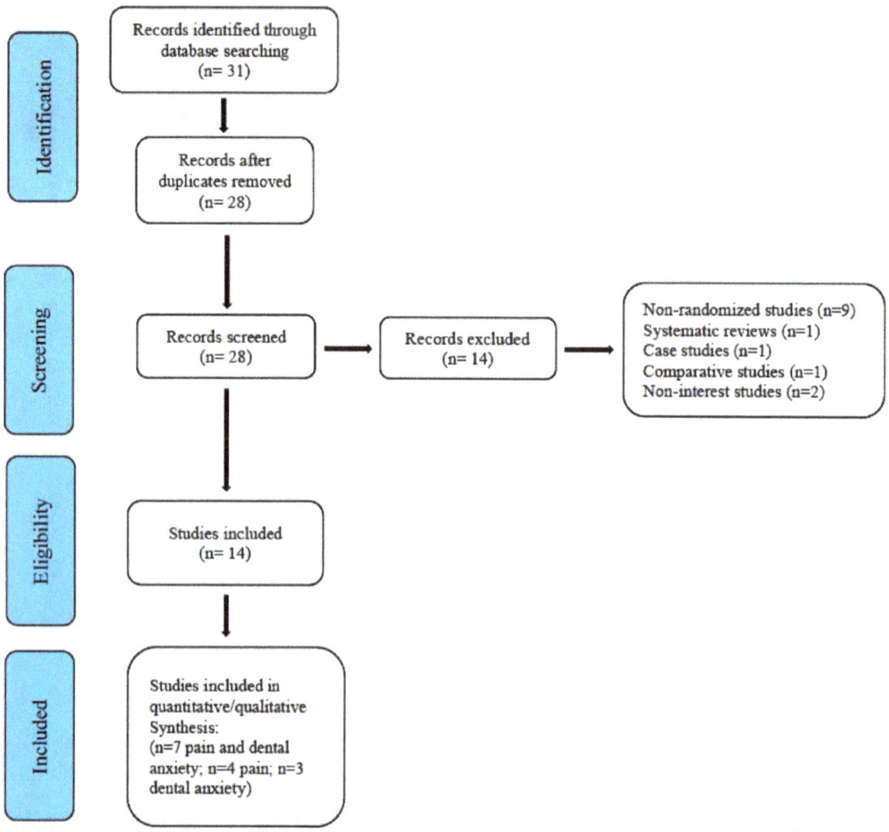

Figure 2. Flow chart of the study selection process. PRISMA (Preferred Reporting Items for Systematic Review and meta Analyses) [16].

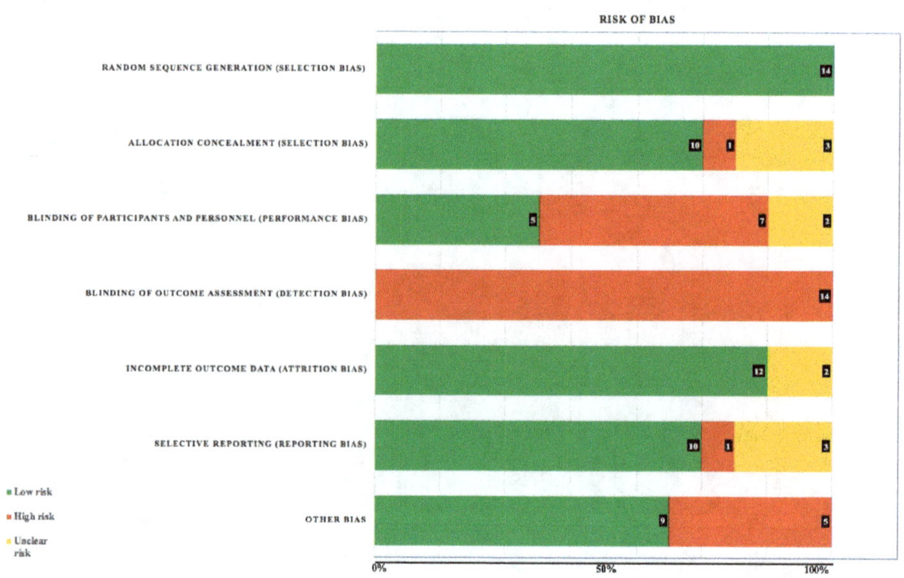

Figure 3. Risk of bias.

The STROBE criteria reported an average score of 27.4 (± 0.85), the maximum scores corresponding to the studies by Al-Halabi et al. [20] and Mitrakul et al. [27]. It is also noteworthy that Item 9 (Bias) was only reported in five studies [21,22,24,26,27], which is also the case with Item 19 (Limitations) [20–22,26,27] (Table 1).

3.2. *VR and Anxiety Management*

Regarding anxiety, the composite measure is not significant, neither for all together (children + adults) (p = 0.302), nor for children (p = 0.243) (Figure 4) nor adults (p = 0.567) (Figure 5). The heterogeneity seems to be moderate (Table 3).

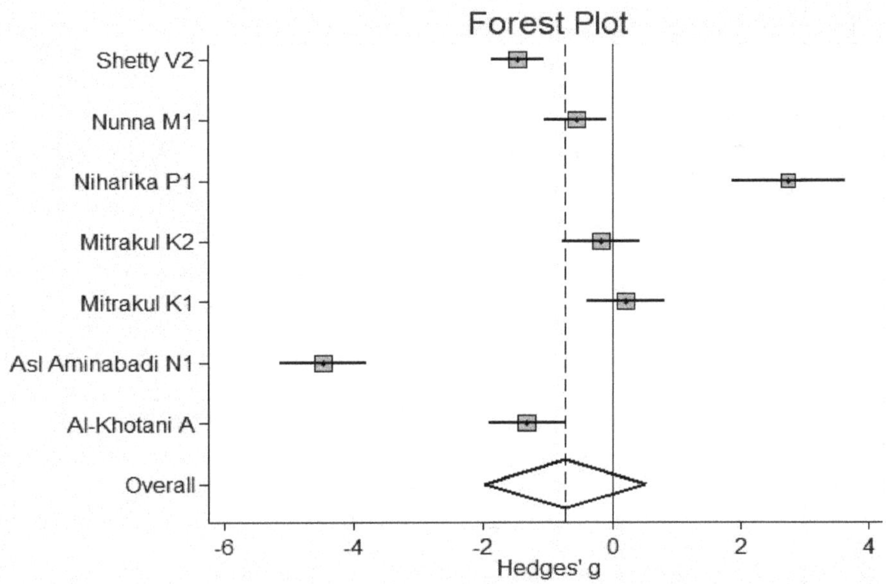

Figure 4. Forest plot for anxiety in Children.

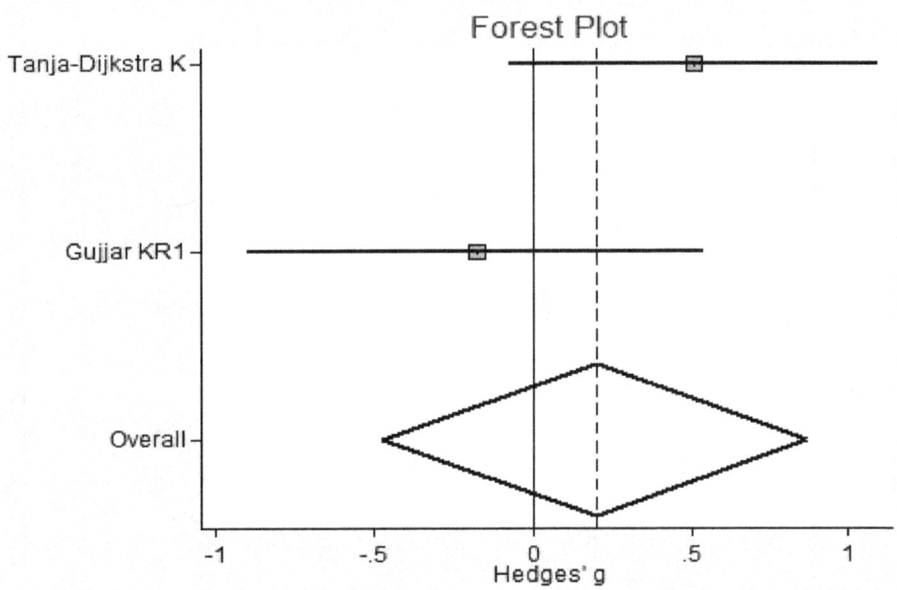

Figure 5. Forest plot for Anxiety in Adults.

Table 3. Meta-analysis of anxiety. Characteristics of individual studies and meta-analysis. a: Standardized difference of means.

Age group/Study	Year	Scale	Test		Control			SMD[a]			Heterogeneity I^2 (p-Value)	Public.bias p-Value (Egger Test)
			n	Mean ± sd	n	Mean ± sd	Weight	Mean	95%-CI	p-Value		
Children + Adults (n = 9)			282		284			−0.54	−1.58 to 0.49	0.302	31% (p = 0.169)	p = 0.399
Children (n = 7) (see Figure 5)												
Shetty V2 [25]	2019	MDAS	60	11.3 ± 3.5	60	16.5 ± 3.5	14.6%	−1.48	−1.88 to −1.07			
Nunna M1 [23]	2019	VCARS	35	0.57 ± 0.61	35	1.00 ± 0.84	14.5%	−0.58	−1.06 to −0.10			
Niharika P1 [24]	2018	MDAS	20	19.6 ± 0.9	20	17.3 ± 0.8	13.8%	2.74	1.86 to 3.63			
Mitrakul K2 [27]	2015	FLACC	21	26.0 ± 9.1	21	28.0 ± 12.0	14.3%	−0.18	−0.79 to 0.43			
Mitrakul K1 [27]	2015	FLACC	21	29.5 ± 11.3	21	27.3 ± 10.6	14.3%	0.20	−0.41 to 0.80			
Asl Aminabadi N1 [22]	2012	MDAS	60	12.6 ± 1.0	60	17.7 ± 1.2	14.2%	−4.46	−5.14 to −3.78			
Al-Khotani A [26]	2016	MDAS	28	0.14 ± 0.36	28	0.75 ± 0.52	14.3%	−1.34	−1.93 to −0.76			
Total			245		245		100%	−0.74	−1.99 to 0.51	0.243	38% (p = 0.139)	p = 0.536
Adults (n = 2) (see Figure 6)												
Tanja-Dijkstra K [9]	2014	MDAS	22	3.73 ± 0.65	24	3.33 ± 0.87	54.6%	0.51	−0.08 to 1.10			
Gujjar KR1 [6]	2019	MDAS	15	18.3 ± 2.6	15	18.8 ± 2.8	45.4%	−0.18	−0.90 to 0.54			
Total			37		39			0.20	−0.48 to 0.87	0.567	0% (p = 0.317)	-

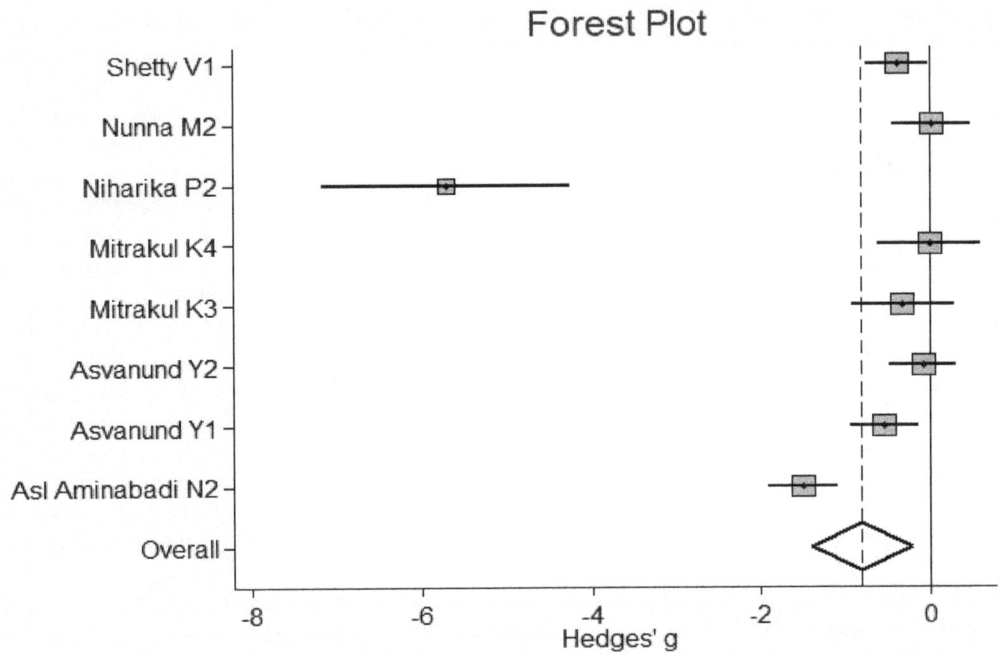

Figure 6. Forest plot for pain in Children.

3.3. *VR and Pain Management*

For pain, there is a significant protection for children (SMD = −0.82, i.e., a substantial effect according to Cohen's scale [29]) (Figure 6), but not for adults (Figure 7), since the 95%-confidence interval (CI) includes the null value 0 (Table 4). Nevertherless, it is based only on two studies.

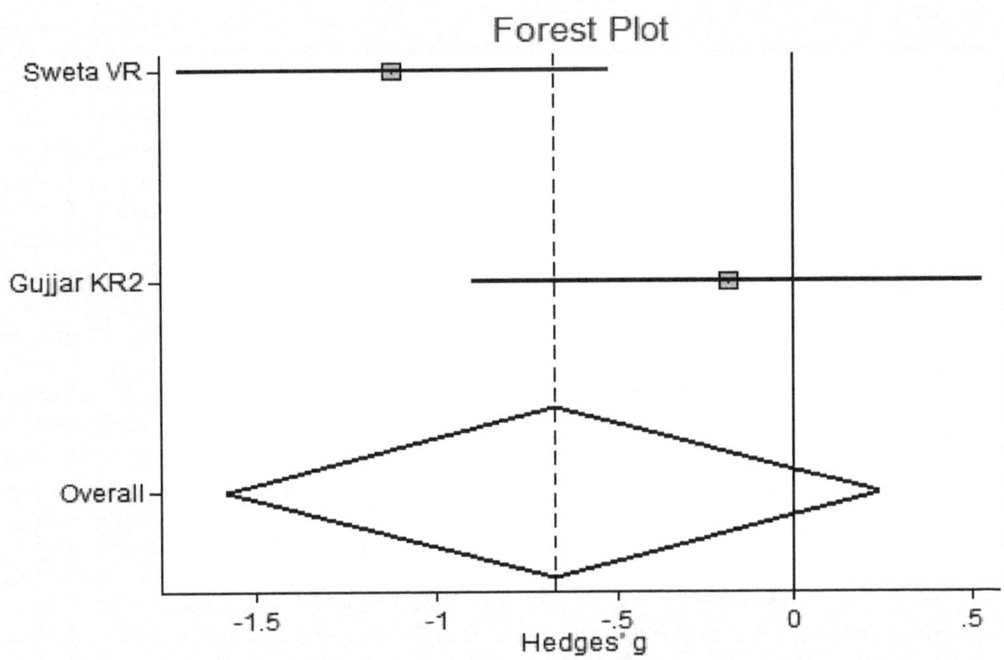

Figure 7. Forest plot for Pain in Adults.

Table 4. Meta-analysis of pain according to random effect models. Characteristics of individual studies and meta-analysis. a: Standardized difference of means.

Age group/Study	Year	Scale	Test		Control			SMD[a]			Heterogeneity I^2 (*p*-Value)	Public.bias *p*-Value (Egger Test)
			n	Mean ± sd	n	Mean ± sd	Weight	Mean	95%-CI	*p*-Value		
Children + Adults (n = 10)			355		355			−0.77	−1.28 to −0.26	0.003	65.8% (0.002)	0.173
Children (n = 8) (see Figure 7)												
Shetty V1 [25]	2019	W-BFS	60	2.00 ± 0.50	60	2.42 ± 1.47	13.6%	−0.38	−0.74 to −0.0			
Nunna M2 [23]	2019	W-BFS	35	3.03 ± 2.22	35	2.97 ± 2.49	13.2%	0.03	−0.44 to 0.49			
Niharika P2 [24]	2018	W-BFS	20	2.56 ± 0.39	20	5.22 ± 0.51	7.8%	−5.71	−7.16 to −4.25			
Mitrakul K4 [27]	2015	FPS-R	21	1.90 ± 2.93	21	1.90 ± 3.32	12.5%	0.00	−0.60 to 0.60			
Mitrakul K3 [27]	2015	FPS-R	21	0.86 ± 1.49	21	1.62 ± 2.94	12.5%	−0.32	−0.93 to 0.29			
Asvanund Y2 [28]	2015	FPS-R	49	2.23 ± 2.29	49	2.46 ± 3.46	13.5%	−0.08	−0.47 to 0.32			
Asvanund Y1 [28]	2015	FPS-R	49	1.57 ± 2.29	49	3.04 ± 3.08	13.5%	−0.54	−0.94 to −0.13			
Asl Aminabadi N2 [22]	2012	W-BFS	60	1.89 ± 0.65	60	3.00 ± 0.81	13.4%	−1.50	−1.91 to −1.10			
Total			315		315		100%	−0.82	−1.42 to −0.22	0.008	71% (p = 0.001)	p = 0.180
Adults (n = 2) (see Figure 7)												
Sweta VR [2]	2019	VAS	25	1.28 ± 0.89	25	2.60 ± 1.38	52.3%	−1.12	−1.72 to −0.52			
Gujjar KR2 [6]	2019	VAS	15	68 ± 10	15	70 ± 14	47.7%	−0.18	−0.90 to 0.53			
Total			40		40			−0.67	−1.58 to 0.24	0.149	0% (p = 0.317)	-

3.4. Publication Bias and Heterogeneity

All estimates seem not to be affected by publication bias, according to the Egger test (Tables 1 and 2), but heterogeneity seems to be substantial.

4. Discussion

While anxiety and pain are usually associated with dental treatments, the number of studies addressing their management, especially during anesthetic block, which is one of the procedures that usually causes great anxiety among patients, is very limited [2,30].

Although most studies are based on pediatric population, fear of dental treatment affects 15%–20% of the population, being recognized by the World Health Organization (WHO) as a real pathology [3,31,32] that leads those who are affected by it to reject even the most basic dental treatments, such as simple dental check-ups or cleanings [33]; thus, its management is essential to improve the patient's quality of life [34].

Despite the existence of rigorous reviews of literature [5], we believe that this is the first systematic review and meta-analysis focused on the efficacy of VR in patients, regardless of age, who suffer from anxiety triggered by dental treatments.

Our meta-analysis is based on 10 studies: two on pain, two on DA and six on DA and P together, and has proved that VR is an effective tool for reducing pain (SMD = −0.82), as reported by child patients during a variety of dental procedures.

Some studies proved that, both for pain and anxiety, the use of VR was more effective in children than in adults. A possible reason for this could be that VR is especially appealing to children, since they become more engaged in whimsical thinking and are fascinated by imaginative play [35].

Nevertheless, regarding age, it should be noted that the differences in the efficacy of VR, in each study, could be due to the interpretive problems to which these analyses are susceptible; such phenomenon, known as ecological fallacies, could be associated either to the heterogeneity of the study's characteristics (methodological diversity), or to the study populations (clinical diversity) [36].

VR was found to be more effective for treating P and DA than conventional treatments; however, it is difficult to assess its efficacy as compared to other types of distraction. Klassen and colleagues [37] conducted a meta-analysis on distraction using music therapy as an alternative method to reduce anxiety and pain in different medical and dental procedures, finding a significant reduction, with an effect size of 0.35. A Cochrane review of psychological interventions using different types of distraction to relieve pain in children and adolescents, published in 2006 and updated in 2013 and 2018 [38–40], reported different distraction techniques such as musical therapy, reading, watching films, hypnosis, breathing techniques and combined cognitive-behavioral strategies, as effective tools to reduce pain and anxiety during needle procedures. However, the reviewers considered the level of certainty of the review to be low, since in most of these studies there was no blinding of participants and assessors. This is consistent with our meta-analysis, according to which only 35% of the studies included met this requirement.

The heterogeneity of VR software and hardware is also relevant to the immersive approach, which is influenced by the interaction with the virtual environment, either through translation or change of position, rotation or change of direction, viewpoint or perspective and visual field. This aspect is difficult to analyze when referred to patients who are undergoing dental treatment (especially in children), since adequate patient immersion is hindered by the fact that they are expected to remain with their heads as still as possible to facilitate the professional's work [41].

Large devices (hardware), also hinder the dentist's work, limiting vision of and access to the dental operation area [42].

Another interesting aspect that has not been given due regard by researchers is gender difference and its significance in terms of fear of dental treatment. Patients who suffer from dental phobia are characterized by a gender-specific brain structure. Such differences have not been sufficiently addressed by researchers and clinicians, and could contribute to greater effectiveness in the management of dental phobia [43].

Likewise, patients' different personality traits were not considered in the studies included, either. Patients with dental fear and a high predisposition to anxiety magnify their pain expectations when they are exposed to critical situations. When patients with dental anxiety undergo dental treatment, their beliefs about the negative consequences of bodily excitement can negatively influence their assessment of pain linked to such treatment [44]. DA as a predisposing factor is associated with a state of anxiety, which has a constant impact on pain during the patient's entire dental treatment; hence, anxiety should be assessed as a critical step not only towards anxiety management in patients with high DA, but also towards P management in all dental patients [45].

On the other hand, the studies included used different pain and DA assessment scales: VAS, W-BFS, FPS-R FLACC, VRS, MDAS, NCAQ and VCARS. Likewise, none of the studies included single scales for joint assessment by dentist and patient. Vital signs as emotional state indicators were also assessed in some of the studies, thus it would be convenient and appropriate to find validated scales that might be used to adequately assess all of these aspects [46].

Eijlers and colleagues [5,47] presented two preparatory studies for pediatric surgery based on VR training programs; however, the use of this type of preparatory program before certain dental procedures is yet to be explored by researchers and, therefore, it is currently not possible to compare effects with and without preparation.

Moreover, none of the studies drew attention to factors that could moderate VR's effectiveness, such as a subject's sensitivity to anxiety or their temperament. Shy and emotional temperaments could be associated with dental anxiety [48–51].

For all these reasons, we believe that this systematic review has certain limitations in terms of number, quality and methodology of the studies included: only three studies in adults were included [2,6,9], which is too scarce to consider them significant in our analysis, the authors themselves even acknowledge the limited sample size in one of them [2], and the existence of major limitations with regard to participant and assessor blinding, in another [6].

Hence, to determine the effects of VR on anxiety and pain in dental treatments, it would be necessary to reduce the risk of bias, to remove confusion factors and to establish a clear definition of the adequate parameters, all with the purpose of obtaining results that can be translated into broad clinical applications, so that the evidence can effectively support the practice of clinical dentistry.

5. Conclusions

This systematic review and meta-analysis leads to the conclusion that VR is a useful tool to reduce P in children undergoing dental treatment. No significant effect was found for DA. Studies in adults are scarce. On the other hand, most of the studies chose to focus on immersion in the pediatric population, neglecting a series of aspects that should be considered, such as training programs, the different types of software and hardware of virtual reality devices, the temperament and patient personality, gender difference and more. Due to all this, the role of virtual reality in the control of anxiety and dental pain in children and adults should be considered as a topic for future research.

Author Contributions: Study concept and design: N.L.-V., A.L.-V., J.M.F.; Acquisition of data (Literature search and Study Selection): N.L.-V., J.F.F., J.M.R.; Analysis and interpretation of data (literature): M.B., L.F.V.J., J.H.P., L.A.B.A.; Drafting of the manuscript: N.L.-V.; A.L.-V., B.M.d.S.; Critical revision of the manuscript for important intellectual content: A.L.-V., M.B. All authors have read and agreed to the published version of the manuscript.

Abbreviations

VR	Virtual Reality
DA	Dental Anxiety
VAS	Visual Analogic Scale
W–BFS	Wong–Baker Faces Scale
FPS-R	Faces Pain Scale-Revise
FLACC	Consolability Scale
VRS	Verbal Rating Scale
MDAS	Modified Dental Anxiety Scale
NCAQ	Norman Corah's anxiety questionnaire
VCARS	Venham's Clinical Anxiety Rating Scale
RoB	Risk of Bias
SDs	Standard Deviation
SMD	Standard Mean Deviation
CI	Confidence Interval

References

1. López-Valverde, A.; Montero, J.; Albaladejo, A.; Gómez de Diego, R. The discovery of surgical anesthesia: Discrepancies regarding its authorship. *J. Dent. Res.* **2011**, *90*, 31–34. [CrossRef] [PubMed]
2. Sweta, V.R.; Abhinav, R.P.; Asha, R. Role of Virtual Reality in Pain Perception of Patients Following the Administration of Local Anesthesia. *Ann. Maxillofac. Surg.* **2019**, *9*, 110–113. [PubMed]
3. Ougradar, A.; Ahmed, B. Patients' perceptions of the benefits of virtual reality during dental extractions. *Br. Dent. J.* **2019**, *227*, 813–816. [CrossRef] [PubMed]
4. Carl, E.; Stein, A.T.; Levihn-Coon, A.; Pogue, J.R.; Rothbaum, B.; Emmelkamp, P.; Asmundson, G.; Carlbring, P.; Powers, M.B. Virtual reality exposure therapy for anxiety and related disorders: A meta-analysis of randomized controlled trials. *J. Anxiety Disord.* **2019**, *61*, 27–36. [CrossRef]
5. Eijlers, R.; Utens, E.; Staals, L.M.; de Nijs, P.F.A.; Berghmans, J.M.; Wijnen, R.M.H.; Hillegers, M.H.J.; Dierckx, B.; Legerstee, J.S. Systematic Review and Meta-analysis of Virtual Reality in Pediatrics: Effects on Pain and Anxiety. *Anesth. Analg.* **2019**, *129*, 1344–1353. [CrossRef]
6. Gujjar, K.R.; van Wijk, A.; Kumar, R.; de Jongh, A. Efficacy of virtual reality exposure therapy for the treatment of dental phobia in adults: A randomized controlled trial. *J. Anxiety Disord.* **2019**, *62*, 100–108. [CrossRef]
7. Raghav, K.; Van Wijk, A.J.; Abdullah, F.; Islam, M.N.; Bernatchez, M.; De Jongh, A. Efficacy of virtual reality exposure therapy for treatment of dental phobia: A randomized control trial. *BMC Oral Health* **2016**, *27*, 25. [CrossRef]
8. Wiederhold, M.D.; Gao, K.; Wiederhold, B.K. Clinical use of virtual reality distraction system to reduce anxiety and pain in dental procedures. *Cyberpsychol. Behav. Soc. Netw.* **2014**, *17*, 359–365. [CrossRef]
9. Tanja-Dijkstra, K.; Pahl, S.; White, M.P.; Andrade, J.; Qian, C.; Bruce, M.; May, J.; Moles, D.R. Improving dental experiences by using virtual reality distraction: A simulation study. *PLoS ONE* **2014**, *2*, e91276. [CrossRef]
10. Dahlquist, L.M.; McKenna, K.D.; Jones, K.K.; Dillinger, L.; Weiss, K.E.; Ackerman, C.S. Active and passive distraction using a head-mounted display helmet: Effects on cold pressor pain in children. *Health Psychol.* **2014**, *26*, 794–801. [CrossRef]
11. Schneider, S.M.; Hood, L.E. Virtual reality: A distraction intervention for chemotherapy. *Oncol. Nurs. Forum* **2007**, *34*, 39–46. [CrossRef] [PubMed]
12. Malloy, K.M.; Milling, L.S. The effectiveness of virtual reality distraction for pain reduction: A systematic review. *Clin. Psychol. Rev.* **2010**, *30*, 1011–1018. [CrossRef] [PubMed]
13. American Society of Anesthesiologists Task Force on Sedation and Analgesia by Non-Anesthesiologists. Practice guidelines for sedation and analgesia by non-anesthesiologists. *Anesthesiology* **2002**, *96*, 1004–1017. [CrossRef] [PubMed]
14. Dixon, R.A.; Kenyon, C.; Marsh, D.R.; Thornton, J.A. Midazolam in conservative dentistry. A cross-over trial. *Anaesthesia* **1986**, *41*, 276–281. [CrossRef]
15. Foley, J. The way forward for dental sedation and primary cares? *Br. Dent. J.* **2002**, *193*, 161–164. [CrossRef]

16. Hutton, B.; Ferrán Catalá-López, F.; Moher, D. The PRISMA statement extension for systematic reviews incorporating network meta-analysis: PRISMA-NMA. *Med. Clin.* **2016**, *16*, 262–266. [CrossRef]
17. Higgins, J.P.T.; Altman, D.G.; Sterne, J.A.C. *Cochrane Handbook for Systematic Reviews of Interventions*, version 5.1.0; Higgins, J.P.T., Green, S., Eds.; The Cochrane Collaboration: London, UK, 2006; Chapter 8; Available online: http://www.cochrane-handbook.org (accessed on 20 October 2019).
18. Vandenbroucke, J.P.; von Elm, E.; Altman, D.G.; Gøtzsche, P.C.; Mulrow, C.D.; Pocock, S.J.; Charles, P.; James, J.S.; Matthias, E. STROBE Initiative. Strengthening the reporting of observational studies in epidemiology (STROBE): Explanation and elaboration. *PLoS Med.* **2007**, *4*, e297. [CrossRef]
19. Tanja-Dijkstra, K.; Pahl, S.; White, M.P.; Andrade, J.; May, J.; Stone, R.J.; Bruce, M.; Mills, I.; Auvray, M.; Gabe, R.; et al. Can virtual nature improve patient experiences and memories of dental treatment? A study protocol for a randomized controlled trial. *Trials* **2014**, *22*, 90. [CrossRef]
20. Al-Halabi, M.N.; Bshara, N.; AlNerabieah, Z. Effectiveness of audio visual distraction using virtual reality eyeglasses versus tablet device in child behavioral management during inferior alveolar nerve block. *Anaesth. Pain Intensive Care* **2018**, *22*, 55–61.
21. Bentsen, B.; Svensson, P.; Wenzel, A. Evaluation of effect of 3D video glasses on perceived pain and unpleasantness induced by restorative dental treatment. *Eur. J. Pain* **2001**, *5*, 373–378. [CrossRef]
22. Asl Aminabadi, N.; Erfanparast, L.; Sohrabi, A.; Ghertasi Oskouei, S.; Naghili, A. The Impact of Virtual Reality Distraction on Pain and Anxiety during Dental Treatment in 4-6 Year-Old Children: A Randomized Controlled Clinical Trial. *J. Dent. Res. Dent. Clin. Dent. Prospect.* **2012**, *6*, 117–124.
23. Nunna, M.; Dasaraju, R.K.; Kamatham, R.; Mallineni, S.K.; Nuvvula, S. Comparative evaluation of virtual reality distraction and counter-stimulation on dental anxiety and pain perception in children. *J. Dent. Anesth. Pain Med.* **2019**, *19*, 277–288. [CrossRef] [PubMed]
24. Niharika, P.; Reddy, N.V.; Srujana, P.; Srikanth, K.; Daneswari, V.; Geetha, K.S. Effects of distraction using virtual reality technology on pain perception and anxiety levels in children during pulp therapy of primary molars. *J. Indian Soc. Pedod. Prev. Dent.* **2018**, *36*, 364–369. [CrossRef] [PubMed]
25. Shetty, V.; Suresh, L.R.; Hegde, A.M. Effect of Virtual Reality Distraction on Pain and Anxiety during Dental Treatment in 5 to 8 Year Old Children. *J. Clin. Pediatr. Dent.* **2019**, *43*, 97–102. [CrossRef]
26. Al-Khotani, A.; Bello, L.A.; Christidis, N. Effects of audiovisual distraction on children's behaviour during dental treatment: A randomized controlled clinical trial. *Acta Odontol. Scand.* **2016**, *74*, 494–501. [CrossRef] [PubMed]
27. Mitrakul, K.; Asvanund, Y.; Arunakul, M.; Paka-Akekaphat, S. Effect of audiovisual eyeglasses during dental treatment in 5–8 year-old children. *Eur. J. Paediatr. Dent.* **2015**, *16*, 239–245. [PubMed]
28. Asvanund, Y.; Mitrakul, K.; Juhong, R.O.; Arunakul, M. Effect of audiovisual eyeglasses during local anesthesia injections in 5- to 8-year-old children. *Quintessence Int.* **2015**, *46*, 513–521.
29. Cohen, J. *Statistical Power Analysis for the Behavioral Sciences*, 2nd ed.; Lawrence Erlbaum Associates: New York, NY, USA, 1988.
30. Yamashita, Y.; Shimohira, D.; Aijima, R.; Mori, K.; Danjo, A. Clinical Effect of Virtual Reality to Relieve Anxiety During Impacted Mandibular Third Molar Extraction Under Local Anesthesia. *J. Oral Maxillofac. Surg.* **2019**, *26*, 31343–31346. [CrossRef]
31. Hill, K.B.; Chadwick, B.; Freeman, R.; O'Sullivan, I.; Murray, J.J. Adult Dental Health Survey 2009: Relationships between dental attendance patterns, oral health behaviour and the current barriers to dental care. *Br. Dent. J.* **2013**, *214*, 25–32. [CrossRef]
32. Seligman, L.D.; Hovey, J.D.; Chacon, K.; Ollendick, T.H. Dental anxiety: An understudied problem in youth. *Clin. Psychol. Rev.* **2017**, *55*, 25–40. [CrossRef]
33. De Stefano, R. Psychological Factors in Dental Patient Care: Odontophobia. *Medicina* **2019**, *8*, 55. [CrossRef] [PubMed]
34. Fiorillo, L. Oral Health: The First Step to Well-Being. *Medicina* **2019**, *7*, 55. [CrossRef] [PubMed]
35. Bolton, D.; Dearsley, P.; Madronal-Luque, R.; Baron-Cohen, S. Magical thinking in childhood and adolescence: Development and relation to obsessive compulsion. *Br. J. Dev. Psychol.* **2002**, *20*, 479–494. [CrossRef]
36. Thompson, S.G.; Higgins, J.P. How should meta-regression analyses be undertaken and interpreted? *Stat. Med.* **2002**, *21*, 559–573. [CrossRef]

37. Klassen, J.A.; Liang, Y.; Tjosvold, L.; Klassen, T.P.; Hartling, L. Music for pain and anxiety in children undergoing medical procedures: A systematic review of randomized controlled trials. *Ambul. Pediatr.* **2008**, *8*, 117–128. [CrossRef]
38. Uman, L.S.; Chambers, C.T.; McGrath, P.J.; Kisely, S. Psychological interventions for needle-related procedural pain and distress in children and adolescents. *Cochrane Database Syst. Rev.* **2006**, *18*. [CrossRef]
39. Uman, S.L.; Birnie, K.A.; Noel, M.; Parker, J.A.; Chambers, C.T.; McGrath, P.J.; Kisely, S.R. Psychological interventions for needle-related procedural pain and distress in children and adolescents. *Cochrane Database Syst. Rev.* **2013**, *10*. [CrossRef]
40. Birnie, K.A.; Noel, M.; Chambers, C.T.; Uman, L.S.; Parker, J.A. Psychological interventions for needle-related procedural pain and distress in children and adolescents. *Cochrane Database Syst. Rev.* **2018**, *10*. [CrossRef]
41. Hoffman, H.G.; Sharar, S.R.; Coda, B.; Everett, J.J.; Ciol, M.; Richards, T.; Patterson, D.R. Manipulating presence influences the magnitude of virtual reality analgesia. *Pain* **2004**, *111*, 162–168. [CrossRef]
42. Yu, M.; Zhou, R.; Wang, H.; Zhao, W. An evaluation for VR glasses system user experience: The influence factors of interactive operation and motion sickness. *Appl. Ergon.* **2019**, *74*, 206–213. [CrossRef]
43. Schienle, A.; Scharmüller, W.; Leutgeb, V.; Schäfer, A.; Stark, R. Sex differences in the functional and structural neuroanatomy of dental phobia. *Brain Struct. Funct.* **2013**, *218*, 779–787. [CrossRef]
44. Klages, U.; Kianifard, S.; Ulusoy, O.; Wehrbein, H. Anxiety sensitivity as predictor of pain in patients undergoing restorative dentalprocedures. *Community Dent. Oral Epidemiol.* **2006**, *34*, 139–145. [CrossRef] [PubMed]
45. Lin, C.S.; Wu, S.Y.; Yi, C.A. Association between Anxiety and Pain in Dental Treatment: A Systematic Review and Meta-analysis. *J. Dent. Res.* **2017**, *96*, 153–162. [CrossRef] [PubMed]
46. Astramskaitė, I.; Juodžbalys, G. Scales used to rate adult patients' psycho-emotional status in tooth extraction procedures: A systematic review. *Int. J. Oral Maxillofac. Surg.* **2017**, *46*, 886–898. [CrossRef] [PubMed]
47. Eijlers, R.; Legerstee, J.S.; Dierckx, B.; Staals, L.M.; Berghmans, J.; van der Schroeff, M.P.; Wijnen, R.M.; Utens, E.M. Development of a Virtual Reality Exposure Tool as Psychological Preparation for Elective Pediatric Day Care Surgery: Methodological Approach for a Randomized Controlled Trial. *JMIR Res. Protoc.* **2017**, *6*, e174. [CrossRef] [PubMed]
48. Jain, A.; Suprabha, B.S.; Shenoy, R.; Rao, A. Association of temperament with dental anxiety and behaviour of the preschool child during the initial dental visit. *Eur. J. Oral Sci.* **2019**, *127*, 147–155. [CrossRef] [PubMed]
49. Stenebrand, A.; Wide Boman, U.; Hakeberg, M. Dental anxiety and temperament in 15-year olds. *Acta Odontol. Scand.* **2013**, *71*, 15–21. [CrossRef]
50. Lundgren, J.; Elfström, M.L.; Berggren, U. The relationship between temperament and fearfulness in adult dental phobic patients. *Int. J. Paediatr. Dent.* **2007**, *17*, 460–468. [CrossRef]
51. Bergdahl, M.; Bergdahl, J. Temperament and character personality dimensions in patients with dental anxiety. *Eur. J. Oral. Sci.* **2003**, *111*, 93–98. [CrossRef]

Permissions

All chapters in this book were first published by MDPI; hereby published with permission under the Creative Commons Attribution License or equivalent. Every chapter published in this book has been scrutinized by our experts. Their significance has been extensively debated. The topics covered herein carry significant findings which will fuel the growth of the discipline. They may even be implemented as practical applications or may be referred to as a beginning point for another development.

The contributors of this book come from diverse backgrounds, making this book a truly international effort. This book will bring forth new frontiers with its revolutionizing research information and detailed analysis of the nascent developments around the world.

We would like to thank all the contributing authors for lending their expertise to make the book truly unique. They have played a crucial role in the development of this book. Without their invaluable contributions this book wouldn't have been possible. They have made vital efforts to compile up to date information on the varied aspects of this subject to make this book a valuable addition to the collection of many professionals and students.

This book was conceptualized with the vision of imparting up-to-date information and advanced data in this field. To ensure the same, a matchless editorial board was set up. Every individual on the board went through rigorous rounds of assessment to prove their worth. After which they invested a large part of their time researching and compiling the most relevant data for our readers.

The editorial board has been involved in producing this book since its inception. They have spent rigorous hours researching and exploring the diverse topics which have resulted in the successful publishing of this book. They have passed on their knowledge of decades through this book. To expedite this challenging task, the publisher supported the team at every step. A small team of assistant editors was also appointed to further simplify the editing procedure and attain best results for the readers.

Apart from the editorial board, the designing team has also invested a significant amount of their time in understanding the subject and creating the most relevant covers. They scrutinized every image to scout for the most suitable representation of the subject and create an appropriate cover for the book.

The publishing team has been an ardent support to the editorial, designing and production team. Their endless efforts to recruit the best for this project, has resulted in the accomplishment of this book. They are a veteran in the field of academics and their pool of knowledge is as vast as their experience in printing. Their expertise and guidance has proved useful at every step. Their uncompromising quality standards have made this book an exceptional effort. Their encouragement from time to time has been an inspiration for everyone.

The publisher and the editorial board hope that this book will prove to be a valuable piece of knowledge for researchers, students, practitioners and scholars across the globe.

List of Contributors

Tanya Guitard and Claude Bélanger
Département de Psychologie, Université du Québec à Montréal, Montréal, QC H3C 3P8, Canada

Stéphane Bouchard
Département de Psychoéducation et de Psychologie, Université du Québec en Outaouais, Gatineau, QC J8X 3X7, Canada
School of Psychology, University of Ottawa, Ottawa, ON K1N 6N5, Canada

Maxine Berthiaume
School of Psychology, University of Ottawa, Ottawa, ON K1N 6N5, Canada

Laura Andreu-Pejó and Verónica Martínez-Borba
Nursing Department, Universitat Jaume I de Castelló, Castelló de la Plana, 12071 Valencia, Spain
Instituto de Investigación Sanitaria de Aragón, 50009 Zaragoza, Spain

Carlos Suso-Ribera
Nursing Department, Universitat Jaume I de Castelló, Castelló de la Plana, 12071 Valencia, Spain

Jorge Osma
Instituto de Investigación Sanitaria de Aragón, 50009 Zaragoza, Spain
Departmento de Psicología y Sociología, Universidad de Zaragoza, 44003 Teruel, Spain

Roberta Bevilacqua, Elvira Maranesi and Fabrizia Lattanzio
Scientific Direction, IRCCS INRCA, 60129 Ancona, Italy

Giovanni Renato Riccardi and Valentina Di Donna
Clinical Unit of Physical Rehabilitation, IRCCS INRCA, 60100 Ancona, Italy

Paolo Pelliccioni
Eye Clinic, Polytechnic University of Marche, 60100 Ancona, Italy

Riccardo Luzi
Medical Direction, IRCCS INRCA, 60100 Ancona, Italy

Giuseppe Pelliccioni
Neurology Unit, IRCCS INRCA, 60100 Ancona, Italy

Tracy Gladstone and Katherine R. Buchholz
The Robert S. and Grace W. Stone Primary Prevention Initiatives, Wellesley Centers for Women, Wellesley College, Wellesley, MA 02481, USA

Marian Fitzgibbon
Department of General Pediatrics, College of Medicine, University of Illinois at Chicago, Chicago, IL 60612, USA
Institute for Health Research and Policy, School of Public Health, University of Illinois at Chicago, Chicago, IL 60608, USA
University of Illinois Cancer Center, University of Illinois at Chicago, Chicago, IL 60612, USA

Linda Schiffer
Institute for Health Research and Policy, School of Public Health, University of Illinois at Chicago, Chicago, IL 60608, USA

Miae Lee and Benjamin W. Van Voorhees
Department of General Pediatrics, College of Medicine, University of Illinois at Chicago, Chicago, IL 60612, USA

Bruno Porras Garcia, Marta Ferrer Garcia, Agata Olszewska, Lena Yilmaz, Cristina González Ibañez, Mireia Gracia Blanes, Gamze Gültekin and José Gutiérrez Maldonado
Department of Clinical Psychology and Psychobiology, University of Barcelona, Passeig de la Vall d'Hebron, 171, 08035 Barcelona, Spain

Eduardo Serrano Troncoso
Child and Adolescent Psychiatry and Psychology Department, Hospital Sant Joan de Déu of Barcelona; Passeig de Sant Joan de Déu, 2, 08950 Esplugues de Llobregat, Barcelona, Spain
Children and Adolescent Mental Health Research Group, Institut de Recerca Sant Joan de Déu, Passeig de Sant Joan de Déu, 2, 08950 Esplugues de Llobregat, Barcelona, Spain

Luca Provenzano, Giuseppina Porciello and Sofia Ciccarone
Department of Psychology, "Sapienza" University of Rome, 00185 Rome, Italy
IRCCS, Santa Lucia Foundation, 00142 Rome, Italy

Bigna Lenggenhager
Department of Psychology, University of Zurich, 8050 Zurich, Switzerland

Gaetano Tieri
IRCCS, Santa Lucia Foundation, 00142 Rome, Italy
Virtual Reality Lab, University of Rome Unitelma-Sapienza, 00161 Rome, Italy

Matteo Marucci
Department of Psychology, "Sapienza" University of Rome, 00185 Rome, Italy
IRCCS, Santa Lucia Foundation, 00142 Rome, Italy
BrainTrends Ltd., Applied Neuroscience, Gallicano nel Lazio (RM), 00010 Rome, Italy

Federico Dazzi
Department of Human Sciences, Lumsa University, 00193 Rome, Italy

Camillo Loriedo
Clinica Psichiatrica, "Sapienza" University of Rome, 00185 Rome, Italy

Ilaria Bufalari
IRCCS, Santa Lucia Foundation, 00142 Rome, Italy
Department of Developmental and Social Psychology, "Sapienza" University of Rome, 00185 Rome, Italy

Artemisa R. Dores
Center for Rehabilitation Research, School of Health, Polytechnic Institute of Porto, 4200-072 Porto, Portugal
Laboratory of Neuropsychophysiology, Faculty of Psychology and Education Sciences of University of Porto, 4200-135 Porto, Portugal

Andreia Geraldo and Fernando Barbosa
Laboratory of Neuropsychophysiology, Faculty of Psychology and Education Sciences of University of Porto, 4200-135 Porto, Portugal

Irene P. Carvalho
CINTESIS and Department of Clinical Neurosciences and Mental Health, School of Medicine, University of Porto (FMUP), 4200-319 Porto, Portugal

Diana Castilla
Department of Personality, Evaluation and Psychological Treatment, University of Valencia, 46010 Valencia, Spain
CIBER of Physiopathology of Obesity and Nutrition (CIBEROBN), ISCIII CB06/03/0052 Instituto Salud Carlos III, 28029 Madrid, Spain

Carlos Suso-Ribera
Department of Basic Psychology, Clinical Psychology and Psychobiology, Universitat Jaume I, 12071 Castellón, Spain

Rahel Bachem and Andreas Maercker
Psychopathology and Clinical Intervention, University of Zürich, 8050 Zürich, Switzerland

Kim Mathiasen
Department of Psychology, Faculty of Health Sciences, University of Southern Denmark, 5230 Odense M, Denmark
Center of Telepsychiatry, University of Southern Denmark, 5000 Odense, Denmark

Karine Chevreul
URC Eco Ile-de-France (AP-HP), Hotel Dieu, 1, Place du Parvis Notre Dame, 75004 Paris, France

Jean Baptiste Hazo
Eceve, Unit 1123, Inserm, University of Paris, Health Economics Research Unit, Assistance Publique-Hôpitaux de Paris, 75004 Paris, France

Jérôme Holtzmann
University Hospital Grenoble Alpes, Mood Disorders and Emotional Pathologies Unit, Pôle de Psychiatrie, Neurologie et Rééducation Neurologique, 38043 Grenoble, France

Mark Hoogendoorn
Department of Computer Science, VU University Amsterdam Faculty of Sciences, De Boelelaan 1081m, 1081 HV Amsterdam, The Netherlands

Annet Kleiboer
Section Clinical Psychology, Faculty of Behavioural and Movement Sciences, Vrije Universiteit Amsterdam and EMGO+ Institute for Health Care and Research, Van der Boechorststraat 1, 1081 BT Amsterdam, The Netherlands

Nadine Friedl and Tobias Krieger
Department of Clinical Psychology, University of Bern, 3012 Bern, Switzerland

Antoine Urech
INSELSPITAL, University Hospital Bern, University Clinic for Neurology, University Acute-Neurorehabilitation Center, 3010 Bern, Switzerland

Heleen Riper
Department of Psychiatry and the Amsterdam Public Health Research Institute, GGZ inGeest/Amsterdam UMC, Vrije Universiteit, de Boelelaan 1117, 1081 HV Amsterdam, The Netherlands
Department of Research and Innovation, GGZ inGeest Specialized Mental Health Care, Oldenaller 1, 1081 HJ Amsterdam, The Netherlands
Department of Clinical, Neuro-and Developmental Psychology and the Amsterdam Public Health Research Institute, Vrije Universiteit Amsterdam, van der Boechorststraat 7, 1081 BT Amsterdam, The Netherlands

Christian Moser and Thomas Berger
Clinical Psychology and Psychotherapy, University of Bern, 3012 Bern, Switzerland

Irene Zaragoza
CIBER of Physiopathology of Obesity and Nutrition (CIBEROBN), ISCIII CB06/03/0052 Instituto Salud Carlos III, 28029 Madrid, Spain

Mª Dolores Vara
Polibienestar Research Institute, University of Valencia, 46022 Valencia, Spain
CIBERObn Physiopathology of Obesity and Nutrition, Instituto de Salud Carlos III, 28029 Madrid, Spain

Adriana Mira
Department of Personality, Evaluation and Psychological Treatment, Faculty of Psychology, University of Valencia, 46010 Valencia, Spain

Marta Miragall
CIBERObn Physiopathology of Obesity and Nutrition, Instituto de Salud Carlos III, 28029 Madrid, Spain
Department of Personality, Evaluation and Psychological Treatment, Faculty of Psychology, University of Valencia, 46010 Valencia, Spain

Azucena García-Palacios and Cristina Botella
CIBERObn Physiopathology of Obesity and Nutrition, Instituto de Salud Carlos III, 28029 Madrid, Spain
Department of Basic and Clinical Psychology and Psychobiology, Faculty of Health Sciences, Jaume I University, 12071 Castellon de la Plana, Spain

Margalida Gili
Institut Universitari d'Investigació en Ciències de la Salut, University of Balearic Islands, E-07122 Palma de Mallorca, Spain
Institut d'Investigació Sanitaria Illes Balears, 07120 Palma de Mallorca, Spain
Primary Care Prevention and Health Promotion Research Network, RedIAPP, 28029 Madrid, Spain

Pau Riera-Serra
Institut Universitari d'Investigació en Ciències de la Salut, University of Balearic Islands, E-07122 Palma de Mallorca, Spain
Institut d'Investigació Sanitaria Illes Balears, 07120 Palma de Mallorca, Spain

Javier García-Campayo
Primary Care Prevention and Health Promotion Research Network, RedIAPP, 28029 Madrid, Spain
Aragon Institute for Health Research (IIS Aragón), Miguel Servet Hospital, University of Zaragoza, 50009 Zaragoza, Spain

Bruno Macedo de Sousa
Institute for Occlusion and Orofacial Pain Faculty of Medicine, University of Coimbra, Polo I - Edifício Central Rua Larga, 3004-504 Coimbra, Portugal

Manuel Bravo
Department of Preventive and Community Dentistry, Facultad de Odontología, Campus de Cartuja s/n, 18071 Granada, Spain

Fermín Mayoral-Cleries
Mental Health Unit, Hospital Regional of Malaga, Biomedicine Research Institute (IBIMA), 29010 Málaga, Spain

Rosa Mª Baños
Clinical Psychology and Psychotherapy, University of Bern, 3012 Bern, Switzerland
CIBERObn Physiopathology of Obesity and Nutrition, Instituto de Salud Carlos III, 28029 Madrid, Spain
Department of Personality, Evaluation and Psychological Treatment, Faculty of Psychology, University of Valencia, 46010 Valencia, Spain

Nickolai Titov, Olav Nielssen and Blake F. Dear
MindSpot Clinic and Department of Psychology, Macquarie University, Sydney, NSW 2109, Australia

Heather D. Hadjistavropoulos
Online Therapy Unit, Department of Psychology, University of Regina, Regina, Saskatchewan, SK S4S 0A2, Canada

David C. Mohr
Center for Behavioral Intervention Technologies, Department of Preventive Medicine, Northwestern University, Chicago, IL 60611, USA

Gerhard Andersson
Department of Behavioural Sciences and Learning, Linköping University, Linköping SE-581 83, Sweden
Department of Clinical Neuroscience, Karolinska Institute, Stockholm 171 77, Sweden

Nansi López-Valverde, Jorge Muriel Fernández, Antonio López-Valverde, Javier Flores Fraile, Julio Herrero Payo and Leticia A. Blanco Antona
Department of Surgery, University of Salamanca, Instituto de Investigación Biomédica de Salamanca (IBSAL), 37007 Salamanca, Spain

Luis F. Valero Juan
Department of Biomedical and Diagnostic Sciences, University of Salamanca, Avda. Alfonso X El Sabio S/N, 37007 Salamanca, Spain

Juan Manuel Ramírez
Department of Morphological Sciences, University of Cordoba, Avenida Menéndez Pidal s/n, 14071 Cordoba, Spain

Index

www.ingramcontent.com/pod-product-compliance
Lightning Source LLC
LaVergne TN
LVHW082222200926
848484LV00008B/2286